Community Quality-of-Life and Well-Being

The Community Quality of Life and Well-being book series is a collection of volumes related to community level research, providing community planners and quality of life researchers involved in community and regional well-being innovative research and application. Formerly entitled, Community Quality of Life Indicators: Best Practices, the series reflects a broad scope of well-being. Next to best practices of community quality-of-life indicators projects the series welcomes a variety of research and practice topics as related to overall community well-being and quality of life dimensions, whether relating to policy, application, research, and/or practice. Research on issues such as societal happiness, quality of life domains in the policy construct, measuring and gauging progress, dimensions of planning and community development, and related topics are anticipated. This series is published by Springer in partnership with the International Society for Quality-of-Life Studies, a global society with the purpose of promoting and encouraging research and collaboration in quality of life and well-being theory and applications.

More information about this series at https://link.springer.com/bookseries/13761

Seung Jong Lee

Public Happiness

Springer

Seung Jong Lee
Graduate School of Public Administration
Seoul National University
Seoul, Korea (Republic of)

This work was supported by the Ministry of Education of the Republic of Korea and the National Research Foundation of Korea (NRF-2015S1A5B1010910).

ISSN 2520-1093 ISSN 2520-1107 (electronic)
Community Quality-of-Life and Well-Being
ISBN 978-3-030-89642-3 ISBN 978-3-030-89643-0 (eBook)
https://doi.org/10.1007/978-3-030-89643-0

This Springer imprint is published by the registered company Springer Nature Switzerland AG
The registered company address is: Gewerbestrasse 11, 6330 Cham, Switzerland

To my parents

Preface

Why happiness? In order to answer this question, one needs to first ask why human beings live. Why do we live? Putting religion aside, life is not a choice, but rather given to us. Thus, why we live is not a fair question. Instead, we should be asking *how* we should live. The answer to this question depends on how an individual wishes to live. Often, humans wish to live happily. There is no need for an explanation. This is obvious and what anybody wants. To live happily while alive, this is a fundamental human demand. We often speak of natural rights as basic rights, but the basic part of basic rights has to do with the right to live happily, and thus, we can interpret happiness as a natural right.

Despite happiness being a basic right, it is impossible for every human being to experience the same level of happiness. This is due to the differences in individual characteristics and living conditions (or social conditions). On the one hand, two individuals with the same living conditions may experience different levels of happiness due to differences in individual personalities. On the other hand, even if two individuals had identical personalities, they may have different living conditions, creating differences in happiness levels. Be that as it may, we cannot accept these differences as normative. An ideal situation is one in which we all live happily without extreme differences in happiness levels.

How shall we accomplish this? Individual personalities are given to us and near impossible to change, but there is hope in improving living conditions to increase happiness levels. These efforts are not wasted. As long as humans are clothed in material goods and live among social relationships, living conditions will have a significant effect on happiness levels. Of course, how much material goods affect happiness levels will differ from one person to another. Some individuals can live happily, despite their living conditions. However, this is merely a difference in the strength of correlation between living conditions and happiness. There is no doubt that living conditions have a certain causal effect on individual happiness. There is no human being whose level of happiness has no correlation with external conditions, and thus, it is reasonable to focus on conditions to create a society in which everybody has a happy life.

The point is society must acknowledge a responsibility to fix conditions that are so deplorable that people are unable to achieve a minimum level of happiness or inequality in conditions that are so extreme that there are extreme levels of inequality in happiness levels. Of course, if these conditions are the result of an individual's choice or due to reasons attributable to others then society is free of responsibility. However, if these differences are not wholly attributable to personal choice or if these conditions are difficult to change or surmount at the individual level, then society has a responsibility to pay attention to these as a social issue. This is where the publicness of happiness or public happiness becomes necessary.

This is the problem this book addresses—the publicness of happiness. That is, rather than treating the problem of happiness as a purely individual one separate from the collective, this book approaches happiness as a collective problem as individuals are the building blocks of communities. In doing so, the book will pay particular attention to policy efforts to increase the happiness of citizens as members of a nation-state. I approach this from a policy perspective because governments arguably have the greatest resources and power to realistically affect citizens' lives. Some argue that the spread of capitalism and globalization has made the meaning of national boundaries weaker, but the nation-state remains a critical unit and agent of groups of people. Nation-states are important actors in the happiness problem from a normative perspective as well. Everyone lives within national boundaries, as a member of nation-states. Regardless of the strength of nation-states, nobody is free from the boundaries of nation-states. Nation-states and citizens are bonded to each other as nation-state citizens. Why does the state exist? A common belief that has endured over centuries is that the state exists to make its citizens happy. From Locke's weak state theory to Hobbes or Hegel's strong state theory, the existence of a state must be based on its citizens to be justified. In other words, a nation-state does not exist for itself, but for its citizens. Especially today, when most countries claim to be a democracy, a democratic state should exist for its citizens and should make an active effort to increase the happiness of its citizens. If a nation-state that purportedly exists for its citizens makes little effort for its citizens' happiness, then this is a denial of its own raison d'etre and gross negligence of its minimum responsibility.

A state's efforts to increase citizen happiness is expressed in its public policies. Public policy is the action that a government adopts to achieve a public goal, and thus, we can understand happiness policy as the policies that a government adopts to increase citizen happiness. What do happiness policies aim for? I have already mentioned the importance of living conditions for happiness and happiness policies should focus on improving the living conditions and thereby increasing happiness, rather than focusing on increasing the perceived happiness of each individual. The reason for this is the relationship between external factors and happiness (which is a personal emotional state) is unclear, and thus, it is nearly impossible for a state to promise happiness through public policies (there is also the question of whether this is desirable). While it is impossible to guarantee a final level of happiness for all individuals however, it would be possible to set the guarantee of an average level of happiness from a collective point of view as a policy goal. Furthermore, happiness policies should include the goal of achieving a certain level of equitable and just distribution of happiness levels among its citizens. The issue of distribution only arises as a collective problem. If individuals simply existed apart from the collective, the issue of distribution would be moot. Thus, public happiness has two faces—level and distribution—and happiness policies should pay attention to both. High levels with highly unequal distribution or low levels with low inequality cannot be an appropriate goal for happiness policies. Happiness policies should thus focus on identifying the conditions that have significant effects on the level and distribution of happiness and try to create conditions for high and equal distributions of happiness.

Meanwhile, the responsibilities of public happiness do not solely belong to the state. As members of a community called nation-state, its citizens must participate in these efforts of public happiness. I mean this in two ways. First, citizens should not simply be consumers of happiness policies, but also be an active participant in policymaking processes. Second, citizens should not only be concerned with their personal level of happiness, but also with the happiness of others. Without these efforts, happiness policies that are dominated by the government are at the risk of creating a mismatch between policies adopted and the policies desired by its citizens, exhaustion of public resources due to extreme demands, and the deterioration of civic culture.

There has been increased attention to happiness since the twenty-first century. Bhutan already introduced the new concept of a happy nation in the early 1970s by discussing Gross National Happiness. However, this small country's efforts did not garner much attention. For the next 30 years, there was a period of challenges and then the leading economies of the western hemisphere began to actively pay attention to happiness in the 2000s. These efforts reflect a national interest in public happiness rather than an individual's happiness and was driven by practitioner demands to address the limitations of the development state and welfare state, rather than scholarly demands. New interests in happiness also appeared in academia. The Easterlin Paradox, referring to the nonlinear relationship between wealth and happiness, inspired the happiness studies and still continues to motivate a growing body of research. Many of these studies focused on measuring happiness, identifying the influencing factors of happiness, and have contributed to making happiness studies more rigorous and scientific. Despite this large body of research, there remains the question of whether there is adequate research to support the practical interests in happiness. Notwithstanding the large body of existing research, happiness studies have (1) focused on individual happiness rather than public happiness, (2) focused on measuring and identifying influencing factors of happiness with scant attention to happiness policies, (3) focused on narrow policy recommendations, failing to address a more comprehensive happiness policy, and (4) paid little attention to the governance problem of happiness policies.

Based on these limitations of previous studies, this book adopts the publicness of happiness as its key assumption and discusses happiness policies (and the governance models for these happiness policies). This approach assumes that happiness studies should ultimately contribute to the practical goal of increasing happiness. In doing so, this book aims to contribute to the previous blind zone and to connect the interest in public happiness to happiness policies and governance. There is another important reason for this book focusing on happiness policies. This is the belief that happiness policies can be a useful tool for policy development. Historically, public policies have claimed to be "for the people" but has been criticized for its government-centric goals and processes. The calls to transform patriarchic policymaking processes to a citizen-centric one to produce citizen-serving policies are the evidence. Despite the many suggestions, changes to the policy process seem difficult. The main agent of public policy remains policy decision-makers, and in reality, citizens are ignored in the policy process and remain its passive recipients. These realities can change with the pursuit of happiness policies. Happiness is what citizens feel, and in the pursuit of happiness as a policy goal, it is inevitable that public policy will become "for the people" and "by the people." Moreover, happiness policies can be a useful tool for making policies more efficient and equitable. Under the common goal of happiness, the various bureaucracies within the government will work together to create better coordinated policies, and the focus on a more equitable distribution of happiness levels within society will make policies more equitable. The challenges of democracy, efficiency, and equity in policy development have existed for a long time, and the active pursuit of happiness policies can bring us closer to achieving these. Nevertheless, the discussion and research on happiness so far has been limited to viewing increases in happiness as a simple tool without recognizing these potential policy development outcomes. In other words, happiness policies can go beyond the basic goal of increasing happiness and act as an important tool in solving the basic problems of public policy. This role should not be treated simply as a secondary effect of happiness policies, but rather as a key impact.

I am very grateful to Minho Choi, Yeong Ah Jeong, Changduck Jo, Jiho Kim, Yeon Kyung Lee, Ji Eun Lee, Suhee Lee, Min Hye Kim, Janice Lee, Jennifer Lee, YH Lee, Inseok Suh and especially Yunji Kim for helping me in the preparation of the manuscripts and to co-researchers of the Global Community Institute, Rhonda Phillips, Yoshiaki Kobayashi, Kai Ludwigs, Young Chul Choi, and Young Kyun Oh for their insightful comments. Last but not least, I thank the Korea Research Foundation for awarding me a research grant for this publication.

Seoul, Korea (Republic of) Seung Jong Lee

Contents

Chapter 1
Introduction

A democratic government should respond to what their citizens want. It is natural that the owner of a country is its people. What do citizens want? Citizens want progress—that is, they want life today to be better than yesterday and tomorrow to be better than today. Knight et al. (2002)'s study based on a survey of 10,000 UK citizens showed that respondents wanted progress and provide strong empirical support for this. Citizens from various backgrounds and environments are mentioning progress.

What is progress? Development (progress) is not a new concept created in the present, but has been pursued from ancient times, and encompasses material, moral, and psychological development (Nisbet, 2009: xiii). The definition of development varies, but is generally understood to refer to an upward change in a desired or desirable direction (Choi, 2006: 64) or a change from inferior to superior (Nisbet, 2009:5). History shows that civilization has not always progressed to a better state. Thus, progress is not natural but requires a certain level of effort. This is why a certain level of artificial effort for life progress is necessary. In making these efforts, an important question is how we understand progress. In modern society, progress has often been understood as economic output, and thus, economic growth (measured by GDP) has been understood as progress. Specifically, after World War II, it was agreed upon at the Bretton Woods conference that GNP would be used as the measure of progress. Afterward, the GNP was replaced by GDP, and both developed and developing countries have competed for the common goal of economic growth. Not only nation-states, but also individuals and corporations set economic growth as an ultimate goal.

However, since the 2000s, with developed western countries at its forefront, there has been a movement to shift the goals of national development through a reinterpretation of progress. There is growing recognition that economic growth as measured by GDP does not guarantee citizen happiness or wellbeing and worldwide efforts to adopt happiness or wellbeing as national goals. In other words, there is more interest in the qualitative aspects (i.e., happiness, wellbeing, QOL) beyond GDP.

S. J. Lee, *Public Happiness*, Community Quality-of-Life and Well-Being,
https://doi.org/10.1007/978-3-030-89643-0_1

These efforts have been called the "beyond GDP" initiative or movement.[1] The beyond GDP movement has many actors, such as central governments, local governments, non-government organizations, and international organizations. Nation-states have competed as developmental states, then as welfare states, and now it seems as happiness states. One could say the twenty-first century is the happiness century.

Characteristics of this movement can be summarized as follows. The national development goal has shifted from economic progress to holistic progress. There is increasing attention to qualitative progress, above and beyond quantitative progress and economic growth. This is a shift from welfare states (quantitative welfare) toward national happiness (qualitative welfare). There is an emphasis on QOL, better life, happiness, wellbeing, community, etc. There is a trend that stresses community wellbeing through local government services. There are pros and cons to these shifts, but these shifts are meaningful in that they are emphasizing goal-oriented government goals, compared to the previous discussion that was more process oriented. This shift is valid because (1) understanding progress in terms of happiness is natural because humans aspire to be happy and (2) human desires are more diverse than just economics. If citizens want progress—not only economic progress but also progress in happiness—nation-states must pay attention to these desires. This shift in national progress goals is efforts to push back against market-centrism and think about a new role for the government and sociopolitical institutions based on human-centrism. These efforts are goal-oriented and value-laden (Woo 2014a, b).

Why these shifts? In terms of the limits of the welfare state, shifts in demography and growth stagnation have created roadblocks to economic growth. On the other hand, despite the economic growth heretofore, there has been increased social inequality and little increase in wellbeing. In other words, growth itself has reached a limit and growth does not guarantee happiness. There are many studies that show economic growth is not linked to increases in overall wellbeing, happiness, quality of life, and/or life satisfaction. There are studies that also support the opposite, but overall, it is difficult to find unequivocal evidence for the guaranteed outcomes of growth. In sum, there is increasing suspicion toward the effects of economic growth from both developing and developed countries (Woo, 2014a, b) and developed countries are leading efforts to reset their national goals that go beyond GDP. Of course, these efforts are still in its early stages and are not at a full-fledged state. Moreover, this new paradigm does not deny the economy, but rather tries to complement the old paradigm (qualitative revision of progress). Thus, the current state is not described as "no GDP" but "beyond GDP."

Happiness is a generic desire that does not require additional explanation. Of course, there is still debate about whether happiness is the ultimate goal of life, and some may consider other goals such as liberty, responsibility, and self-realization to be more important (Frey & Stutzer, 2002: 3). An individual may even opt for the

[1] The Beyond GDP initiative is about developing indicators that are as clear and appealing as GDP, but more inclusive of environmental and social aspects of progress. Economic indicators such as GDP were never designed to be comprehensive measures of prosperity and wellbeing. We need adequate indicators to address global challenges of the twenty-first century such as climate change, poverty, resource depletion, health, and quality of life (European Commission 2020).

freedom to choose unhappiness. For most people, however, happiness is an important and fundamental life goal. The following statement, "How to gain, how to keep, how to recover happiness is in fact for most men at all times the secret motive for all they do" (James 1902: 76, recited from Frey & Stutzer, 2002: 3) does not seem so objectionable.

If happiness is so important to an individual, the state (whose constituents are individuals) should have an active interest for the happiness of these individuals. In this regard, Musikanski et al., (2019: 25) argued that the primary purpose of government is to secure equal opportunities for people to pursue happiness and governments are to create the circumstances that allow each person to pursue happiness per their unique definition. Jeong Yak-yong, an old prominent scholar and magistrate of the Josun Dynasty, an ancient Korean regime, argued that the state should actively provide for the needs of those who are vulnerable in society, such as the poor, elderly, orphans, and those with illnesses, for the happiness of the public. Moreover, he argued there has to be promotion of technology to support the material abundance and increase in comfort and tools to protect human rights (Jang, 2017: 77–84).

In fact, happiness has been regarded as an ideal goal for governments and a value that governments have a responsibility for. Modern examples include the United States' Declaration of Independence, French Declaration of Revolution, and the UN resolution for the Day of International Happiness that codify the public right to happiness. Many national constitutions also recognize the right to pursue happiness. For example, Article 10 of the Constitution of the Republic of Korea states, "All citizens have dignity and value as human beings and have the right to pursue happiness. The State has a responsibility to guarantee these inviolable basic human rights of individuals." Happiness is also mentioned in Japan's Constitution and the idea of "buen vivir" is mentioned in the constitutions of Bolivia and Ecuador. As such, several important statements have explained that happiness goes beyond individual responsibility to public responsibility. Happiness has been a normative demand of humanity, apart from its survival. Despite this, it has been difficult to find the practice of this national responsibility toward public happiness. Finally, with the changes in context, happiness has become today's most urgent task.

Efforts to increase citizen happiness, however, is a more difficult and ambitious goal than the previous efforts toward economic growth. The economic growth state of the past only had to focus on the economy, and the welfare state only had to focus on the welfare levels that were a result of the economy. However, the happiness state has to focus on other elements in addition to the economy. Furthermore, the happiness state now has to pay attention to how economic elements are connected to happiness. This is even more difficult because the causal relationship between economy and happiness is unclear. Despite this difficulty, as long as citizens want happiness, the state has a responsibility to work toward citizen happiness, even if that is not their national goal. This is because the state has a responsibility to work toward what citizens want. A government that does not pay attention to what its citizens want lacks its raison d'etre and citizen trust. The decline in trust in government in the twenty-first century can be seen as evidence that governments are failing to meet citizens' demands (Nye et al., 1997).

Overall, the interest that the state is showing in citizen happiness is premised on the realization of public responsibility for happiness, and thus, we should start from a discussion of public happiness. In other words, the increased interest of the state and public institutions in happiness is a recognition that happiness is no longer a private issue but a public issue. This increased attention to happiness can contribute to the happiness of marginalized populations that lack private resources and capabilities to achieve happiness.

Along with the interest of practitioners, there has been renewed interest in happiness research. For example, the research of Easterlin and others have increased the quantity of happiness research. This academic research is not completely separate from practice. The research outputs of happiness studies motivate national interest in happiness, and the practical interest in happiness also motivates research. Notwithstanding these outputs and meanings, the happiness research so far has some limitations from the perspective of public happiness. The background of recent happiness research tends to focus on public happiness beyond private happiness and is related to the theory of public happiness. Still, existing research tends to focus on private/individual happiness while discussing individual, community, and nations and thus has made limited contributions to the needs of public happiness.

Based on this observation, this book offers a discussion of public happiness above and beyond private happiness. Specifically, the book has the following goals. First, this book purports to deal with theory and practice of public happiness to which adequate attention has not been paid since the upsurge of happiness research in the early twenty-first century. In doing so, it emphasizes that happiness is the ideal goal to be pursued as a public responsibility and national goal on the one hand. On the other hand, it suggests how policy for happiness should be redirected and governance systems for enacting happiness policy should be renovated. This book also emphasizes that the primary goal of happiness policy should have as its final goal not promising individual happiness as an outcome, but rather the construction of the basic social conditions that support individuals pursue their happiness according to their own preferences and values. This approach signifies that actors in happiness policies include not only the state but also citizens as members of that state. This is an effort to redress the shortcomings of existing literature that has never adequately dealt with the relationship among public policy, governance, and public happiness.

Second, it introduces the recent efforts to change national development goals among developed countries based on reinterpretation of progress and explicates that this is a shift from welfare states (quantitative welfare) toward national happiness states (qualitative welfare) where social wellbeing (happiness, quality of life) rather than social welfare is considered important. This shift away from the traditional indicator for progress, GDP, can be called the "beyond GDP" movement. This book will introduce in detail the beyond GDP movements of various countries, local governments, and international organizations.

Thirdly, this book will suggest basic orientations for happiness-driven public policy and governance restructuring for happiness policy. Given the recent movements to adopt public happiness as national goals, if the movement wants to contribute to the change in national development goals, there must be a change in policy implementation and the governance that is pursuing these policies. In other words, governance innovation (structure and role) is necessary and related studies should support this innovation. While previous happiness studies focused on measuring happiness levels and extracting influencing factors, they lacked equivalent attention to reorienting policy paradigms and restructuring governance which are necessary for promoting happiness. As of yet, "Beyond GDP" movement is in its early stages and there has not been a serious recognition that happiness should be a national development goal that should be connected to policy. With this in mind, this study will go beyond the discussion of happiness measurement and influencing factors to include the reorienting of policy (government innovation) and restructuring governance to address the limitations of previous studies. In doing so, this study will critically review the previous process-oriented governance (government) paradigms (e.g., traditional government, New Public Management, and New Public Service) and present a new goal-oriented paradigm for national development. Unlike the process-oriented governance paradigm, in goal-oriented governance paradigm, there is no pre-determined distribution of roles for policy actors and there is the acknowledgement that this can change fluidly depending on the potential for achieving the intended outcome. With this flexibility, the goal-oriented paradigm resolves the incompatibility with the previous paradigm, motivates theoretical studies, and can give comprehensive directions for the new policies and governance systems that focus on a new developmental goal. This has never been dealt with in the previous literature of happiness or wellbeing.

This book starts from the decision model of public happiness. Figure 1 summarizes how public happiness is determined by private activities stemming from individual and social conditions.

As shown in Fig. 1, government activity following public responsibility (happiness policy and governance) affects individual and social conditions. Here, individual conditions refer to the resources, capabilities, and values of individuals and social conditions (living conditions for individuals) include physical (e.g., SOC and welfare) and non-physical (e.g., culture, social capital, social values). Individual and social conditions affect each other (Chaps. 6 and 7).

Individual and social conditions affect an individual's actions in the pursuit of happiness, both separately and/or together (Chap. 5). The achievement of happiness will differ by the contents and intensity of an individual's pursuit of happiness. This achievement can be evaluated by its level and distribution (Chap. 4). The final evaluation for happiness achievement will depend on the components of happiness such as feelings, evaluations, and life meaning (Chaps. 2 and 3).

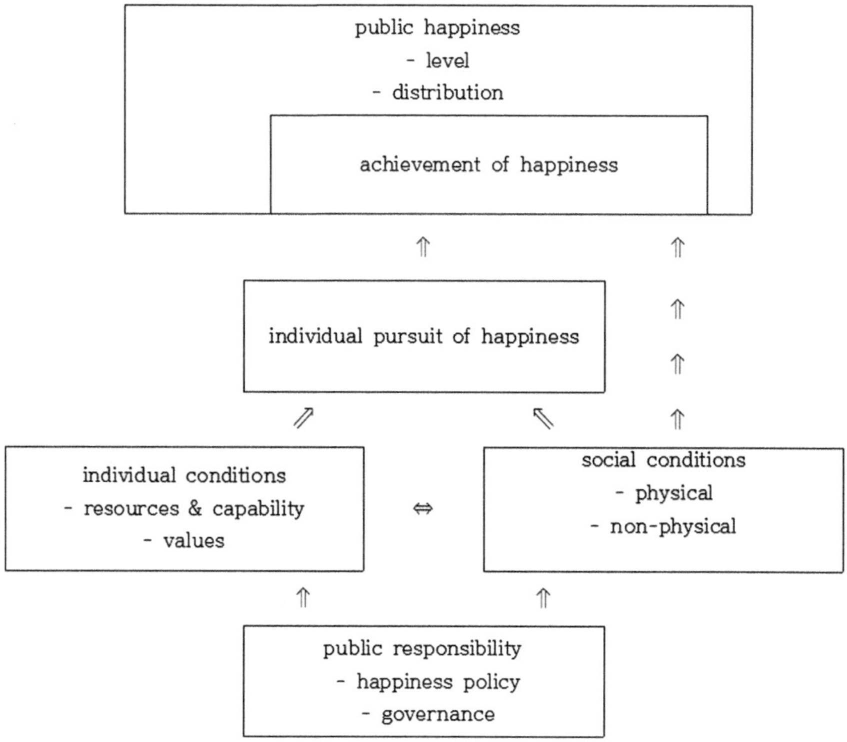

Fig. 1 Determining public happiness

References

Choi, H. (2006). *Development administration.* Shinwon Culture Co. (Korean).

EC (European Commission). (2020). Beyond GDP. https://ec.europa.eu/environment/beyond_gdp/background_en.html. Accessed June 15, 2020.

Jang, S. (2017). *Dasan, Technique of happiness.* Communication Books. (Korean).

Frey, B., & Stutzer, A. (2002). *Happiness and economics: How the economy and institutions affect human well-being.* Princeton University Press.

Knight, B., Ghigudu, H., & Tandon, R. (2002). *Reviving democracy—Citizens at the heart of governance.* Earthscan Publications.

Musikanski, L., Phillips, R., & Crowder, J. (2019). *The happiness policy handbook: How to make happiness and well-being the purpose of your government.* New Society Publishers.

Nisbet, R. (2009). *History of the idea of progress.* Transaction Publishers.

Nye, J. S., Zelikow, P. D., & King, D. C. (1997). *Why people don't trust government.* Harvard University Press.

Woo, C. (2014a). Exploring an alternative approach to the global development: Theoretical foundation and policy implications of happiness approach in the context of global development. *Korean Society and Public Administration, 24*(4), 411–434. (Korean).

Woo, C. (2014b). The effect of good governance on happiness of the people: Does technical quality precedes democracy? *Korean Journal of Public Administration, 52*(1), 219–246. (Korean).

Chapter 2
Theoretical Backgrounds of Public Happiness

1 Conceptualization of Happiness

Any human being wants to be happy and thus makes efforts to be happy while living. They earn money, love, and/or hold on to a religion. They even choose death when they are unhappy. The problem of happiness follows us like a shadow during our life. There is no need to question why happiness and why humans pursue happiness. Happiness is an absolute good in life that does not require any explanation (Layard, 2005). It is the ultimate goal of life and the resolution of other values. The following lyrics from a Korean pop song describes how much humans want happiness:

> If I could only live one day, but be happy, I would choose that path (from Jong Hwan Kim "For Love").

What is happiness? The question of what is happiness or what is a good life has been asked for a long time in western philosophy.[1] In ancient Greece, Aristotle said happiness, the raison d'etre of life and life's most important goal, can be achieved with the correct desires (cited in Ludwigs, 2018). For Aristotle, happiness or a good life is eudaimonia (Prior 1991: 148). Epicurians defined the goal of life as pleasure and defined the pursuit of pleasure and avoidance of pain as an ethical principle. In general, the pleasures that Epicurians valued are mental pleasures, but some (e.g., Cyreneans) pursued physical pleasures. While Aristotle emphasized fulfillment of the correct desire, Epicurians discussed fulfillment of general desires and the ancient Stoics argued for the suppression of desire (Bok 2010: 50). In the ancient times, happiness was seen as something given by a god or other external agent, akin to luck or blessing. For example, Aristotle used eudaimonia (good spirit) interchangeably with "makario (blessed)" in Greek (Miao et al., 2013).

This perspective became more widespread in the middle ages and the belief that happiness is given to a select few through faith in god. This traditional perspective on

[1] In general, Western happiness studies were actively dealt with in three periods: ancient Greek philosophy, post-enlightenment philosophy in Europe, and current Quality of Life research (Veenhoven 1991a, b).

S. J. Lee, *Public Happiness*, Community Quality-of-Life and Well-Being,
https://doi.org/10.1007/978-3-030-89643-0_2

happiness changed in the thirteenth century through the ideas of Tomas Aquinas that individuals can become happy with their efforts (Koo et al., 2015). This emphasis on an individual's efforts for happiness became stronger in the seventeenth and eighteenth century Enlightenment era and led to ideas that personal pleasure is a key factor of happiness and that happiness is internal and thus something that an individual can achieve with effort. This was the beginning of a shift from a happiness of fortune to a happiness of pleasure (Miao et al., 2013). This perspective is well represented in the eighteenth century philosophy of utilitarianism that equated happiness with pleasure. In contrast, there is deontoligism that is best represented by Kant. Understanding of happiness based on Kant's ethical philosophy assumes that there is an absolute ethical standard that all humans ascribe to. Thus, pleasure that ignores ethics was not recognized as happiness (Koo et al., 2015).

As much as happiness is an interest of western civilization, it was also discussed in Eastern philosophy from the early ages. Confucius, in West Scripture (西經), defines five blessings for happiness, which are physical and mental wellbeing (康寧); long life (壽); wealth (富); taking pleasure in following ethical norms and sharing with one's neighbors (攸好德); and to accomplish one's responsibility and mission with diligence (考終命). This happiness perspective highlights the important components of a happy life and not only shows an individual perspective but also includes the community that one belongs to for a comprehensive perspective on happiness. It is said that the word "happiness" cannot be found in the traditional Confucian text, but it can be said that the Confucian perspective approaches happiness through the word "blessing". Happiness can be defined as freedom, comfort, or a condition where all deficiencies are fulfilled. Confucians emphasize that to be happy we should get rid of selfishness or the ego. Doing so leads to the highest sense of joy from the inside, motivating love and life. Wealth and honor are something everybody desires, but if it comes without morals, then this is not genuine happiness. Similarly, Jeong Yak-yong (1762–1836), an ancient Korean scholar, defined a happy life as a moral and meaningful life. He believed that the subjective attitude of accepting with joy is more important for happiness than the objective blessing itself (Jang, 2017: 53). In general, the Eastern view of happiness can be traced from a Confucian approach that pursues a virtuous equilibrium that is neither excessive nor insufficient (Xi, 1999) and Lao-tzu's Taoism that emphasizes conforming to the non-artificial form in nature is the basis of a happy life (Lao-tzu 2007: 174; Jiwook 2018: 104).

Overall, in eastern culture, the concepts of fortune (福), pleasure (樂), and flourishing (吉) have been used in discussions of a good life, and these can be seen as representing happiness. There are some clear differences in eastern and western perspectives on happiness. While the western perspective can be broadly divided into hedonistic and eudaimonic views, in the eastern perspective the emphasis on virtue is more widely accepted than pleasure. Eastern philosophy views happiness as an enduring trait that arises from a mind in a state of equilibrium and entails a conceptually unstructured and unfiltered awareness of the true nature of reality, rather than a momentary emotion aroused by sensory or conceptual stimuli (Crum & Salovey, 2013). In other words, the perspective of happiness in eastern culture usually means the achievement of human nature through practice.

These days, happiness has a strong hedonistic bend as it is not seen as something given externally but something that can be pursued with one's own efforts internally and is seen as a subjective emotion and evaluation (Koo et al., 2015). However, the question of whether happiness should be viewed as a momentary pleasure or whether the satisfaction or evaluation stemming from a mistaken perception can be viewed as genuine happiness remains. The notion that life without morality and virtue cannot be a good life is also strong (e.g., Kesebir & Diener, 2008). Increasingly, the perspective of balancing this with eudaimonism—a meaningful life—and focusing on an individual's capacity to pursue this type of life is becoming more important. The inclusion of both hedonistic and eudaimonic components in many surveys and indicators is one evidence (Koo et al., 2017: 17).

How is the concept of happiness defined? Across eastern and western philosophy, happiness has been understood in various ways, and as a result, there is no unified definition of happiness in modern day. In fact, the confusion of the concept of happiness is common, and some even say this is an important roadblock to understanding happiness (Cummins, 2013). Some exemplary definitions are as follows. Veenhoven (1991a, b, a leading happiness scholar, equates satisfaction to happiness. For him, life satisfaction, i.e., happiness is conceived as "the degree to which an individual judges the overall quality of his life-as-a-whole-favorably". In other words, "how well he likes the life he leads". This is basically subjective satisfaction and aligns with the hedonic aspect of happiness.[2] Likewise, some scholars like Tatarkiewicz (1966: 1) and Michalos (1985) equate happiness as satisfaction with one's life.

Other scholars prefer satisfaction to happiness. Campbell et al. (1976) say life satisfaction is a more reliable concept than happiness because it is a cognitive judgment, whereas happiness refers to a feeling or affect. Lane and Terry (2000) say happiness is a mood, while satisfaction with life is a more cognitive evaluation. Helliwell and Putnam (2004) say the life satisfaction measure seems marginally better than the happiness measure in terms of social context.

As such, while the two concepts are recognized as related (Yeh et al., 2015), there are criticisms to it. Feldman (2010: 5) is specific at this point. He gives an example of the Eurobarometer which asks two questions about life satisfaction. One is "On the whole, are you very satisfied, fairly satisfied, not very satisfied, or not at all satisfied with the life that you lead?", and the other is "If you had the opportunity to live your life over, would you want to change many things in your life, or some things, or nothing at all?". Regarding this, Feldman indicates that one is satisfied but may not be happy and that one may not want to change her life again but may not be happy. In other words, life satisfaction and happiness are not the same. Relatedly, Haybron (2016) found that the judgment of respondents' satisfaction in the survey is arbitrary, and the relationship between life satisfaction and happiness is weak because satisfaction actually represents the good-enoughness of a life rather than the goodness of a life. However, it is not possible to entirely deny the relationship

[2] The reason Veenhoven (1991a, b) pays attention to satisfaction is that life satisfaction is ① quite precisely defined, ② fairly well measured, ③ empirical data is accumulated, and ④ various difficulties exist in employing an objective conception.

between satisfaction and happiness. Although one may be satisfied but not happy, or dissatisfied but happy, it is more common that one is satisfied and happy, and dissatisfied and unhappy. Therefore, it is reasonable to understand that both are related. The general view on this is to see satisfaction as a sub-concept of happiness, as explicated later.

Wellbeing is often used interchangeably with happiness (Musikanski et al., 2019: 19). In psychology texts, happiness is the common sensical, wellbeing is a representative name for human wellness (David et al., 2013). According to Diener et al. (2009: 9), wellbeing is an individual's global evaluation of his or her life across a variety of different aspects of life. Thus, wellbeing refers to being well in general rather than within any specific area of life. That is wellbeing is an overall evaluation of an individual's life in all its aspects. From this perspective, it is difficult to distinguish happiness from wellbeing.

However, there are some limitations to treating wellbeing and happiness as synonyms. In this regard, Thin (2012: 34) argues that feeling well is not the same as feeling happy. He explains, "Happiness is in practice a much more expansive, complex, and motivating term, including numerous linked concepts that together combine to form much more holistic, narrative evaluations of lives. He indicates that without the 'subjective' prefix, 'wellbeing' is too easily understood in expert-led, paternalist ways that disregard people's own preferences and feelings." He also indicates that wellbeing contains the concept of subjective wellbeing, which is often used interchangeably with happiness, but in practice, the word emphasizes the body, basic provisioning, and illbeing, and thus, some say it is a narrower concept than happiness. Graham (2011: 25) also defines happiness as a comprehensive concept. According to her, happiness is a catch-all term including wellbeing as an overall evaluation of one's life, wellbeing as experienced in day-to-day living, wellbeing as influenced by innate character traits, and wellbeing as quality of life broadly defined. In addition, she argues that happiness is more useful than wellbeing in daily conversations because the latter is often understood in expert-led, paternalist ways that disregard peoples' own preferences and feelings.

What then is the concept of happiness here? I prefer a holistic definition of happiness that helps to capture its complexity: how positively people feel about their lives (Pfeiffer & Cloutier, 2016). That is, happiness equals the goodness of one's life. The level of good life is defined by the individual's comprehensive evaluation. If we use the term wellbeing, happiness is the same as subjective wellbeing. While wellbeing is an umbrella term for a number of concepts related to human wellness and includes subjective wellbeing (David et al., 2013), subjective wellbeing is how people evaluate their own lives in terms of both affective and cognitive components (Diener et al., 1999). However, happiness is not the same as satisfaction. As I will explain later, if subjective wellbeing includes feeling, satisfaction, and meaning, then subjective wellbeing becomes a broader concept than satisfaction. In sum, as long as we see happiness and subjective wellbeing as synonymous, we cannot treat happiness and satisfaction as synonyms.

Which term (between happiness and subjective wellbeing) shall we use then? As Seligman and Csikszentmihalyi (2000) noted, subjective wellbeing is the more scientific-sounding term that generally means happiness. Nevertheless, this book prefers to use the term "happiness" for the following reasons. First, happiness more effectively calls the attention of people and the media (Musikanski et al., 2019: 20), making it easier to gather support for happiness policies. Second, given that the purpose of happiness studies is not limited to scholarly discussion but also includes practical contributions, it is better to use the term that is often used in casual discussions of the good life. Third, the scope of happiness is broader, allowing for more flexibility in its implementation.

On the one hand, despite the diverse meanings of happiness, the insistence on a single, unified conceptualization of happiness may be unnecessary. In fact, Alexandrova (2012) is wary of the over-generalization or attempts to arrive at a single definition of happiness. Such a focus requires a general evaluation, considering all the relevant aspects, adding and weighing them appropriately. According to Alexandrova (2012), previous conceptualizations have the limit of invariantism. A single concept of wellbeing applies to all, irrespective of moral or other considerations, where the construct of wellbeing does not vary with circumstances. Thus, Alexandrova calls for a more variant definition than the current fixed, generalized conceptualization. Of the variantist view, there are many concepts of wellbeing, some general and some very contextual. These new definitions of wellbeing are less universal but actually usable.

While we should remain wary of a simplistic, singular conceptualization, the happiness dialogue would benefit from a certain level of shared understanding of the concept. As Alexandrova (2012) also acknowledges, there exists already an overlap with the previous conceptualizations, and context is a realistic issue to be considered when applying the concept. Therefore, we maintain the aforementioned definition of happiness as "a positive evaluation of life." This definition sees happiness as a subjective feeling that includes positive feelings, evaluations, and life meaning. It excludes the objective conditions that motivate happiness. If we see happiness as a resultant of the individual's position on two independent dimensions of positive affect and negative affect as Bradburn (1969: 9), then we can include negative feelings as a component of happiness.

2 Perspectives of Happiness

It is difficult to find a unified definition of happiness because happiness is understood as being synonymous to a good life (Vittersø 2013a, b) and the understanding of what is a good life is not neutral but connected to philosophical views (Veenhoven 1991a, b). As aforementioned, the philosophical views of happiness or a good life include the hedonistic view that focuses on feeling (pleasure) or satisfaction and the eudaimonic view that focuses on virtue and morals (Ryan & Deci, 2001).

2.1 Hedonistic View

Strong support for the hedonistic view stems from utilitarianism. In general, utilitarianism sees the pursuit of surplus of happiness over suffering as "good" (Katarzyna and Singer 2017: xix). Thus, they argue for maximizing utility by producing benefit, advantage, pleasure, good, or happiness and preventing mischief, pain, evil, or unhappiness. This view of utilitarianism can be traced back to Epicuros of ancient Greece who considered pleasure as the measure of happiness, but the systematic logic of this view started with the late eighteenth century English scholar Bentham. Bentham considered utility the measure of morality and that any pleasure that increases utility is good, while any pain that decreases utility is evil. Furthermore, Bentham believed that when individuals seek to maximize their own utility, the total sum of these individuals' utility or social utility also becomes maximized. This key idea of utilitarianism can be seen in Bentham (1748–1832)'s rhetoric of "greatest happiness of the greatest number." In other words, maximizing the contentment (satisfaction) and pleasure of the greatest number of individuals as they experienced their lives is the goal. The evaluation criteria for a state (law, institutions, and administration) or individual when deciding what is beneficial become the total sum happiness of the greatest number. Dewey (1963) explains that Bentham's utilitarianism "made the wellbeing of the individual the norm of political action in every area in which it operates." Bentham's theory defines an individual's pleasure and pain, which is the evaluation criteria of individuals' actions, as elemental units that can be summed algebraically and each individual's happiness is assigned the same weight. Bentham's utilitarianism is considered to be the foundation of classical English economic theory and capitalism (Kang, 2013).

John Stuart Mill (1806–1873) is also a leading utilitarian. He also responded to the criticism that utilitarianism diminishes the sanctity of humans by defining humans as animals that only pursue pleasure. The saying, "Dissatisfied human beings are better than satisfied pigs, and Socrates is better than satisfied fools" shows his perspective. Basically, Mill sees humans as being able to constrain their pleasure, unlike other animals, and that the pleasure that humans pursue is qualitatively different from the pleasure that other animals pursue. Another criticism of utilitarianism is that the pursuit of pleasure is nothing more than selfishness. This is really a question of whether to recognize unethical pleasure. Regarding this, Mill points out that "we need to separate the argument that pleasure or pain by itself is good or evil and the argument that every pleasure or pain is good or evil." For example, even if an unethical act brings pleasure to an individual, this can bring great pain to the collective group and thus should be criticized. In sum, the interpretation of an individual's momentary pleasure is a simplistic interpretation of the greatest happiness of the greatest number principle of utilitarianism (Kim & Chung, 2003: 15). If we see Bentham's perspective as quantitative utilitarianism that sees pleasure as quantifiable and measurable, Mill's perspective can be seen as qualitative utilitarianism that goes beyond materialistic pleasure to mental pleasure. Still, they share the idea that pleasure is happiness.

Utilitarianism encourages individuals to make the right decision for the greatest happiness of the greatest number, and thus the individual becomes the sole agent that has the responsibility and authority for happiness. This is related to the liberal perspective that emphasizes an individual's capacity and characteristics. We see this reflected in the key principles of liberalism, such as prioritization of individual rights, inviolability of basic rights, and minimization of government intervention (Daly, 1994).

2.2 *Eudaimonism*

In contrast to utilitarianism, eudaimonism emphasizes virtue or character. The Greek word eudaimonia is a combination of "eu (good)" and "daimon (spirit)" and generally means good spirit or flourishing. This is applied to life overall, rather than a specific feeling or moment (Graham, 2011). The origins of eudaimonism can be traced to Aristotle of ancient Greece. In regards to the question of what is a good life, he says a virtuous life is a good life and a happy life. A good life is the achievement of Eudaimonia, and this is in line with happiness, prosperity that human beings ultimately desire (Park, 2012). Aristotle sees happiness as being determined in the process of training for virtue within a local, political community. This is related to his belief that "man is a political animal" and therefore the appropriate goal of people's lives is determined within the local political unit (Friedman, 1994). In sum, the meaning of Eudaimonia is goal-oriented and unifies community life with a meaningful life. For Aristotle, communal life has important meaning for achieving happiness. Here, community is not the simple sum of individuals. The state is an organic order consisting of diverse citizens who exist together for a common good (Lee, 1998). Considering that virtue exists in social relationships, Aristotle's eudaimonia should of course be related closely to community.

In general, unlike the hedonic approach that sees pleasure as the core value of happiness, the eudaimonic approach aims for an evaluation of life overall. This approach does not deny pleasures, but emphasizes the meaning or fulfillment of life. Moreover, it emphasizes the social approval and moral evaluation of different pleasures (Thin, 2012: 35). The eudaimonic approach makes an ethical evaluation of pleasure because eudaimonia is created within the relationships in a community. On the other hand, as liberalism forms the basis for hedonism (Daly, 1994), communitarianism forms the basis for eudaimonism. We can see this in communitarianism's emphasis on equality over individual freedom and its emphasis on social responsibility and value judgments. It is notable that Thin (2012: 35) suggests a pathophobic approach as a third approach. Instead of actively pursuing a good life, this approach passively pursues a good life by minimizing unpleasantness. In contrast to the utilitarian approach that highlights active pursuit of utility, the pathophobic approach can be seen as a negative utilitarian approach. Regardless of the direction of utility pursuit, however, this basically belongs to the hedonistic approach because the ultimate goal is hedonistic.

3 Components of Happiness

To understand happiness, we need to go beyond defining the concept and discuss the components of happiness. This is necessary to operationalize the abstract concept on a practical level and to develop happiness policies. Similar to the conceptualization of happiness, the approaches to defining the components of happiness are also closely related to philosophical views. The two main opposing viewpoints are the hedonic perspective and eudaimonic perspective.

Broadly speaking, the hedonic perspective suggests affect and cognition as components of happiness, while the eudaimonic perspective suggests the eudaimonic component. The affective (or hedonic) component is "the degree to which the various affects a person experiences are pleasant: in other words: how well he usually feels." The relative balance of positive and negative feelings determines a person's overall level of affective experience. The affective component refers to both moods and emotions associated with experiencing momentary events. The cognitive (or evaluative) components is "the degree to which an individual perceives his aspirations to have been met. In other words: to what extent one thinks oneself to have got what one wants in life." When this evaluation process is directed toward an overall judgment of life as a whole, it is life satisfaction. The eudaimonic component consists of a more enduring sense of purpose, fulfillment, and self-realization. It is also called flourishing (David et al., 2013; Pavot & Diener, 2013; Ryan & Deci, 2001).

Thus, happiness studies so far suggest three components of happiness: affective, cognitive, and eudaimonic components. These are mutually distinctive but not entirely exclusive and do overlap. They may be considered to exist on a continuum (National Research Council, 2013: 15). Below, I discuss the components of happiness according to the two philosophical views.

3.1 Hedonic Perspective

The hedonic perspective sees happiness as a subjective state of joyful and satisfactory life (pleasure, satisfaction) and suggests two aspects—affect and cognition—as the components of happiness. For example, Venhoveen (1991a, b) sees happiness as a synonym for life satisfaction. Satisfaction includes an affective aspect (hedonic level) and a cognitive aspect (contentment). Similarly, Diener (2000: 34) stated that happiness is people's cognitive and affective evaluation of their lives, and Ludwigs (2018: 25) defines happiness as "overall enjoyment of one's life as-a-whole" and includes affective and cognitive aspects as components of happiness. The OECD (2013: 29) says happiness refers to good mental states, including all of the various evaluations, positive and negative, that people make of their lives, and the affective reactions of people to their experiences. McAslan et al., (2013: 156) employed two types of happiness measures: life satisfaction and emotional wellbeing. While life satisfaction reflects how satisfied people are when they think or reflect on their life, emotional wellbeing measures the momentary experiences of happiness, worry, stress, and other emotional states. While life satisfaction refers to being happy "about" your life, emotional wellbeing refers to being happy "in" your life.

In this regard, Pavot and Diener (2013) present a three-component model and four-component model of subjective wellbeing. The three-component model includes positive affect and negative affect that are often experienced relatively independently of each other. They indicate that with this distinction many regard SWB as having three components: two affects (positive and negative) and life satisfaction (cognitive). The four-component model divides the satisfaction component of SWB into two parts: life satisfaction and domain satisfaction. They explain that specific life domains (e.g., marital, work, housing or health) can provide a more specific and detailed view of the experience of SWB for each individual or for particular groups of individuals.

There is some confusion in the hedonic perspective's components of happiness. While some studies like the above adopt a hedonic perspective that include affect and cognition component (e.g., Ryan & Deci, 2001), other studies consider cognition as an element of evaluative perspective, rather than hedonic (Pavot & Diener, 2013; National Research Council, 2013; Thin, 2012: 36). For example, the National Research Council (2013) suggests experienced (hedonic), evaluative, and eudaimonic wellbeing as the components of subjective wellbeing. This is the same as the hedonic point of view in that it is limited to the experience (affect) and the evaluation is presented as a separate element. Similarly, Thin (2012: 36) distinguishes evaluative (cognitive) components from hedonic components by presenting three components of happiness: hedonic, evaluative, and existential components.

The reason for this confusion around the range of hedonic dimension or the nature of cognitive (evaluative) component may be that evaluation lies somewhere between pleasure and eudaimonia. In fact, it is not easy to conceptually differentiate eudaimonic and evaluation, and in measurement, it is difficult to separate life satisfaction and meaningful life. For example, the World Value Survey's question about life satisfaction, "Overall, how satisfied are you with life as a whole nowadays?" (OECD, 2013: 254), and the eudaimonic question from the Annual Population Survey, "Overall, to what extent do you feel the things you do in your life are worthwhile" (National Research Council, 2013: 19), are very similar. Nevertheless, presenting the evaluation dimension parallel to the hedonic, eudaimonic dimension without a discussion of how the evaluation dimension is related to the previous two perspectives hinders the understanding of happiness perspectives and its components.

3.2 Eudaimonic Perspective

The eudaimonic perspective values eudaimonic components, such as meaningfulness, sense of purpose, and life value as the components of happiness. However, today it is difficult to find studies that only present the eudaimonic components. Instead, several studies criticize the narrow approach to happiness that only focuses on pleasure or satisfaction and present pleasure (feeling), satisfaction, and meaning together as components of happiness from a perspective that comprises both eudaimonic and hedonic. For example, Vittersø (2013a, b) says that the combination of good feelings and favorable evaluations, i.e., the duality of experiences and evaluations, has dominated modern happiness research and argues that there are limits to defining happiness narrowly as hedonic balance and life satisfaction. He explains.

> The study of happiness is reduced to simply asking people if they are happy (emotion) or satisfied with their life (satisfaction). .... Feelings and evaluations make little sense if they are isolated from the goals and plans held by those who experience the feeling and make the evaluations.

He then suggests a functional wellbeing model that incorporates good feelings and positive evaluations and in addition includes the idea of good functioning.

Bruni (2016: 272–4) says that subjective wellbeing centered on pleasure does not include flourishing (eudaimonic aspect) and thus is limited. He argues that from the interpretation of happiness as goodness of life, subjective wellbeing should be flourishing per the Aristotelian tradition and argues that relational goods (such as family, friends, and community) should receive more attention in the happiness concept. Relatedly, he criticizes that current measures of subjective wellbeing are limited in two ways: (1) cognitive errors occur because an evaluation of the objective conditions is infeasible due to adaptation of the respondent and (2) respondents tend to prefer consumption goods to creative goods in measuring happiness. In sum, subjective wellbeing is important, but like GDP, it is not enough for measuring the goodness of life.

In a similar vein, many studies have presented the components of happiness from a comprehensive perspective (Diener & Biswas-Diener, 2019; Diener & Suh, 1997; Diener & Seligman, 2004; Dolan et al., 2011; Fowers et al., 2010; Frey, 2008; Huta & Waterman, 2014; Kraut, 1979; Pfeiffer & Cloutier, 2016; Ryan & Deci, 2001; Straume & Vittersø, 2012; Tiberius & Hall, 2010; Thin, 2012; Waterman et al., 2008). In particular, the OECD (2013: 29–32) presented affect, life evaluation, and eudaimonia as the survey guidelines for measuring happiness.

Additional studies go beyond checking the affect, cognition, and eudaimonic components and have identified their specific components. For example, according to Ryan and Deci (2001: 144), the happiness that we study is the combination of the ideal experience and functioning that come from the hedonic perspective and eudaimonic perspective. The hedonic perspective has been understood by psychologists as physical or mental happiness or preference and thus includes as its components, subjective items such as pleasure attainment or pain avoidance. In particular, these are the key components of the likes and dislikes in life. In contrast, the eudaimonic components include self-realization and the degree to which a person is fully functioning. From the eudaimonic perspective, happiness is living peacefully with one's original self and becomes possible through self-determination. In order to accomplish this, one needs autonomy and competence—which are connected to growth, integrity, wellbeing (life satisfaction and happiness), and self-congruence (Ryan & Deci, 2001: 147).

Table 1 Components of happiness

Components of eudaimonism	Components of hedonism
Growth/self-realization/self-actualization/development of potentials/full functioning/maturity	Pleasure/enjoyment/life satisfaction/happiness
Meaning/purpose/long-term perspective/caring about and contributing to the broader context	Low distress/comfort/relaxation
Authenticity/identity/personal expressiveness/autonomy/constitutive goals/integrity	Evaluative mind-set
Excellence/virtue/using the best in oneself/reaching a high standard/ signature strengths)	Engagement/interest/flow
	Pursuit of homeostasis
Relatedness/positive relationships/social wellbeing	
Competence/environmental mastery	
Awareness/contemplation/mindfulness	
Acceptance/self-acceptance	
Effort/engaging with challenge	
Subjective wellbeing	

Source Huta and Waterman (2014: 1435)

Straume and Vittersø (2012) described the two perspectives as a state and personal traits. In terms of a state, hedonism includes feeling or the achievement of life goals as components, and eudaimonism includes the inspiration or challenges in the process of pursuing goals. In terms of trait, eudaimonism links to personal growth and optimal functioning, while hedonism links to pleasant feelings. Fowers et al. (2010) present fun, challenge, positive feelings, negative feelings, and satisfaction with life as the components of hedonism and integrity, personal expression, purpose in life, self-actualization, and positive relationships as the components of eudaimonism.

Meanwhile, Huta and Waterman (2014: 1425) point out that while previous studies have tried to identify the components of happiness according to the two perspectives, there has not been an effort to make a systematic evaluation or distinction that combines the two perspectives. Accordingly, they suggest a combined list of the components for eudaimonism and hedonism. As seen in Table 1, they identify ten components in the eudaimonic perspective and five components in the hedonic perspective.

3.3 Summary

So far, we have seen how the components of happiness are related to the philosophies of hedonism and eudaimonism. In general, the hedonistic perspective presents affect and satisfaction as the components of happiness and the eudaimonic perspective presents meaning as the main component.

We cannot say which perspective on happiness is right or wrong, but rather that each perspective shows an important component of happiness. Thus, it is appropriate to operationalize happiness by including the components from both perspectives. Likewise, many studies have shown a tendency to include affect, satisfaction, and life meaning as the components of happiness reflecting both perspectives. Of course, pleasure and satisfaction are understood as hedonic components and fulfillment as a eudaimonic component. As mentioned above, however, some understand evaluative components like life satisfaction as an intermediate position between the hedonic and the components.

The relationship among the three components cannot be defined singularly. As mentioned, the three components can be distinguished, but they are related and partly overlapping. Eudaimonic components such as fulfillment and virtuous activities tend to bring more pleasure, more sustainability than disapproved short-term gratifications. Thus, we cannot see happiness as merely pleasure. There are various forms of pleasure, and many are virtuous, pro-social, beautiful, and admirable activities (Thin, 2012: 46). In terms of measuring happiness, the measurement of the eudaimonic aspect is related to measure of affective and cognitive aspects (National Research Council, 2013: 41). In other words, the components of happiness are interrelated, and we should be wary of defining these as being exclusive and definitive. Nettle (2006) combines the concepts of hedonism and eudaimonism by dividing happiness into three levels (Fig. 1). Level 1 is the personal, momentary emotion, and the judgment of these emotions leads to level 3 that includes quality of life,

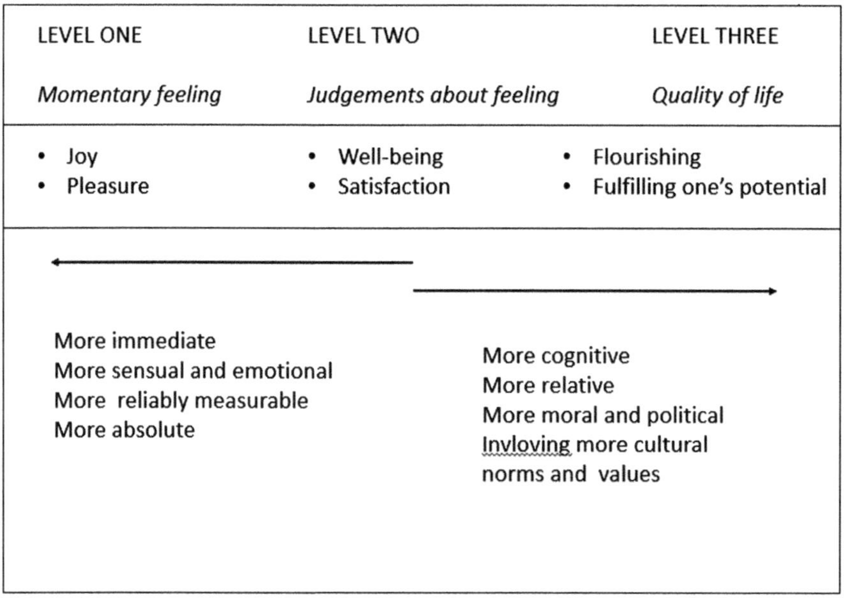

Fig. 1 Levels of happiness components. *Source* Nettle (2006: 18)

prosperity, and self-realization. By doing so, he shows the connection between the hedonic component and the eudaimonic component.

4 Related Concepts

Happiness is used interchangeably with several concepts, such as wellbeing, welfare, utility, pleasure, life satisfaction, meaningful life, and contentment. While some researchers and policymakers differentiate between the terms happiness and other related concepts, such as wellbeing, quality of life, and emotions, many scholars do not differentiate happiness from related concepts, such as pleasure, satisfaction, and welfare. For example, Oswald (1997) defines happiness as pleasure or satisfaction. Easterlin (2001: 465) uses happiness, subjective wellbeing, satisfaction, utility, well-being, and welfare interchangeably. Economists are more concerned with measuring happiness than defining it. Many happiness studies use the World Values Survey that measure happiness ("how happy are you?") and life satisfaction ("how satisfied are you with your life?")—both of which are considered measures of happiness. Many other scholars have similar tendencies (Adler et al., 2017; Bruni & Porta, 2007; Diener, 2006; Forgeard et al., 2011; Frey, 2008; Frey & Stutzer, 2002; Veenhoven, 2015). That is, in the happiness discussion, there is not a strict distinction between happiness and its related concepts. However, it is necessary to address this confusion to move the happiness discussion forward. A discussion of these related concepts follows.

4.1 Wellbeing

Wellbeing (WB) means the good life and is a comprehensive evaluation of life. It is often used interchangeably with happiness, but to be precise, we can differentiate the two concepts. Happiness is emotional, but wellbeing includes an objectively good life (Woo, 2014) and is based in flourishing. Abundance affects happiness, but happiness is not necessarily based on abundance. We see this from the fact that happiness can accompany physical or mental disabilities, but not wellbeing (Raibley, 2012).

Wellbeing can be divided into objective and subjective wellbeing, and the former can be seen as the objective life conditions, while the latter is the personal, qualitative evaluation of life. For example, Kim (2009: 7) said wellbeing can be divided into an objective aspect (objective wellbeing, quality of life) and subjective aspect (subjective wellbeing, life satisfaction, and happiness). Objective wellbeing means the objective point of view that is independent of an individual's own subjective values and norms. Subjective wellbeing requires a reference to the individual's own interests, needs, preferences, or desires (Diener et al., 2009: 9). Some calculate subjective wellbeing by subtracting negative affect from positive affect plus life satisfaction and flourishing (Diener & Biswas-Diener, 2008: 249).

Subjective wellbeing (SWB) and happiness are both related to human emotions, and thus, the distinction between the two is a key point of interest. Examining several studies, we see that some studies understand SWB from a hedonic perspective and argue that it falls under happiness—a higher-level concept (e.g., Bruni & Porta, 2007; Diener et al., 1999; Frey & Stutzer, 2010; Lane et al., 2009; Nettle, 2006). For them, SWB is a concept encompassing how people evaluate their own lives in terms of both affective (how we feel) and cognitive (how we think) components (Diener et al., 1999). The affective component refers to both moods and emotions associated with the experiencing of momentary events. The cognitive component, represented by life satisfaction, relates to the way individuals perceive their lives and refers to a discrepancy between the present situation and what is thought to be the ideal or deserved standard. Life satisfaction is the degree to which individuals judge their lives favorably (David et al., 2013), which is similar to happiness defined by Veenhoven (1991a, b). The "subjective" in SWB means the subjective approach allows individuals to judge how their life is according to what they themselves find important for happiness. This differs from the eudaimonic approach which specifies in advance the human potentials that we all have to realize. SWB includes at least two components. SWB includes both happiness at the level of experience and active reflective evaluation, i.e., life satisfaction. In other words, SWB includes experience and attitude (Alexandrova, 2005: 302).

Some other studies adopt an eudaimonic perspective which is connected to a meaningful life and understand SWB as equivalent to happiness (Frank, 1997; Layard, 2005; OECD, 2013; Ryan & Deci, 2001). They understand SWB as a wider, all-encompassing concept that includes the eudaimonic component of meaningful life with the hedonic affects and satisfaction.

Which position should we adopt? There are benefits to interpreting SWB from the standpoint of the hedonistic perspective. According to Veenhoven (1991a, b), the hedonic level is less vulnerable to cognitive adaptation, because it is a direct experience and is less open to defensive distortion and because it is less threatening to admit that one feels bad sometimes than to admit to being disappointed in life. Both overall happiness and hedonic level have been found to be highly correlated can be also taken into account.

Despite such benefits, this interpretation of SWB is too narrow. This concept only includes the hedonic aspects and excludes the important eudaimonic aspect. Considering the mainstream understanding of happiness as more than emotion or satisfaction (Feldman, 2010) and the general tendency to use SWB and happiness interchangeably, there is a need to add the eudaimonic approach here. In this case, SWB comprises affect (experience), evaluation (attitude), and life meaning and then becomes equivalent to happiness. Of course, this is a broader meaning of SWB than the narrow one that excludes eudaimonia. But there are benefits to using this expanded concept of SWB. When using the narrow SWB, there remains the problem of what to call the eudaimonic concept. If this is not SWB, then it has to fall under objective wellbeing or intersubjective wellbeing. However, it is impossible to objectively define or evaluate a meaningful life. How can one person define and evaluate what is a meaningful life for another? Therefore, it is impossible to include the eudaimonic component under objective wellbeing. The best way to minimize confusion is to call the physical conditions necessary for SWB as objective wellbeing. That is, defining SWB in a narrow way erases the name for an important element of happiness—the eudaimonic component. This does not mean there have not been perspectives that see the eudaimonic component as an objective component. For example, Alexandrova (2012) sees the components defined by eudaimonic as non-subjective. This is probably because he sees the virtues defined in eudaimonism as the generally accepted virtues. However, whether there are generally accepted virtues is questionable, and even with a generally accepted set of virtues, ultimately an individual has to make a subjective judgment about those virtues. The existence of virtues and following those virtues and what one feels from it are different issues. The latter is subjective at its core. This is the same for experiences or attitudes. Two individuals may have the same conditions of life, but what each individual feels or their attitudes may be different. Basically, happiness is about mental states toward the good life (Feldman, 2010: 5). Similarly, SWB is about mental states, and there is enough reason to connect the two.

As such, we see SWB as synonymous to happiness, including affect, satisfaction, and meaning. Affect, satisfaction, and meaning all require an individual judgment. Affect is an evaluation of joy or pain. Satisfaction is an evaluation of satisfaction. And meaning is an evaluation of moral, value, and meaning. The object is the same, but the evaluation aspect differs. Related, Alexandrova (2012) criticized Kahneman (1999)'s objective happiness and argued for the reevaluation of experiences with a value base, and this argument shows the limits of a narrow definition of SWB.

Some see SWB as a higher-level concept of happiness. Diener (2006) defines SWB as a higher-level concept that includes the following six lower-level concepts: (1) positive affect (2) negative affect (3) happiness (4) life satisfaction (5) life domain satisfaction 6) quality of life. Here, happiness is defined as "a general positive mood," "a global evaluation of life satisfaction," or "living a good life." An important point is unlike other studies, Diener (2006: 401) explains that SWB is the component of overall life events that includes positive and negative affect, cognitive evaluation, satisfaction, and interest and is the mind-set and environment. In sum, SWB includes both subjective and objective elements.[3] Most studies differentiate wellbeing and SWB. However, Diener (2006:399) uses wellbeing and SWB interchangeably to avoid the confusion around the word subjective. Thus, Diener is in fact attempting to conceptualize wellbeing rather than SWB, and this places happiness under the concept of SWB.

4.2 Community Wellbeing (CWB)

Recently, a research project on community wellbeing is being conducted based on the assumption that individual and collective aspects of wellbeing differ and that

[3] However, meaningful life elements were excluded from subjective wellbeing.

there is a need to build wellbeing from a community aspect. This research project was conducted from 2010 to 2020 by the Community WellBeing Research Center of the Seoul National University with the Global Community Institute, a collaborative research institute in Korea. Several researchers, including the author, from the United States, United Kingdom, Australia, Italy, Canada, Germany, China, Japan, and South Korea participated.

What is community wellbeing (CWB)? CWB refers to wellbeing at the community (or collective) level, which is distinct from individual-level wellbeing. Lee and Kim (2016) present Fig. 2 which shows the location of CWB with regard to several wellbeing concepts using two crossing axes of individual-collective and subjective–objective. Broadly speaking, wellbeing can be divided into individual wellbeing and community wellbeing. Individual wellbeing (IWB) can be further divided into objective IWB and subjective IWB. Here, objective IWB refers to the resources that an individual has. Subjective IWB is the subjective evaluation (satisfaction) of the individual's state of life. Overall, objective wellbeing acts as a condition that contributes to subjective wellbeing.

Community wellbeing (CWB) refers to the community level of wellbeing and includes objective, subjective, and intersubjective community wellbeing. Here, objective CWB refers to the resources that a community has. Subjective CWB is the individual's subjective evaluation (satisfaction) of the resources that the community has. The newly added intersubjective community wellbeing refers to the individual's subjective evaluation of the resource levels that a community has. In other words, it is the subjective evaluation of objective conditions, or objective conditions reflected in the individual cognition and have both characteristics of subjective and objective wellbeing. This intersubjective evaluation is a subjective evaluation of objective

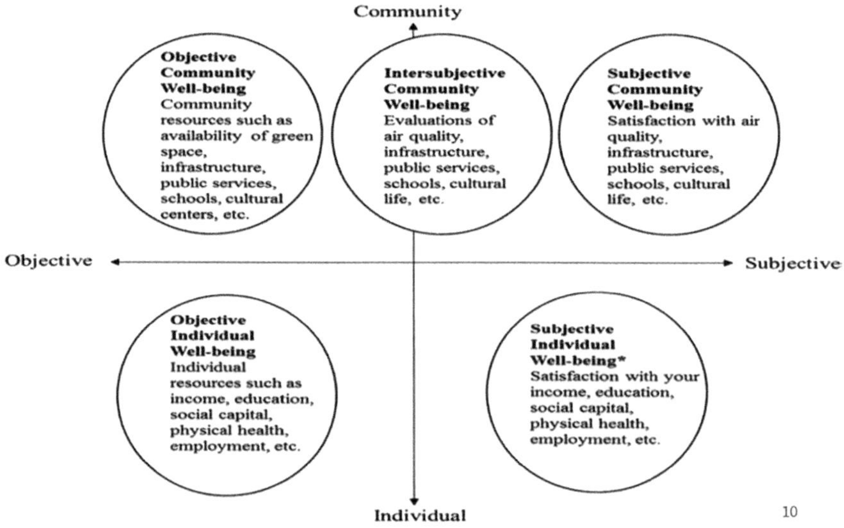

Fig. 2 Dimensions of wellbeing. *Source* Lee and Kim (2016)

conditions of a community and thus has the characteristic of an estimate, but the two are not equal. Estimate is the effort to get close to objectivity, while evaluation considers objectivity but goes through a subjective interpretation stage. Of course, both estimate and evaluation are attempts to consider the objective level and thus are related to each other, but they are not equal.

Lee et al. (2013) suggested intersubjective wellbeing as a new construct to overcome the limitations of previous subjective or objective measurements of community wellbeing and thus does not exist as a separate domain from objective or subjective community wellbeing, but rather it is an invention that helps measurement.

On the one hand, many studies treat wellbeing and happiness as similar concepts, and thus, it is necessary to discuss the relationship between the two. Often, happiness is understood to be synonymous with subjective wellbeing. This book also follows this interpretation. However, objective wellbeing is not equal to happiness, but rather a condition of happiness. Therefore, wellbeing, which includes subjective and objective wellbeing, should be understood as a broader concept than happiness. Happiness includes subjective individual wellbeing and subjective community wellbeing. Community wellbeing is more related to happiness as subjective wellbeing when its subjectivity is emphasized and is more related to the condition of happiness than happiness when its objectivity is emphasized.

Beyond the issue of clarification of related concepts to happiness, there is a practical benefit to paying attention to community wellbeing. It provides useful implications for public policy to promote the wellbeing of residents (Kim and Lee 2014). The improvement of individual wellbeing does not only come from an individual's efforts and capability, but is also affected by public policy. Public policy should ultimately improve individual wellbeing. But first, public policy should focus on community wellbeing, rather than individual wellbeing. This is because public policy is often implemented in units of geographic boundaries or functional groups. This also applies when a policy (or service) is targeted at an individual—a geographic or functional boundary is the basic unit for policy implementation and evaluation. Also, a consideration of both individual wellbeing and community wellbeing gives a more comprehensive evaluation of wellbeing. The information about community wellbeing can be useful for policies that improve individual wellbeing. Nonetheless, wellbeing studies have mostly been focused on the individual level, because it is based on the subjective feelings of an individual. But it is more appropriate to deal with wellbeing at the collective level beyond the individual level.

4.3 Objective Happiness

Daniel Kahneman (1999) argues for objective happiness. According to Kahneman, objective happiness is the extent to which one wants the experience he is having at that moment to continue. The objective happiness of a certain period is measured by a temporal integral of instant utility. This method includes repeated assessment, such as instant records of blood pressure, pain, and happiness. Instant utility is the subjective evaluation—good or bad—of specific moments. A temporal integral approximates the product of average instant utility and duration and is considered a measure of total utility. In sum, Kahneman's objective happiness is a moment-based hedonic evaluation of happiness (Alexandrova, 2012). In any case, the idea of objective happiness received much attention because it objectifies happiness which has been heretofore considered fully subjective. However, there have also been various critiques of this idea.

For example, Alexandrova (2005) strongly criticized this idea saying that objective happiness is not an appropriate indicator of SWB. Assuming that memory-based measurement tools like surveys contain errors, Kahneman tries to use instant records to measure SWB, rather than retrospective judgements. And because these responses are not based on the respondent's subjective, retrospective judgments, he calls it objective happiness. However, what Kahneman presents as "objective happiness" is not really objective. On the one hand, it does not include the conditions of one's life or society, and it still relies on the subjective report of an individual. Furthermore, Kahneman's method excludes the information that only the respondent can know retrospectively and thus violates the basic assumption of the subjective approach—that the authority to evaluate the diverse aspects of life and experiences in the process of measuring happiness belongs to the respondent. Not only is retrospection unavoidable when measuring wellbeing, it is ideal, and thus, retrospection should not be avoided. Of course, objective happiness is context-dependent. That is, in specific situations, objective happiness can become an appropriate indicator of SWB. However, as to what those situations are, scientific verification and ethical consideration are required. Alexandrova (2005) says, "Each person is the best judge of her own wellbeing is widely used as the main reason to prefer the subjective to the objective approach" and supports the subjective approach that emphasizes the individual's subjective, retrospective evaluation. There is another critique on objective happiness. Feldman (2010: 37) is also critical to the idea of objective happiness. He indicates that "it is doubtful that objective happiness is closely related to anything we would ordinarily call happiness and is also doubtful that it is related in any interesting way to welfare. A person can be very happy and doing well at a time even though she does not want her experience to continue."[4]

---

[4] In a sense, Feldman (2010: 241)'s approach to happiness is similar to Kahneman's in that he argues that "A person's happiness for an interval is the integral of his momentary happiness levels for all the moments in the interval." This approach is not very different from Kahneman's objective happiness in that it collects the moment-to-moment happiness and sees the sum of it as happiness. In other words, Feldman's approach also takes on a moment-based approach like Kahneman's "objective happiness". However, unlike Kahneman, who insists on objectivity by denying the respondent's recollection, Feldman accepts the bias according to recollection as it is.

4.4 Quality of Life

Quality of life (QOL) refers to the conditions that need to be improved to increase happiness. It is an overarching term for the quality of the various domains in life. It is a standard level that reflects the expectations of an individual or society for a good life. These expectations are guided by the values, goals, and sociocultural context in which an individual life. It is a subjective, multidimensional concept which includes a standard level for emotional, material and social wellbeing. It serves as a reference against which an individual or society can measure the different domains of one's own life. The degree to which expectations for these factors are met in an individual's life is defined as life satisfaction.

Quality of life research began after the 1960s and includes the objective and subjective dimensions of social indicators to capture quality of life (Kroll, 2008: 25). There are basically two approaches to quality of life. One is the approach to favor objective measures of wellbeing to assess one's level of living. In this approach, if an individual possesses high levels of income, wealth, knowledge, and skills, this is considered a high quality of life. For example, Santos and Martins (2013: 80) introduce four conditions of quality of life: environmental (green spaces, climate, noise, air quality, water, energy, and waste management), collective material (cultural facilities, sports facilities, educational facilities, social and health facilities, built environment, mobility, retail, and services), economic (income and consumption, labor market, housing market, and economic dynamism), and society (population, education, cultural dynamism, civic participation, health, safety, and information society). That is, they understand quality of life as objective quality of life.

The other approach focuses on subjective measures of wellbeing as indicators for life quality. Under this approach, an individual's satisfaction is quality of life rather than the possession of resources. For example, McAslan et al., (2013: 149) defines QOL as the level of enjoyment and fulfillment derived by humans from the life they live within their local economic, cultural, social, and environmental conditions. That is, their understanding is based on subjective dimensions of quality of life.

There is a more comprehensive approach comprising the two approaches. For example, Erik Allardt (1993: 89) defines quality of life in terms of having, loving, being, i.e., the sum of material security, social relationships, and personal self-expressions. Similarly, Zapf (1984) defines QoL as "good living conditions which go together with positive subjective wellbeing." Amartya Sen (1999) defines high quality of life as a life wherein an individual can express their capabilities. Capabilities are defined as the freedom a person has to choose certain combinations of functionings, i.e., the various doings and beings of a person that enable her to live a thriving life.

Veenhoven (2013) distinguishes between life chances and life outcomes and between external qualities (social quality) and internal qualities (personal quality). A combination of the two dichotomy yields a fourfold matrix (Table 2). This shows the relationship between quality of life and happiness. He explains that happiness

Table 2 Four qualities of life

	External qualities	Internal qualities
Life chances	*Livability of environment*	*Life-ability of the person*
Life outcomes	*Utility of life*	*Appreciation of life*

Source Veenhoven (2013)

includes all four qualitative characteristics of life, but that the fourth quadrant (appreciation of life) is the strongest, while the second quadrant (livability of environment) is the weakest.

It should be noted that all quadrants are related to happiness, but not all are happiness. Excluding the fourth quadrant (appreciation of life), the rest are not happiness but rather the conditions that affect happiness. In terms of quality of life, these can all be seen as lower elements, but not in terms of happiness. From this perspective, quality of life is a broader concept than happiness, and along with the good life, it emphasizes both subjective and objective elements.

5 Conditions of Happiness

While the conditions (or influencing factors) for happiness are not similar to happiness, they are often used interchangeably. Frequently, most studies include the conditions for happiness when measuring happiness. In this regard, Alexandrova (2012: 680) indicates the problem arising from it: "Depending on the object of inquiry, we use objective or subjective indicators, but because of this complexity, it is difficult to evaluate the validity of the constructs of wellbeing for given circumstances every time we contemplate relying on claims involving a different construct."

It should be noted that perceived happiness and happiness conditions are different. As Feldman (2010: 9) points out, happiness is a mental state, and the conditions that affect it should be differentiated. Of course, the objective conditions of happiness are potential conditions that will have a significant effect on happiness. That is, objective conditions are also potential happiness. Thus, notwithstanding that potential happiness cannot be seen as the achievement of happiness, many scholars have studied it as the necessary conditions of happiness, and these have become studies of happiness factors at the individual, social, national, and local levels. Nevertheless, it is clear that conditions or potential happiness is not perceived happiness. In addition, the attempts to objectively measure happiness, such as objective happiness, have not been successful so far.

When trying to differentiate perceived happiness from the conditions of happiness in psychology studies, scholars differentiate happiness into experiential and evaluative aspects. The experiential aspect refers to objective happiness and is based on the question of "how good or bad is your current experience?"[5] In particular, for an individual to fully realize their potential, the conditions are important elements, and this can be seen as objective conditions of happiness. Thus, the discussion of what are the basic conditions for a human life, conditions for a rich life, and the elements to improve quality of life has become more important. In contrast, the evaluative aspect is based in the retrospective methods of evaluating someone's subjective emotion of happiness. The happiness evaluations that we currently use are generally based on an evaluative context and mean happiness or subjective wellbeing.

Then what is perceived happiness? According to McDowell (2010), perceived happiness is acquired through the filter of personality, cognition, and emotional judgment and implies positive self-evaluation. Perceived happiness is similar to subjective happiness and subjective wellbeing and can be used interchangeably. Among the three, subjective wellbeing is used most often. SWB appeared because scholars recognized that previous happiness studies that try to study the effect of objective indicators, such as demographic variables, on happiness were limited in explaining happiness (Lyubomirsky & Lepper, 1999). One can be miserable even with a lot of wealth, one can be happy even in poor conditions, and thus, the subjective process of happiness is important. According to Diener (2000), Diener et al. (2009), the core of subjective wellbeing is "whether people themselves believe that they are living a good life in terms of the conditions that make up a good life."

What are the conditions of happiness? The conditions of happiness are the elements that affect happiness and include individual and collective elements. These conditions affect happiness by affecting the individual's efforts to pursue happiness. Many studies present a list of conditions for happiness. For example, Welsch (2009) divides happiness into a micro- and macro-level and categorize them. The micro-level refers to individual conditions such as employment or wages.

The macro-level includes public bads like corruption or terrorism, institutional conditions like political freedom, democracy, rule of law, environmental amenities like policy evaluation and satisfaction, and macro-economic conditions like unemployment, inflation, and growth. Other examples include the Better Life Index (BLI), World Value Survey, and Community Wellbeing Survey. The items in these surveys, excluding happiness or subjective wellbeing, may be considered the conditions of happiness.

Let us take the OECD's Better Life Index (BLI) as an example. BLI divides indicators of wellbeing into quality of life and material conditions. The former consists of health status, work–life balance, education and skills, social connection, civic engagement and governance, environmental quality, personal security, and subjective wellbeing, and the latter consists of income and wealth, jobs and earnings, and housing. Of the 11 components of BLI, all indicators except subjective wellbeing can be considered conditions for happiness.

Every condition has the potential to affect happiness, so it can be called potential happiness. However, not all conditions significantly affect happiness to the same

[5] Basically, objective happiness is to see happiness as a matter of measurement rather than conceptualization.

degree or through the same path. Also, the conditions of happiness and their association with happiness may vary depending on the object and time. While the conditions of happiness were discussed here with a focus on conceptual distinction between happiness per se and the conditions of happiness, Chap. 5 focuses on the relationship with happiness and discusses it in more detail with related theories.

6 Effects of Happiness

Happiness is important as a goal of human beings. Thus, Bruni (2006: 19) even asserts "Happiness…is never a means; on the contrary it is the only goal which is impossible to instrumentalise." With the same perspective, most happiness studies have treated happiness as a goal and exhibit little attention to the effect or outcomes of happiness. However, happiness is important not only because of its purpose value, but also because of its instrumental value that has a positive influence on individuals and society (Diener & Biswas-Diener, 2019).

In general, better outcomes can be expected from happy people. The effects of happiness have been reported in many aspects: health, life longevity (Diener & Chan, 2011; Veenhoven 1991a, b, strong families and relationships (Diener & Seligman, 2002), success and better outcome (Boehm & Lyubomirsky, 2008; Lyubomirsky et al., 2005), workplace productivity (Diener et al., 2017), pro-social behaviors such as charitability, cooperativeness, creativity, innovation (Greater Good Science Center, 2018), creativity and adaptivity (Fredrickson 1998), self-control and psychological resilience (Fredrickson & Joiner, 2002), sociability, activity, altruism, self-confidence, positive perceptions of others, flexible thinking (Diener & Scollon, 2003: 13–14), community and social support (Diener et al., 2018), democracy (Inglehart 2009: 2), etc. Diener and Biswas-Diener (2019) provide a summary list of the benefits of happiness: higher life expectancy, health behavior such as wearing seat belts and exercising, better immune system functioning, better organizational citizenship behaviors, better supervisor and customer ratings, earning higher incomes, longer and healthier marriage, donating more money to charity and volunteering, social activism to solve societal problems, and resilience-bouncing back more quickly from stress and adverse events. Such an effect of happiness is not only beneficial to individuals, but contributes to the formation of a better, stronger, and more caring society at the collective level (Bok 2010: 30; Thin, 2012: 56).

Some are skeptical about the functions of happiness. It is said that the pursuit of happiness leads to economic and political decline by expanding apathetic, easy-going, or irresponsible optimism and also increases individualism and egotism, causing weaker moral consciousness, disrupting social bonds, and causing social harm. However, there is not much evidence for such a criticism, but rather positive findings. Finucane et al. (2010) seem to be one of the exceptional studies which are pessimistic on the effects of happiness. Through a study in which 180 subjects were analyzed and divided into happy, sad, or control groups, happiness did not significantly affect positive behaviors such as alerting, orienting, and executive attention, and sadness did not affect other factors, but decreased intrinsic alertness. The findings show that the effects of happiness or unhappiness are limited, while at the same time showing that happiness does not at least have negative social effects. The argument of Veenhoven (1991a, b) is also a good reference. He introduces that several modern psychology studies support positive effects. For example, humanist psychologists believe that happiness leads to active involvement, creativity, and better personal relations, stress theory emphasizes that positive attitudes such as happiness buffer the impact of negative life events, and psychosomatic theory supports that chronic dissatisfaction increases vulnerability to disease and premature death. He continues: "These results suggest that a positive appreciation of life tends to broaden perception rather than paralyze it, to encourage active living rather than inducing apathy and to foster social contact rather than lead to selfish individualism. There are strong indications that happiness fosters health and even lengthens lives somewhat. These findings do not conclude the whole discussion of whether happiness should be promoted or not; they simply do away with the argument that happiness is harmful."

Recently, increasingly more studies are beginning to pay attention to the outcomes of happiness, and these studies find that happiness leads to positive outcomes. Studies reporting the negative effects of happiness are hard to find. Of course, it is not clear whether the same causality can be established in different cultural contexts. Although there may be differences in degree, it seems that basically happiness has a considerable degree of positive effect at both the individual and the social level. If so, we can expect a virtuous cycle wherein happiness leads to good outcomes and good outcomes lead to more happiness. It is a good reason to pay attention to happiness, whether for purpose value or for instrumental value.

References

Adler, A., Boniwell, I., Gibson, E., Metz, T., Seligman, M. E. P., Uchida, Y., & Xing, Z. (2017). Definitions of terms. In Centre for Bhutan Studies and GNH (Ed.), *Happiness: Transforming the development landscape*. (pp. 21–38). The Centre for Bhutan Studies and GNH.

Alexandrova, A. (2005). Subjective well-being and Kahneman's 'objective happiness.' *Journal of Happiness Studies, 6*(3), 301–324.

Alexandrova, A. (2012). Well-being as an object of science. *Philosophy of Science, 79*(5), 678–689.

Allardt, E. (1993). Having, loving, being: An alternative to the Swedish model of welfare research in M. Nussbaum, & A. Sen (Eds.), *The quality of life* (pp. 88–95). Clarendon.

Boehm, J. K., & Lyubomirsky, S. (2008). Does happiness promote career success? *Journal of Career Assessment, 16*(1), 101–116.

Bok, D. (2010). *The politics of happiness: What government can learn from the new research on well-being*. Princeton University Press.

Bradburn, N. M. (1969). *The structure of psychological well-being*. Aldine Publishing Company.

Bruni, L. (2006). *Civil happiness: Economics and human flourishing in historical perspective*. Routledge.

Bruni, L. (2016). Public happiness and relational goods. In S. Bartolini, E. Bilancini, L. Bruni, & P. L. Porta (Eds.), *Policies for happiness* (pp. 263–282). Oxford University Press.

Bruni, L., & Porta, P. L. (2007). *Economics and happiness: Framing the analysis*. Oxford University Press.

Campbell, A., Converse, P. E., & Rodgers, W. L. (1976). *The quality of American life: Perceptions, evaluations, and satisfactions*. Russell Sage Foundation.

Crum, A. J., & Salovey, P. (2013). Emotionally intelligent happiness. In S. A. David, I. Boniwell, & A. Conley Ayers (Eds.), *Oxford handbook of happiness* (pp. 73–87). Oxford University Press.

Cummins, R. A. (2013). Measuring happiness and subjective well-being. In S. A. David, I. Boniwell, & A. Conley Ayers (Eds.), *Oxford handbook of happiness* (pp. 185–200). Oxford University Press.

Daly, M. (Ed.). (1994). *Communitarianism: A New Public Ethics*. Wadsworth.

David, S. A., Boniwell, I., & Ayers, A. C. (Eds.). (2013). *Oxford handbook of happiness*. Oxford University Press.

Dewey, J. (1963). *Liberalism and social action*. Putnam Sons.

Diener, E., & Scollon, C. (2003). Subjective well-being is desirable, but not the summum bonum. *Paper to be delivered at the University of Minnesota Interdisciplinary Workshop on Well-Being*, Minneapolis.

Diener, E. (2000). Subjective well-being: The science of happiness and a proposal for a national index. *American Psychologist, 55*(1), 34–43.

Diener, E. (2006). Guidelines for national indicators of subjective well-being and ill-being. *Journal of Happiness Studies, 7*(4), 397–404.

Diener, E., & Biswas-Diener, R. (2008). *Happiness: Unlocking the mysteries of psychological wealth*. Wiley-Blackwell.

Diener, E., & Biswas-Diener, R. (2019). Well-being interventions to improve societies. In J. Sachs, R. Layard, & J. F. Helliwell (Eds.), *Global happiness and well-being policy report 2019* (pp. 95–110). Sustainable Development Solutions Network.

Diener, E., & Chan, M. Y. (2011). Happy people live longer: Subjective well-being contributes to health and longevity. *Applied Psychology: Health and Well-Being, 3*(1), 1–43.

Diener, E., Heintzelman, S. J., Kushlev, K., Tay, L., Wirtz, D., Lutes, L. D., & Oishi, S. (2017). Findings all psychologists should know from the new science on subjective well-being. *Canadian Psychology/psychologie Canadienne, 58*(2), 87–104.

Diener, E., Lucas, R., Schimmack, U., & Helliwell, J. (2009). *Well-being for public policy*. Oxford University Press.

Diener, E., & Seligman, M. E. P. (2002). Very happy people. *Psychological Science, 13*(1), 81–84.

Diener, E., & Seligman, M. E. P. (2004). Beyond money: Toward an economy of well-being. *Psychological Science in the Public Interest, 5*(1), 1–31.

Diener, E., Seligman, M. E. P., Choi, H., & Oishi, S. (2018). Happiest people revisited. *Perspectives on Psychological Science, 13*(2), 176–184.

Diener, E., & Suh, E. (1997). Measuring quality of life: Economic, social, and subjective indicators. *Social Indicators Research, 40*(1), 189–216.

Diener, E., Suh, E. M., Lucas, R. E., & Smith, H. L. (1999). Subjective well-being: Three decades of progress. *Psychological Bulletin, 125*(2), 276–302.

Dolan, P., Layard, R., & Metcalfe, R. (2011). Measuring subjective well-being for public policy: Recommendations on measures. *Centre for Economic Performance, Special Papers, 23*, 1–20.

Easterlin, R. A. (2001). Income and happiness: Towards a unified theory. *The Economic Journal, 111*(473), 465–484.

Feldman, F. (2010). *What is this thing called happiness?* Oxford University Press.

Finucane, A. M., Whiteman, M. C., & Power, M. J. (2010). The effect of happiness and sadness on alerting, orienting, and executive attention. *Journal of Attention Disorders, 13*(6), 629–639.

Forgeard, M. J., Jayawickreme, E., Kern, M. L., & Seligman, M. E. P. (2011). Doing the right thing: Measuring well-being for public policy. *International Journal of Well-being, 1*(1), 79–106.

Fowers, B. J., Mollica, C. O., & Procacci, E. N. (2010). Constitutive and instrumental goal orientations and their relations with eudaimonic and hedonic well-being. *The Journal of Positive Psychology, 5*(2), 139–153.

Frank, R. H. (1997). The frame of reference as a public good. *The Economic Journal, 107*(445), 1832–1847.

Fredrickson, B. L. (1998). What good are positive emotions? *Review of General Psychology, 2*(3), 300–319.
Fredrickson, B. L., & Joiner, T. (2002). Positive emotions trigger upward spirals toward emotional well-being. *Psychological Science, 13*(2), 172–175.
Frey, B. S. (2008). *Happiness: A revolution in economics*. MIT Press.
Frey, B. S., & Stutzer, A. (2002). What can economists learn from happiness research? *Journal of Economic Literature, 40*(2), 402–435.
Frey, B. S., & Stutzer, A. (2010). *Happiness and economics: How the economy and institutions affect human well-being*. Princeton University Press.
Friedman, J. (1994). The politics of communitarianism. *Critical Review, 8*(2), 297–340.
Graham, C. (2011). *The pursuit of happiness: An economy of well-being*. Brookings Institution Press.
Greater Good Science Center. (2018). The science of happiness. https://ggsc.berkeley.edu/what_we_do/event/the_science_of_happiness. Accessed June 15, 2020.
Haybron, D. M. (2016). Mental state approaches to well-being. In M. D. Adler & M. Fleurbaey (Eds.), *The oxford handbook of well-being and public policy* (pp. 347–378). Oxford University Press.
Helliwell, J. F., & Putnam, R. D. (2004). The social context of well-being. *Philosophical Transactions of the Royal Society of London Series B Biological Sciences, 359*(1449), 1435–1446.
Huta, V., & Waterman, A. S. (2014). Eudaimonia and its distinction from hedonia: Developing a classification and terminology for understanding conceptual and operational definitions. *Journal of Happiness Studies, 15*(6), 1425–1456.
Inglehart, R. (2009). Democracy and happiness: what causes what? Resource document. Notre Dame University. https://www3.nd.edu/~adutt/activities/documents/InglehartHappinessandDemocracy1.pdf. Accessed June 15, 2020.
Jang, S. (2017). *Dasan, Technique of happiness*. Seoul: Communication Books. (Korean).
Jiwook, J. (2018). *Wealth and philosophy: From the Eastern perspective*. Sechang Media.
Kahneman, D. (1999). Objective happiness. In D. Kahneman, E. Diener, & N. Schwarz (Eds.), *Well-being: The foundations of hedonic psychology* (pp. 3–25). Russell Sage Foundation.
Kang, J. (2013). On the concept of liberty in Bentham's Utilitarianism. *Philosophical Studies, 100*, 103–159. (Korean).
Katarzyna, D. L., & Singer, P. (2017). *Utilitarianism: A very short introduction*. Oxford University Press.
Kesebir, P., & Diener, E. (2008). In pursuit of happiness: Empirical answers to philosophical questions. *Perspectives on Psychological Science, 3*(2), 117–125.
Kim, Y. (2009). Happiness index and sociological approach. *The Korean Sociological Association*, 75–90. (Korean).
Kim, Y., & Chung, W. (2003). Mill's Utilitarianism. *Journal of Philosophical Ideas, 16(spc2–9)*, 1–95 (Korean).
Kim, Y., & Lee, S. J. (2014). The development and application of a community well-being index in Korean metropolitan cities. *Social Indicators Research, 119*(2), 533–558.
Koo, K., Lim, J., & Choi, S. (2015). A synoptic review of the research on happiness. *Journal of Governmental Studies, 21*(2), 95–130. (Korean).
Koo, K., Lim, J., & Choi, S. (2017). *What makes us happy?* Jipmoondang. (Korean).
Kraut, R. (1979). Two conceptions of happiness. *The Philosophical Review, 88*(2), 167–197.
Kroll, C. (2008). *Social capital and the happiness of nations: The importance of trust and networks for life satisfaction in a cross-national perspective*. Peter Lang.
Lane, A. M., & Terry, P. C. (2000). The nature of mood: Development of a conceptual model with a focus on depression. *Journal of Applied Sport Psychology, 12*(1), 16–33.
Lane, R. D., Reis, H. T., Peterson, D. R., Zareba, W., & Moss, A. J. (2009). Happiness and stress alter susceptibility to cardiac events in Long QT Syndrome. *Annals of Noninvasive Electrocardiology, 14*(2), 193–200.
Lao-tzu (unknown), *Lao-tzu*, Lee, K. S. Trans. (2007). Gil Publishing. (Korean).

Layard, R. (2005). *Happiness: Lessons from a new science*. Penguin Books/Penguin Group.
Lee, J. (1998). Philosophical transformation of communitarianism, *Philosophical Studies, 42*, 243–273. (Korean).
Lee, S. J., Kee. Y., Kim, Y., & Kim, N. (2013). A comparative analysis of the measures for community well-being based on the opinions of public officials and experts. *Korean Public Administration Review, 47*(2), 313–337. (Korean).
Lee, S. J., & Kim, Y. (2016). Structure of well-being: An exploratory study of the distinction between individual well-being and community well-being and the importance of intersubjective community well-being. In Y. Kee, S. J. Lee, & R. Phillips (Eds.), *Social factors and community well-being* (pp. 13–37). Springer.
Ludwigs, K. (2018). *The happiness analyzer: A new technique for measuring subjective well-being*. Erasmus University Rotterdam.
Lyubomirsky, S., King, L., & Diener, E. (2005). The benefits of frequent positive affect: Does happiness lead to success? *Psychological Bulletin, 131*(6), 803–855.
Lyubomirsky, S., & Lepper, H. S. (1999). A measure of subjective happiness: Preliminary reliability and construct validation. *Social Indicators Research, 46*(2), 137–155.
McAslan, D., Prakash, M., Pijawka, D., Guhathakurta, S., & Sadalla, E. (2013). Measuring quality of life in border cities: The border observatory project in the US-Mexico border region. In M. J. Sirgy, R. Phillips, & D. Rahtz (Eds.), *Community quality-of-life indicators: Best cases VI* (pp. 143–169). Springer.
McDowell, I. (2010). Measures of self-perceived well-being. *Journal of Psychosomatic Research, 69*(1), 69–79.
Miao, F. F., Koo, M., & Oishi, S. (2013). Subjective well-being. In S. A. David, I. Boniwell, & A. Conley Ayers (Eds.), *Oxford handbook of happiness* (pp. 175–184). Oxford University Press.
Michalos, A. C. (1985). Multiple discrepancies theory (MDT). *Social Indicators Research, 16*(4), 347–413.
Musikanski, L., Phillips, R., & Crowder, J. (2019). *The happiness policy handbook: How to make happiness and well-being the purpose of your government*. New Society Publishers.
National Research Council. (2013). *Subjective well-being: Measuring happiness, suffering, and other dimensions of experience*. National Academy Press.
Nettle, D. (2006). *Happiness: The science behind your smile*. Oxford University Press.
OECD. (2013). *OECD guidelines on measuring subjective well-being*. OECD Publishing.
Oswald, A. J. (1997). Happiness and economic performance. *The Economic Journal, 107*(445), 1815–1831.
Park, S. (2012). Aristotle's teleology advocated by McIntyre. *Journal of the New Korean Philosophical Association, 67*(1), 133–144. (Korean).
Pavot, W., & Diener, E. (2013). Happiness experienced: The science of subjective well-being. In S. A. David, I. Boniwell, & A. Conley Ayers (Eds.), *Oxford handbook of happiness* (pp. 134–151). Oxford University Press.
Pfeiffer, D., & Cloutier, S. (2016). Planning for happy neighborhoods. *Journal of the American Planning Association, 82*(3), 267–279.
Prior, William J. (1991)s. *Virtue and knowledge: Introduction to Ancient Greek ethics*. Routledge.
Raibley, J. R. (2012). Happiness is not well-being. *Journal of Happiness Studies, 13*(6), 1105–1129.
Ryan, R. M., & Deci, E. L. (2001). On happiness and human potentials: A review of research on hedonic and eudaimonic well-being. *Annual Review of Psychology, 52*(1), 141–166.
Santos, L. D., & Martins, I. (2013). The monitoring system on quality of life of the city of Porto. In M. J. Sirgy, R. Phillips, & D. Rahtz (Eds.), *Community quality-of-life indicators: Best cases VI* (pp. 77–98). Springer.
Seligman, M. E. P., & Csikszentmihalyi, M. (2000). Positive psychology: An introduction. *American Psychologist, 55*(1), 5–14.
Sen, A. (1999). *Development as freedom*. Anchor Books.

Straume, L. V., & Vittersø, J. (2012). Happiness, inspiration and the fully functioning person: Separating hedonic and eudaimonic well-being in the workplace. *The Journal of Positive Psychology, 7*(5), 387–398.

Tatarkiewicz, W. (1966). Happiness and time. *Philosophy and Phenomenological Research, 27*(1), 1–10.

Thin, N. (2012). *Social happiness: Theory into policy and practice*. Policy Press.

Tiberius, V., & Hall, A. (2010). Normative theory and psychological research: Hedonism, eudaimonism, and why it matters. *The Journal of Positive Psychology, 5*(3), 212–225.

Veenhoven, R. (2013). Notions of the good life. In S. A. David, I. Boniwell, & A. Conley Ayers (Eds.), *Oxford handbook of happiness* (pp. 161–173). Oxford University Press.

Veenhoven, R. (1991a). Questions on happiness: Classical topics, modern answers, blind spots. In F. Strack, M. Argyle, & N. Schwarz (Eds.), *Subjective well-being: An interdisciplinary perspective* (pp. 7–26). Pergamon Press.

Veenhoven, R. (1991b). Is happiness relative? *Social Indicators Research, 24*, 1–34.

Veenhoven, R. (2015). The overall satisfaction with life: Subjective approaches (1). In W. Glatzer, L. Camfield, V. Møller, & M. Rojas (Eds.), *Global handbook of quality of life* (pp. 207–238). Springer.

Vittersø, J. (2013). Introduction to psychological definitions of happiness. In S. A. David, I. Boniwell, & A. Conley Ayers (Eds.), *Oxford handbook of happiness* (pp. 155–160). Oxford University Press.

Vittersø, J. (2013). Functional well-being: Happiness as feelings, evaluations, and functioning. In S. A. David, I. Boniwell, & A. Conley Ayers (Eds.), *Oxford handbook of happiness* (pp. 227–244). Oxford University Press.

Waterman, A. S., Schwartz, S. J., & Conti, R. (2008). The implications of two conceptions of happiness (hedonic enjoyment and eudaimonia) for the understanding of intrinsic motivation. *Journal of Happiness Studies, 9*(1), 41–79.

Welsch, H. (2009). Implications of happiness research for environmental economics. *Ecological Economics, 68*(11), 2735–2742.

Woo, C. (2014). Exploring an alternative approach to the global development: Theoretical foundation and policy implications of happiness approach in the context of global development. *Korean Society and Public Administration, 24*(4), 411–434 (Korean).

Xi, Z. (1999). *Daxue, Zhongyong*, (M. Y. Kim, Trans.). Hongik Publishing (Korean).

Yeh, H.-J., Hsieh, Y.-S., & Tsay, R.-M. (2015). Self-evaluation affects subjective well-being: The effects of socioeconomic status and personality in Taiwan. In F. Maggino (Ed.), *A new research agenda for improvements in quality of life* (pp. 109–134). Springer.

Zapf, W. (1984). Individuelle Wohlfahrt: Lebensbedingungen und wahrgenommene Lebensqualität. Lebensqualität in der Bundesrepublik. In W. Glatzer, & W. Zapf. (Eds.), *Lebensqualität in der Bundesrepublik (Objektive Lebensbedingungen und subjektives Wohlbefinden* (pp. 13–26). Campus Verlag.

Chapter 3
A Theory of Public Happiness

1 Current Trends

The increased attention on happiness since the 1960s has been spreading simultaneously in both the practical and academic dimensions, which can be called the beyond GDP movement. Why such changes? In practice, as nations are experiencing social instability and polarization, the limits of a growth-centric state and welfare state are becoming clearer, and nations are trying to think about national development in new ways. In academia, the Easterlin paradox which negates the relation between income and happiness became a meaningful triggering point for new interest in happiness. As such, the twenty-first century has become the age of happiness. This change can be interpreted as a new interest in public happiness that goes beyond personal happiness to a national or collective level of concern in its members' happiness. In the following, the current trends of interest in happiness are examined by dividing them into practical and academic areas.

1.1 Practice

Is happiness a private issue? For a long time, happiness has been considered a private issue. Accordingly, nation-states pursued law and order, economic growth, and protection of limited groups (i.e., welfare improvement) as its role, instead of a direct interest in happiness. But as we entered the twenty-first century, many countries have been paying attention to public happiness (or wellbeing) based on the reinterpretation of progress (Bok, 2010; Diener, 2009; Kelly, 2012; Pfeiffer & Cloutier, 2016; Thin, 2012). In the past, economic growth was the measure of progress but with the recognition that economic growth is not genuine progress, there are attempts to find non-economic measures of progress like happiness or wellbeing.

It is notable that Thin (2012: 81) interprets the recent movement as a transition of the national view of happiness from the utilitarian to the eudaimonic approach.

S. J. Lee, *Public Happiness*, Community Quality-of-Life and Well-Being,
https://doi.org/10.1007/978-3-030-89643-0_3

According to him, nation-states in the past were actually adopting a utilitarian approach in pursuing GDP from the economy aspect. Bentham, a representative utilitarian, views happiness as “a sum of pleasures minus the pains” while arguing for the maximization of happiness, and each country has embraced this utilitarian position and focused attention on the accumulation of economic results enabling the accumulation of pleasure. In terms of social policy, countries have adopted a negative utilitarianism approach by focusing on eliminating social ills. These approaches can also be seen in efforts to eliminate crime, improve mental health, and education. In contrast, both developed and developing countries today are showing more direct and explicit interest in happiness than the past. This change can be interpreted as a move beyond the nanny state or therapeutic state toward eudaimonic states, facilitating happiness rather than just minimizing suffering.

Movements in the practical field include activities of central and local governments, the private sector as well as international organizations. We first look into the movement at the national level. Bhutan is widely known as the first country to show a national interest in happiness. And Bhutan is perhaps the only country that has fully adopted a happiness policy. Some nations are showing a political interest in happiness, but these interests have not been expanded to national policies. The fourth king of Bhutan Jigme Singye Wanchuk suggested using the Gross National Happiness (GNH) as the measure of national progress in 1972. GNH emphasizes the balance between economic values and non-economic values and includes indicators of the following four areas—sustainable and equitable socioeconomic development, conservation of the environment, preservation and promotion of culture, and good governance. He believed that a government that does not create happiness for its citizens does not have a reason to exist and presented a new perspective on progress by arguing that if in pursuing Bhutan’s 5-year development plan, its citizens do not become happier, then he would consider this a failed plan (Bok, 2010: 1). This was a meaningful moment in that it transformed happiness, which used to be perceived as an individual responsibility, to a matter of public responsibility. However, it was difficult to find developed countries paying attention to the declaration of this small country. Finally, in the 2000s, developed countries began to show interest in their attempt to reinterpret progress that goes beyond economic growth (Bok, 2010; Diener, 2000; Kelly, 2012; Large, 2010; Thin, 2012). These interests include efforts to measure happiness and develop happiness policies with the belief that happiness is an important element of national progress (Pfeiffer & Cloutier, 2016).

The following section will introduce the important cases other than Bhutan in national trends. First, in 2009, the President Sarkozy of France invited famous scholars, such as Stiglitz, to form the Commission on the Measurement of Economic Performance and Social Progress and to develop an indicator of national progress beyond GDP. Widely known as The Stiglitz Report. “Reforming the International Monetary and Financial Systems in the Wake of the Global Crisis Report” by the Commission On the Measurement of Economic Performance and Social Progress strongly recommended adopting wellbeing or happiness in addition to or in place of GDP (Stiglitz et al. 2009a, b). In the United Kingdom, Prime Minister Cameron commissioned the Office of National Statistics to publish an annual report of the General Wellbeing Index (GWB) and the New Economics Foundation (a private organization) has published the Happy Planet Index since 2011. The Canadian Index of Wellbeing (CIW, 2012) differs from Bhutan, the UK, France, and Australia in that this effort was led by citizens, rather than the national government. The CIW includes eight key domains of life, such as Healthy Populations, Democratic Engagement, Community Vitality, Environment, Leisure and Culture, Time Use, Education, and Living Standards. Japan has adopted the People's Life Index that includes subjective indicators and international standards of happiness and the Life Reform Index that sets public happiness as a goal. Moreover, in 2011, Japan founded a committee on wellbeing measurement that motivated new studies on happiness from a national perspective. Korea government adopted national happiness as one of the keynotes for the national agenda and pursued happiness policies at the entire government level under President Park Geun-hye (2013–2017). With the exception of Bhutan, this may be an exceptional case of adopting the happiness policy as the policy base at the national level. However, as the government was stranded due to the impeachment of the president Park, the promotion of the happiness policy lost its momentum.

Other cases include Australia's Measures of Australia's Progress, China's declaration of the Chinese Dream as a national goal under Xi Jinping, and Dubai's creation of a happiness ministry. Many countries, including Bhutan, Bolivia, Ecuador, Japan, South Korea, and the United States of America, include happiness in their constitution (Pellerin, 2016), and even more countries have been collecting data on happiness or wellbeing (Durand, 2018; Musikanski & Polley, 2016; O'Donnell et al., 2014).

The local and non-government/private sector actors are also making efforts on the topic of happiness. Some examples are the Community Indicators Consortium (US), Young Foundation (UK), PEKEA (Political and Ethical Knowledge on Economic Activities Research Programme) (France), Tasmania Together, Community Indicators Victoria, CI Queensland (all Australia), Major Cities Indicators Project (New Zealand), Happiness League (Japan), and Happy Village (Korea). The Community Indicators Consortium (CIS) (US) is a global community of practitioners and scholars involved in arts, scientific and social movements, and quality of life measurement research (Holden & Phillips, 2010). CIS helps a community to know whether they are measuring what they are interested in and whether the community is on an ideal path. The Young Foundation (YK) of the UK is the Institute for Community Studies that was founded by Michael Young—a social activist—in 1954. This Foundation leads various activities, such as Inequality, Places, Youth & Education, Health & Wellbeing for the progress of communities and connects happiness or quality of life research to local communities in order to solve social problems. Political and Ethical Knowledge on Economic Activities Research Programme (PEKEA) of France is an NGO that creates an open network of researchers and local governments from various sectors. Specific projects include the PEKEA Local Government Club Project. This project helps researchers to assist local governments that lack research capacity. By connecting experts from various fields, it helps local governments to develop policies that increase the level of societal wellbeing. Currently, over 1000 people are directly connected to the network of NGO PEKEA, and some thousands are connected indirectly via partnerships with organizations in over 60 countries. In Australia, there are several local government cases, such as Tasmania Together, Community Indicators Victoria, and Community Indicators Queensland. First, Tasmania Together was created from local residents' efforts to resolve local issues. It is a community effort of the Tasmania state government and citizens to resolve social, economic, and environmental issues together. Community Indicators Victoria (CIV) or Community Indicators Queensland is a collaborative effort between the public and private sector to develop and apply a community wellbeing index. The Happiness League of Japan is a private–public partnership project led by the local government. In June 2013, the 52 local governments of Japan created the Happiness League that focuses on the happiness of residents (Kim, D.H., 2016), and in 2017, 91 local governments were participating. Happiness Village of Korea is a village regeneration project led by village residents and supported by local governments. The project began in 2010 and aims to create physical, economic, and cultural vitality at the village level.

Not only nation-states and local governments, but also international organizations are active. Some examples are OECD's Measuring the Progress of Societies (Better Life Index in 2011), EU's Beyond GDP, UNDP's Human Development Index (HDI, 2004), and UN's International Day of Happiness (2013.3.20). These are international efforts to overcome the limits of GDP as the measure of progress.

The The Organisation for Economic Cooperation and Development (OECD) has called attention to the importance of measuring happiness with a series of OECD World Forum on Statistics, Knowledge and Policy beginning in 2005, its issuance of the OECD Guidelines for Measuring Subjective Wellbeing in 2013, and its Better Life Index issued in 2011. EU has been intensively searching for an alternative to GDP since 2009 under the heading "beyond GDP' (Weimann et al., 2015: 77). In 2011, the European Union created the Bringing Alternative Indicators into Policy (BRAINPOoL) Project and concluded its final report, The BRAINPOoL Project: Beyond GDP—From Measurement to Politics and Policy. It includes policies and practices in various countries as well as issues that may be better understood using "beyond GDP" indicators and policy framework (Musikanski, 2014: 57).

The UN has especially been active. In 2011, the United Nations (UN) General Assembly advised its members to adopt happiness of wellbeing as a development goal in the UN General Assembly resolution: Happiness: Towards a Holistic Definition of Development. More specifically, on July 19, 2011, the United Nations General Assembly adopted a resolution asserting that the pursuit of happiness is a fundamental human goal, suggesting member states to elaborate measures of happiness and wellbeing in guiding their public policies for the promotion of the economic advancement and social progress (Resolution 65/309. https://undocs.org/en/A/RES/65/309). This is evidence of accepting the global trend of valuing citizen happiness or quality of life that goes "beyond GDP" and that the old measure of national progress as economic growth (especially, GDP) is limited. Moreover, the UN declared March 20, 2014, as the International Day of Happiness to show that happiness is an appropriate goal for human civilization. Since 2012, the UN has published the World Happiness Report (issued by the Sustainable Development Solutions Network) every year. The World

Happiness Report measures and reports the happiness level of more than 150 countries. In 2018, the first Global Happiness Policy Report, also issued by the SDSN, was published with support of the United Arab Emirates at the World Government Summit held in Dubai. In particular, the latter draws attention as a movement to show more active interest in policies beyond measuring happiness.

The UN officially included wellbeing in the SDGs (2016–2030). SDGs are the continuation of the Millennium Development Goals (MDGs) and set eradication of poverty (the original goal of MDGs) as the most urgent goal but also include global cooperative agenda and action plans for each nation to address the socioeconomic polarization, exacerbation of social inequality, and destruction of the environment that threated sustainable growth. Among the total 17 goals, health and wellbeing are the third goal. The MDGs (2000–2015) of the past did not include happiness as a goal, and this shows the international community's increased interest in happiness.

In sum, above-mentioned movements can be seen reflecting a paradigm shift from measuring national progress from an economic standpoint through GDP to a more holistic standpoint that includes happiness or wellbeing and can be collectively called the "beyond GDP movement." This movement is also related to the efforts to develop a measure that is as simple and attractive as GDP, but also includes the environmental and social aspects of progress to address the twenty-first century problems of climate change, poverty, resource depletion, health, and quality of life. Of course, these efforts do not argue for throwing away the GDP and replacing it with happiness or wellbeing as the only developmental goal. The GDP remains an important developmental goal. Nevertheless, given that the economy does not guarantee happiness or wellbeing, there is a demand for diversifying policy goals to go beyond "GDP only".

1.2 Research

Although reflection on happiness dates back more than 2,500 years to the ideas of Aristotle, Confucius, Buddha, and so on, modern happiness research was dominated by the scholars of the eighteenth century Enlightment Era (Bruni & Zamagni, 2007; Crum & Salovey, 2013). The early Enlightenment scholars who were influenced by the ancient Greek philosophical ideas viewed the right to happiness as a basic human right and a normative social goal. In that period, happiness was widely used in civil society and was mentioned as the ultimate life goal, but there was limited knowledge about the concept of happiness and its influencing factors, and thus, the term was used mostly as a slogan (Prycker, 2010). Scholarly interest of that era in happiness, however, was not connected to the twentieth century and was revived in the 1990s. Developed countries were focusing on self-help, while developing countries were focusing on more urgent problems, such as food, justice, and peace, but as many of these problems have improved, there has been an increase in attention to happiness. It is expected that there will be increased attention to wellbeing from all fields (Thin, 2012: 7).

The main interest of modern happiness research is on the relationship between wealth and happiness. Until the mid-twentieth century, the assumption that material affluence increases happiness dominated the political economy field from Smith, Genovasi, Marshall, to Keynes. In the late twentieth century, the positive relationship between income and happiness began to be questioned by Galbraith, Scitovsky, Hirshmann, etc. However, these questions did not receive much attention from mainstream economists until Easterlin (1974) empirically analyzed the relationship between economic growth and happiness in 1974 (Bartolini et al., 2016: 1). The study examined survey data (1946–1970) of 19 countries and found a positive relationship between income and happiness in cross-sectional data, but looking at change over time, did not find significant change in happiness despite the increase in GDP over time. This was named the Easterlin Paradox. The Easterlin Paradox went beyond an economics discussion and challenged modern culture's beliefs that economic growth is a tool for improving individuals' lives (Bartolini et al., 2016: 2). Easterlin's study is considered a tipping point to the resurgence of happiness studies by presenting the relationship between income's marginal utility and happiness from a different perspective.

The Easterlin Paradox is not generally valid. It is about the relationship between happiness and income level among countries, not about the relationship within a country. It showed a positive relationship between happiness and income within a country, though not across countries. That is, there is a limit to the applicability. Graham (2011: 17) attempts to explain this more precisely. She first acknowledges that in most studies reported that within countries, the wealthy countries are happier than the poor. But she indicates that in studies comparing countries, it is difficult to find a significant relationship between income and happiness. Wealthy countries tend to be happier than poor countries. Happiness tends to increase to a certain level, but after that level, it does not increase. However, within the country groups (wealthy, poor), it is difficult to find a significant relationship between income and happiness. She postulates that after basic needs are met, factors other than income (e.g., aspirations, income distribution, and income stability) become increasingly more important.

There are also contradictory or corrective findings in subsequent analyses. Several studies (e.g., Kroll, 2008; Sacks et al., 2010; Stevenson & Wolfers, 2008) empirically show that there is a positive relationship between GDP and happiness. These results show that in the short term there is a positive relationship, but the Easterlin Paradox still remains valid in the long term (Di Tella et al., 2001; Easterlin & Angelescu, 2009; Easterlin et al., 2010). Despite some critical findings, Easterlin's study is meaningful for advancement of happiness studies: (1) It was a catalyst for subsequent happiness research overall. (2) It called attention to the limited effect of economic growth for happiness. (3) It stimulated many countries' efforts to redefine their development goals that go beyond GDP (Woo, 2014a, b).

Research on happiness is being developed in various fields of study.Philosophers, psychologists, and educators were already interested in happiness, but social scientists, including economists, also began to take an interest after Easterlin's study (Clark, 2016; Pugno, 2009; Sacks et al., 2012). In particular, arguments that a narrow focus on economic growth can bring negative effects as the increase in individual income or national wealth above a certain level does not affect happiness level begin to appear (Boyce et al., 2010; Cho, 2013; Frijter et al. 2004; Kim, 2013). This was meaningful because it modified or complemented the old approach of economics evaluating happiness with an economic measure universally, despite the different conditions across nations and regions. These trends increased attention to non-economic factors in national development and offered a new perspective in research by re-defining a successful government and the value of life goals (Eren & Aşıcı, 2016; Mizobuchi, 2017; Nettle, 2006; Oshio, 2017).

In sociology, there are studies that focus on the relationship between social capital and health, wealth, economic growth, and see social capital as indirectly affecting happiness through these variables. For example, Helliwell and Putnam (2004) argue that social capital increases health, which then increases life satisfaction. Zak and Knack (2001) argue that social capital acts as the engine for economic growth that increases happiness. Rodrik (1999) argues that social capital protects one from external stress and thus affects happiness. In contrast, Ram (2010) reported that the relationship between social capital and happiness is unstable.

Interest in happiness studies has expanded to politics and administration. Today, there are discussions about political factors (such as the form and size of government), government factors (such as the role of government and policy), and topics related to social progress and happiness. Radcliff (2001) showed that political factors, such as ideology of multiple parties and the quality and extent of welfare regime, affect satisfaction at the national level. This means that political regimes can increase citizen wellbeing through social policies (Lapinski et al., 1998). Inglehart et al. (2008) found that happiness levels increased when democratization increased people's perception of the freedom of choice. Di Tella and MacCulloch (2005) suggested the concept of partisan social happiness that agreement in ideology between individuals and the government increases happiness. Dreher and Öhler (2011) argued that the ideology of governments affects happiness and that left-leaning individuals are happier under leftist governments and right-leaning individuals are happier under rightist governments.

There are studies that consider government size as a political factor of happiness. Utilitarians believe that the government should have the ambition to create happiness for the greatest number (Ott, 2013). This received a lot of interest from researchers as we entered the 2000s, and government was highlighted as a key influencing factor of quality of life (Bjørnskov et al., 2007; Coggburn & Schneider, 2003; Di Tella & MacCulloch, 2005; Kim & Kim, 2012; Ng & Ho, 2006; Ott, 2005; Veenhoven, 2005; Zorondo-Rodríguez et al., 2014). Bjørnskov et al. (2007) showed a negative correlation between government size (as measured by the size of public expenditure as a percentage of GDP) and life satisfaction. Other studies have found similar negative effects of large government expenditures. Ott (2005) argued that as government expenditures via redistribution and subsidies increase, happiness decreases and Eiji (2009) found in a case study of Japan that government size has a negative effect on happiness. These quantitative studies support the "small government is beautiful" belief of neoliberals.

On the contrary, Kacapyr (2008) also presented research that found no significant relationship between life satisfaction and government expenditure per GDP. Some studies preach caution in including government size as an influencing factor of happiness. Ott (2011) analyzed 130 countries and found that the relationship between the size of government and happiness is largely determined by the quality of government. Relatedly, Coggburn and Schneider (2003) argued that quality of life is an appropriate measure for government performance and that governments have a direct effect on quality of life. This is because governments affect public policies in health, education, and environment that have a direct effect on quality of life.

Despite these couple of studies that examined the relationship between happiness and some governmental factors, there are few studies that systematically examine the qualitative or quantitative aspects of government and its effect on happiness (Kim & Kim, 2012). With the exception of a few studies, the participation of political science or public administration scholars in happiness studies is rather late, and as a result, the government factor has been an almost forgotten variable. Considering that the happiness policy is indispensable for the promotion of happiness, and the decision and implementation of the happiness policy is carried out by the government, more research on government factors in happiness studies is necessary.

Basically, the national interest in happiness is a recent phenomenon, and happiness research, in comparison with other old disciplines, is still in its early stages. Despite this short time frame, happiness-related research has become an important research field and has become an important academic foundation for the rise of the national happiness issue.

In general, the reports that economic performance has limitations in securing happiness or wellbeing seem to be more dominant. Stiglitz et al. (2009a, b) argued that the gap between GDP and human wellbeing is widening. Schumacher (1973), Scitovsky (1976), Carson (2002), and Hirsch (2005) critiqued the limits of GDP as a measure of progress and motivated research interest in non-economic values. As an extension, Stevenson and Wolfers (2008), Kahneman and Deaton (2010), Luttmer (2004), in addition to Easterlin (1974) tried to prove that economic income does not entirely determine wellbeing. Other studies expanded the discussion of wellbeing factors beyond income. For example, Clark and Oswald (1996), Alesina et al. (2004) looked at inequality, Helliwell (2006) looked at social capital, Frey et al. (2004) looked at citizen participation, and Welsch (2009) looked at the environment and its effects on happiness or wellbeing. Recently, with the accumulation of research, there are publications that discuss the conceptualization and influencing factors of happiness or wellbeing. Some examples include Brooks (2008), Diener (2009), Stiglitz et al. (2010), Bok (2010), Halpern (2010), Layard and Layard (2011), and Allin and Hand (2014).

Happiness studies are meaningful for two reasons. First, they altogether formed the basis for the shift of the old economy-centric growth paradigm to a happiness paradigm with the reinterpretation of development that goes beyond GDP. Second, from a practical standpoint, these studies have moved the old discussion that used to be normative to a more objective measure and evaluation of happiness, thus creating the opportunity for happiness to become a policy goal and increasing the possibility of creating policies for happiness by identifying the influencing factors of happiness (Dutt & Radcliff, 2009).

Nevertheless, many studies remain in the domain of individual happiness and have not progressed to the domain of public happiness. In particular, the efforts to measure happiness and identify its influencing factors have not expanded to a discussion of changing policy frame or governance for public happiness. In order to resolve this problem, it is necessary for future research to pay more attention to public policy and governance issues for the standpoint of public happiness.

As an exception, some studies focus on happiness policies. For example, Layard (2005) argues that happiness maximization, rather than income maximization, should be a policy goal and that improvements in educational curriculum, psychological health, tax policy, and welfare programs are necessary. Di Tella et al. (2001) argued that happiness data should be used to shape government policy, Veenhoven (2004a, b, 2010) suggested that government policy can create the conditions for increasing happiness, and thus, happiness should be a policy goal. More specifically, Frank (1999) and Layard (1980) argued for heavy taxation on high-income earners to decrease income inequality under the assumption that relative welfare is important and Graham and Haidt (2010) recommended policies to encourage local festivals to increase happiness.

Apart from these studies, however, there is also a critical stance on the study of happiness policy or governance. Duncan (2005) is a key example. He argues for a careful examination of how the findings of happiness studies become a happiness maximization goal of public policies. This is because the translation of research findings into policy is not so simple. Moreover, the public expectations and trust in government can act as barriers to policy change that happiness studies recommend and can even have a negative effect on happier people. However, it should be noted that his argument emphasizes the constraints of research on happiness policy, but does not deny the necessity of research on happiness policy related to the promotion of happiness.

The discussion above can be summarized as follows: Promoting public happiness through government policy is necessary and feasible, and accordingly, research that considers government and policy as major variables in happiness studies should be actively conducted. Contrary to this necessity, discussions of "happiness policy" and "governance" in happiness studies have been insufficient to date. In particular, despite the fact that there are a number of previous studies revealing that government factors such as government structure, government regime, and size of government affect happiness (e.g., Coggburn & Schneider, 2003), it is regrettable that there has not been sufficient research on government policies or governance variables (e.g., Coggburn & Schneider, 2003). This is the purpose of this book.

2 Public Happiness: The Publicness of Happiness

2.1 The Concept of Public Happiness

What is public happiness? Happiness includes both the individual and collective domain. In general, if happiness means individual or personal happiness, then public happiness refers to the happiness at the community level. Here, community refers to the collectivity of sharing space, interests, or relationships with other members. In general, the concept of community tends to be understood as referring to a collectivity with stronger shared attributes than the concept of group. In addition, since the shared properties of a collectivity are often expressed in the collectivity of small units rather than a large unit, the concept community tends to be understood as a term referring to a collectivity of small units. However, such a difference is not clear or is only a difference in degree. In view of this, this book does not distinguish between community and group and uses them interchangeably. Also, the size of the collective is not defined and can range from family, neighborhood, district, and nation-state to global society. Among these, the nation-state, which has the effective power and resources, can have the biggest influence on members' happiness.

More specifically, public happiness is the happiness at the community dimension that a member of the community enjoys in connection to other members, while individual happiness is the private dimension of happiness, unrelated to the community. In both terms, the agent of happiness is the individual, but there are differences in the unit of analysis, the agent of enjoyment, and public responsibility. As shown in Table 1, in terms of unit of analysis, the individual is the unit for individual happiness, and the collective is the unit for public happiness. In terms of the standing of the individual, in the former, it is the atomic individual, and in the former, it is the collective individual. In terms of responsibility, it is the individual's responsibility for private happiness unrelated to the collective, while the happiness one enjoys as a member of a collective is subject to public responsibility. In terms of the issue of interest, the level of happiness becomes a key issue for individual happiness, while in the case

Table 1 Individual happiness and public happiness

	Individual happiness (private happiness)	Public happiness
Unit of analysis	Individual dimension	Collective dimension
Agent of enjoyment of happiness	Atomic individual	Collective individual
Responsibility of happiness	Individual responsibility	Individual and public responsibility
Main interest	Level of happiness	Level and distribution of happiness

of public happiness, the issue of distribution of happiness in addition to the level becomes a key issue. Therefore, when comparing happiness between countries, for example, simply comparing the level of happiness does not match the perspective of public happiness. A minimum requirement from the viewpoint of public happiness is to consider both the level of happiness and the distribution of the level of happiness among members.

Furthermore, individual happiness is related to the sphere of feelings and moral sentiments, and public happiness is the summation of individual happiness that individuals enjoy as members of a community. Therefore, public happiness is also related to individual members' emotions and moral feelings. It is difficult to find explicit references to personal and public happiness. To my knowledge, Porta and Scazzieri (2007) is the only example. Initially, they classify happiness into individual and social levels. According to them, individual happiness is related to feelings, satisfaction, or moral sentiments, while the social dimension of happiness is related to moral sentiments and enabling conditions of a society. Such an explanation is somewhat confusing because happiness at the collective level can be misunderstood as not related to feelings but only to moral sentiments. It should be indicated that collective happiness is also related to both emotions and moral sentiments, because happiness, whether at the individual level or at the collective level, is basically what the individual enjoys. It can also be pointed out that enabling conditions are not content factors of happiness, but influencing factors.

Public happiness relates to social conditions (or living conditions).[1] What are social conditions? Here, social conditions refer to the situation of a community that affects an individual's activities of pursuit of happiness. Since the individuals' activities for pursuing happiness are centered on the individual's life, social conditions can be also expressed as living conditions. Social conditions (or living conditions) include tangible and intangible conditions. The tangible conditions refer to physical conditions such as social welfare, housing, transportation, infrastructure, and subsidies, and the intangible conditions refer to non-material conditions such as institutions, policies, and culture including social capital and social ethics.

How do these social conditions affect individuals' happiness-pursuing activities? To borrow the explanation of Porta and Scazzieri (2007), who express a direct interest in public happiness, social conditions affect public happiness by (1) supporting members to find their purposes that are mutually respected and (2) transforming their capabilities into actual functionings for such purposes. In other words, the former refers to social admissibility of individual preferences, and the latter refers

[1] Strictly speaking, social conditions and living conditions are not the same. Social conditions are collective conditions that are generally applied to the members of a community. Living conditions are conditions related to the lives of individuals and include exclusive conditions at the individual level and shared conditions at the societal level. That is, social conditions are collective-level conditions and do not include individual-level conditions, and living conditions include individual-level and collective-level conditions. However, conditions at the individual level and conditions at the social level are closely related. For example, personal income and housing are affected by social conditions such as employment and housing systems. Therefore, it makes more sense to use them interchangeably here.

to providing opportunities to pursue such preferences (social opportunities). Then, the happiness achievement of members will increase as the social admissibility of individual values increases and opportunities to achieve socially accepted individual goals are provided.

Social conditions can enable or disable the pursuit of happiness of an individual. It is notable that Porta and Scazzieri (2007) refer to social conditions as enabling conditions, focusing on contributions to happiness. However, the meaning of the enabling condition is somewhat limited. Of course, if enabling and disabling are viewed as a single dimension, such an approach that focuses solely on enabling is also safe. This is because conditions above an appropriate level become enabling factors and conditions below an appropriate level become disabling factors of the happiness-pursuing activities of individuals. However, as Herzberg et al. (1959)'s motivation-hygiene theory suggests, when enabling and disabling are not a single dimension, but a separate dimension, the approach emphasizing only the contributing aspect has a limitation as a partial approach. In view of this, we use social conditions as a more neutral term comprising both enabling and disabling conditions.

In the above discussion, we acknowledge that individual and public happiness are not separate but a dimension of happiness that are connected through social conditions. That is, the social conditions of a community enable or limit the happiness-pursuing activities of individuals and connect individual happiness and public happiness. In particular, moral sentiments connect individual happiness and public happiness by enabling or limiting the happiness-pursuing activities of individuals, depending on the congruence of individual values with social values. Of course, conceptually, one can pursue happiness separate from society based on private resources only and can make an individual value judgment of happiness. An example is an individual's criminal activity that is pursued irrespective of social admissibility. Criminal activities with high social aversion are likely to result in lower happiness than those with low social disgust.

However, even such activities are affected by social admissibility of the activities. As such, it is difficult to conceive conditions wherein there is complete separation between an individual's efforts and values and social conditions (Lee, 2019). Therefore, one should be careful not to ignore the possible connection between the two when discussing public happiness. With regard to individual happiness, we may distinguish between individual happiness that is not connected to the public and individual happiness that is connected to the public and use the term private happiness for the former. Nevertheless, given that individual happiness is used with the concept of private happiness, this book will use the two interchangeably.

On the other hand, not all social conditions will have a significant effect on individual happiness activities to the same extent. Some conditions may have a more significant effect than others. In this regard, among social conditions, a constellation of conditions that is of greater importance to individual happiness-pursuing activities can be classified as basic conditions. Such attempts to distinguish basic social conditions from general social conditions are meaningful in relation to the effectiveness of public policies for promoting happiness. This is because when the state makes policy efforts to improve social conditions in order to promote public happiness, it is difficult to target the improvement of all social conditions with limited resources, and it may be undesirable in terms of the effectiveness of resource allocation. We cannot make a predefined list of which social conditions are basic conditions. This is because the list of basic conditions cannot be defined by innate characteristics of social conditions but rather should be defined by its relation to happiness. Furthermore, the list of basic conditions is not static but variable. Even under the same conditions, the influence of social conditions on happiness achievement may vary depending on the time, region, or cultural ethical factors. Nevertheless, efforts to establish a list of basic conditions are still needed to implement the happiness policy. In this regard, it can be expected that consensus on the list of basic social conditions can progress further as knowledge about the relationship between social conditions and happiness is accumulated through future happiness research and policy experiences. Various current surveys related to happiness indicators or studies on influencing factors of happiness are also linked to efforts to identify basic social conditions from a list of general social conditions. It should be noted that in doing so, efforts to promote understanding of cultural and periodic deviations in social conditions should be increased. As Frawley (2015), Cummins (2013), and others have appropriately indicated, efforts to broaden the understanding of cultural and historical contexts beyond standardization tailored to Western culture and context are required. Such a request should be applied equally not only to studies related to happiness, but also to policy cooperation related to happiness policies between countries or between central and local governments at home.

Public happiness has two meanings. First, as mentioned above, in terms of the unit of analysis, it means the total happiness of constituents that exists within the connections among the collective members, and not as atomic or private individuals. It is the collective happiness of constituents of a community. Second, in terms of responsibility, as constituents of a community, individual happiness is subject to public responsibility. From these two meanings, we see that public happiness is related to individual happiness and has the collective characteristic of individual happiness, but also is not the simple sum of individual happiness. Public happiness is not the total sum of unrelated individuals' enjoyment of happiness, but rather the sum of happiness of individuals that are related to each other as constituents. There is a difference between individual private happiness and public happiness in that the former will be determined by one's own subjective preference and standing unrelated to others, but the latter will be determined in relationship to other members at the community level. In other words, unlike personal happiness, which is determined irrespective of social conditions, public happiness is influenced by the social conditions of the individual's community. Therefore, public happiness affected by social conditions may be greater or smaller than the summation of simple individual happiness. It can also be different in content. Depending on social conditions, moral sentiments may have a higher or lower share of happiness than feelings. An individual's private happiness may be exempt from public responsibility, but an individual's happiness as a member of the community cannot be exempt from public responsibility. To summarize, public happiness means happiness that a constituent enjoys as a member of the community and also means happiness that is supported publicly. In short, public happiness is the total sum of individual happiness of constituents that is subject to public responsibility.

Public happiness thus defined is different from collective happiness. Collective happiness is the simple total sum of the happiness of each member and is a neutral concept that is unrelated to public responsibility. In contrast, public happiness does not define the responsibility for a constituent's happiness as completely private and is a value-laden concept that sees this as being subject to public responsibility. Also, public happiness should not be misunderstood as the happiness of a state or certain community. For example, national happiness is the happiness of citizens that constitute a community called a nation, but it is not happiness of the state as an abstract concept. Happiness is something humans feel as an agent and states or communities as impersonal actors cannot enjoy happiness. Thus, national (or citizen) happiness exists, but state happiness does not. However, the state is closely related to national happiness (or citizen happiness). The nation-state possesses the most power and resources and has the greatest potential to increase citizen happiness, exists for citizens and not for itself, and thus has the responsibility for citizen happiness. We can call nation-states that actively make such efforts the happiness state. The same applies to different units of analysis. For example, if we call public happiness at the local unit as local happiness, this means the happiness of residents that live in a certain area and not of the local government or authority.

Moreover, national happiness is not always public happiness. If a nation-state is a happiness state that makes decisions based on a sense of responsibility for national happiness, national happiness has the nature of public happiness. However, if citizen happiness simply means the sum of individual happiness in a neutral way, then this is simply collective happiness, not public happiness. This is because "public" means constituents or collectivity on the one hand and publicness or public character on the other hand. Therefore, if we say public happiness after defining the nation as the unit, then this simultaneously means the sum of individual happiness and the public responsibility of the nation for that happiness. If we acknowledge the nation's public responsibility, then we should also recognize a certain level of corresponding citizens' responsibility. That is, as a constituent, one has the responsibility to pursue individual happiness within the boundary of not severely harming the public interest. Thus, the pursuit of happiness beyond social norms and laws can be restricted for public interest. Figure 1 summarizes the nature of public happiness discussed above.

2.2 *Why Public Happiness: The Public Responsibility for Happiness*

As mentioned previously, public happiness has to assume public responsibility for the happiness of its constituents, and this requires a discussion of why we should acknowledge public responsibility for individual happiness. Heretofore, happiness was considered a private problem, and there was an unspoken assumption that public

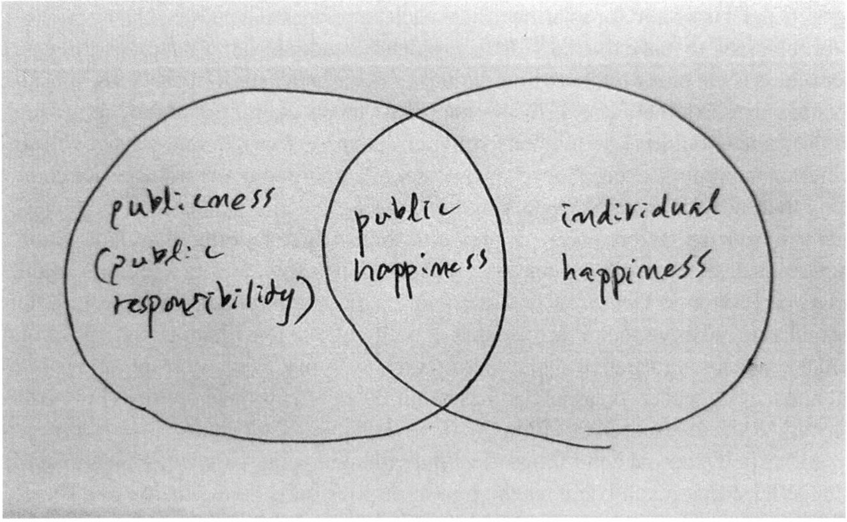

Fig. 1 Nature of public happiness

happiness is simply an element of private happiness and limited the discussion of public happiness (Bruni & Zamagni, 2007). However, this view should be revised from a perspective of public happiness.

There is no consensus on the publicness (or public responsibility) of happiness. From a liberal perspective, an individual's happiness is a purely private matter that a nation cannot and should not be responsible for (Frey et al., 2004; Duncan 2010). Duncan (2010) argued that the emphasis on public responsibility of happiness will only make public policy more complicated. In particular, he argues that maximization of happiness can be a public goal but not a responsibility of government. A similar concern is that increasing individual happiness will become an excuse for big government, nanny state, happiness police, or bureaucrats of bliss (Kim et al., 2015). In contrast, a communitarian perspective sees public responsibility for the happiness of community members because individual happiness is affected by the conditions of the community (Raz, 1994). Lane (1994)'s research also finds that a happy life, high quality of life is impossible without human development, and when the governments ignores this responsibility, it leads to policy failure. Veenhoven (2004a, b) also finds government with a certain level of authority and control affects the social factors (rule of law, economic freedom, acceptance of minorities, etc.) that have a positive impact on citizen happiness levels. Thus, the happiness of society should be subject to an appropriate level of public policy and responsibility.

Which position should we take? Apart from how we define happiness, it is basically a subjective emotion that an individual feels. Therefore, in principle, the individual should take responsibility for his or her happiness or misery. This is clear when we see that even within the same conditions, happiness levels differ by individual characteristics (traits and efforts). Based on this view, happiness is defined as a private matter, and it is invalid for a nation to approach happiness as a public goal. However, it is problematic to make the individual completely responsible for happiness. Because happiness is not only affected by individual characteristics (traits and efforts), but also by objective, external factors. Just as happiness levels may differ among individuals in the same conditions, individuals with similar subjective happiness traits will feel different happiness levels depending on external conditions. Accordingly, we cannot deny that individual happiness is simultaneously affected by individual characteristics and external factors. Related, previous studies have reported that demographic factors such as age, sex, education level, marital status, family relations, health, religion; economic factors such as income, employment, unemployment, inflation, growth rate; positive social factors such as political freedom, democracy, rule of law, and social capital; negative social factors such as crime, terror, corruption; environmental factors such as pleasantness have significant effects on happiness (Frey 2008; Layard, 2005; Welsch, 2009; Bok, 2010, etc.).

As such, if external conditions affect individual happiness (whether big or small), then at least that much becomes the public responsibility of the nation and society, and thus, the government should make efforts to establish the basic conditions for happiness through public policies. Despite this, if we define the responsibility for improving external conditions as fully individual, then the potential for individuals to pursue their happiness goals will shrink. Accordingly, it should be noted that neglecting such policy efforts is not only normatively unjust, but is also undesirable because individuals lack the ability to transform social conditions that affect their happiness-pursuing activities. Moreover, because the resources and efforts of individuals are unequal, without social efforts to improve the basic conditions of happiness, social inequality will grow. This is another reason for public efforts to improve basic conditions for happiness.

It appears that the position of the state's responsibility for happiness seems to create a sharp division between liberals and communitarians. However, the two are not exactly opposed. Even from a liberal perspective, it simply cautions against the unrestricted intervention of the state, but recognizes a minimum level of state intervention, such as the protection of property rights. We can say that the protection of property rights is also ultimately for individual happiness and thus liberals cannot completely be against any public efforts to establish the basic social conditions for citizen happiness. The communitarian perspective does not argue for the guarantee of a final happiness level for each and every individual, but rather focuses on improving the structural socioeconomic inequality such that each individual has the potential for an equal level of happiness. That is, the two opposing perspectives have a quantitative difference, rather than a qualitative difference, and we can find common ground for supporting the social conditions that enable individuals to pursue happiness. Considering that most humans are ultimately interested in happiness (Salichs & Malfaz, 2006; Sheldon & Houser-Marko, 2001), if a nation that exists for its citizens ignores the happiness of its citizens, it lacks the reason for existence. As such, the need for public happiness that requires public efforts for citizen happiness is obvious.

In doing so, there should be equal caution against over-emphasizing public responsibility for happiness as caution against over-emphasizing private responsibility for happiness. The latter can lead to social inequality, while the former can lead to an over-sized government or over-protection of the state. Related, on the one hand, we should be wary of group think in the manner of sacrificing one's personal interest for public good, and on the other hand, be wary of individualistic thinking and thereby combining the two perspectives and foster both the public and private (Kim, 2011). Basically, happiness has both a private dimension and a public dimension, and thus, a balanced perspective is ideal.

2.3 The Scope of Public Happiness

If we accept public responsibility for the happiness of constituents, then how wide is the scope of responsibility? This is the same question as whether public responsibility for happiness means responsibility for the resulting happiness of individuals or the responsibility for creating the basic conditions of happiness. In other words, the question is about giving opportunities or outputs. In general, the liberal perspective supports the former, and the communitarian perspective supports the latter. However, the basic discussion of welfare policies cannot be directly applied to happiness policies. Happiness is an emotion, and taking responsibility for an emotional output is realistically impossible, even if it can be normatively accepted.

This book presents a modest opinion on the scope of public responsibility for happiness. That is, public responsibility for national happiness should not focus on the final happiness achievement of individuals, but the enabling social conditions or living conditions that can support individual activities for happiness. Even if a certain part of happiness is a public issue, a significant part of happiness is determined by individual characteristics, and thus, there is a limit to policy efforts for pubic happiness. Moreover, it is difficult to guarantee a causal relationship between policy efforts and individual happiness, and there are limits to government capacity. Therefore, the ideal and realistic policy goal for public happiness should not be the guarantee of ultimate happiness levels of individuals, but rather creating the social conditions to support individuals' pursuit of happiness. For these reasons, this book understands the public responsibility for happiness as creating the enabling social conditions for national happiness and creating a society wherein individuals realize their happiness based on these conditions.

Related, we should not confuse establishing or improving the enabling conditions for happiness as a national goal with the ultimate national objective.[2] Of course, the

[2] Strictly speaking, objectives are concepts distinguishable from goals. Objectives provide a series of quantifiable milestone or benchmark to pursue. Objectives are means to achieve goals. The objective, as a higher concept of goals, presents a direction of action, but does not specifically present the course of action. The goal, as a higher-level concept of the objective, presents the direction of actions, but does not provide a concrete action process. Also, in general, the goal is rarely defined operationally, but the objective is often defined operationally in order to be used as a means to measure effectiveness (Park 2008; Gulati et al., 2017: 97). However, the distinction between the two is relative. Both refer to the desired state to be achieved and can only be identified

state cannot guarantee final happiness levels of each individual, but the ultimate goal is to increase happiness, and the enabling conditions are the conditions necessary for increasing happiness. Thus, the basic conditions for happiness only have meaning when they are connected to happiness. If not, the social conditions are no different from the list of welfare state items that sees welfare increase as its goal. This requires the state to carefully distinguish the enabling conditions that support happiness in a statistically significant way in the policy efforts for social conditions.

3 Essential Principles of Public Happiness

As mentioned above, there is the need for public efforts to increase public happiness that has a collective characteristic, and as such, the major principles that one should be aware of when pursuing public policy for increasing public happiness are as follows. These principles are the minimum requirements for having a shared understanding of the nature of public happiness and effective public policies.

3.1 Public Responsibility for the Happiness of Constituents

Public responsibility for happiness is imperative. Following this responsibility, the government should accept public happiness as a basic goal (or one of several basic goals) and draft and actively pursue public policies. This public responsibility for happiness is a precondition that takes preference over other principles.

The meaning of public responsibility for happiness is twofold. One is the awareness of public responsibility, and the other is the subject of public responsibility. First, it means the nation should accept national or citizen happiness as a public goal and actively work toward increasing happiness. Of course, happiness is at its basis an individual subjective feeling, the state cannot determine the psychological factors at the individual level, and thus, individual efforts are important. However, external conditions contribute significantly to individual happiness, there are limits to individual efforts for happiness, and thus, we need the state's policy efforts to establish the enabling conditions for individuals to pursue happiness. At this point, the level of national responsibility for individual happiness will differ by ideological paradigms. From a communitarian perspective, it will be expansive, while from a liberal or conservative perspective, it will be diminutive. On the one hand, there are concerns that the process of pursuing happiness will sacrifice other social values (e.g., growth, freedom, equality, justice, stability, peace, democracy, etc.) or that it will lead to a big government or over-protective government (see Woo, 2013). However, even when acknowledging the difference in the level of government intervention, it is difficult

as a chain relationship of the goal and the means depending on the difference of specificity. Thus, we use them interchangeably.

to deny minimal policy efforts for the happiness of citizens who are the members of democratic states. Moreover, happiness need not replace growth, freedom, peace, or other goals as the only public goal. That is, when adopting happiness as a national goal, it can be the only goal, but also stand next to other goals depending on the circumstances. In this way, public responsibility for happiness presented here differs from the utilitarian perspective that emphasizes utility as the only measure and goal (Woo, 2014a, b). Basically, the public responsibility for happiness presented here is a modest proposal that there should be public support for each citizen to pursue happiness, rather than guaranteeing a final level of happiness. At this level, a nation that does not have an active interest in citizen happiness can be seen as having lost its minimum dignity as a nation.

On the one hand, we should understand public responsibility for public happiness as applying not only to the state but also to individuals. That is, individuals should make an effort toward their own happiness, but have the right to demand an appropriate level of support from the state. This right falls under the citizens' right to happiness and is also a government's responsibility. Furthermore, as members of a nation-state, individuals should have a sense of responsibility for the happiness of other members as well. Because happiness in public happiness has both private and public characteristics.

Second, the public responsibility for happiness is not for the happiness of an atomic individual (individual happiness), but for the happiness of a public individual (public happiness) as a member of a community (nation, society, and region). There can be differences between the happiness constituent factors of an atomic individuals' happiness and that of a related individual. For example, from the perspective of an individual separate from others, hedonic components are valued, while from the perspective of an individual in relationship with others, eudaimonic components are more valued. Related to this, as I will explain below, the state should not only establish the social conditions that connect the two, but also show interest in the moral sentiments of the happiness elements.

Who is the agent of public responsibility? If we take the state as our unit, the primary agent of public responsibility is the government that decides public policies. Citizens are, by principle, the subject of public responsibility. But if we acknowledge the publicness of happiness, then the public responsibility of public happiness can also be applied to individuals, and in this case, citizens also become agents of public responsibility. As already explained, citizens have the right to demand the government's active policy efforts and also have a duty to be concerned with the happiness of other constituents and thus become a responsible agent of public happiness. This perception has important meaning for policies aimed at increasing public happiness. What if we narrowly defined public responsibility for public happiness to the state and define citizens as passive consumers of public policy? On the one hand, there is little reason for arguing against the government when it makes a poor policy effort to support happiness, and on the other hand, we can have happiness selfishness that only focuses on individual happiness, and when there is an over-demand for happiness, then there is the risk of depleting public resources. In order to prevent these problems and to make the process of policymaking for public happiness as smooth as possible, we should acknowledge the government as the primary agent, but also emphasize that citizens are agents of public responsibility.

Today, there is government failure on the one hand, and the maturation of civil society creating the need for new governance on the other hand. When we define governance as the cooperation between government and citizens in the policy process, this demand for governance is greater in the policy process for public happiness, than the generic policy process. Happiness is experienced by individuals, as agents of happiness, individual voices should be reflected in the policy process, and for this, individual participation in the policy process should become expanded. With the progress of governance, the role of participating citizens changes from a one-way recipient or consumer of policy to a coproducer or prosumer. This means that the title of individuals changes from object to subject. From an implementation perspective, citizens become an agent of public responsibility for happiness through participating in governance.

3.2 Balanced Consideration of the Level and Distribution of Happiness

In policy efforts for the happiness of constituents, there should not only be a focus on the level of happiness, but also an equal focus on the distribution of happiness. The level and distribution of happiness should be perceived as two faces of public happiness.

For individual happiness, only the level of happiness may be considered, but for public happiness that approaches happiness as existing in the relationships within a community, there should be a consideration for the distribution of happiness as well. On a basic level, both the absolute and relative level of human happiness matter (Clark, 2016). Public happiness, in particular, is about every constituent of a community and thus does not accept a high level of happiness for some and a low level for others. Even if the level of happiness for citizens increases through the government's establishment of a happiness baseline, if there are large inequalities in happiness levels across individuals, then that happiness policy is not a successful one. Happiness inequality will become a social instability factor and will ultimately harm overall citizens' happiness. The increase in happiness levels without an equal distribution of happiness can be a necessary condition for public happiness, but not a sufficient condition, and vice versa. Therefore, a government should set as a policy goal for every citizen to have a high and similar level of happiness. Nevertheless, the majority of discussion around happiness is focused on the level of happiness and ignores the distribution of happiness. This is because of the focus on the individual aspect of happiness.

Between the level and distribution of happiness, which one should be the more important goal? All else being equal, as a principle, a balance between the two is ideal. However, we cannot pre-define the balanced condition. This will differ by sociocultural elements and the situation of balance between the two. Moreover, the balanced perspective between the level and distribution of happiness can make it difficult to compare happiness among communities. As most comparative studies of happiness have done so far, the direct comparison of happiness levels among communities with sociocultural differences has been widely accepted. This is because of the belief that every human being pursues happiness and there are some common happiness factors. However, when it is difficult to define a balanced point between the level and distribution of happiness, the comparison of both at the same time becomes even more difficult. This is because the standard point changes for every comparison. However, from a different perspective, this challenge can also be a solution. This is because it will either suppress the efforts to compare something that is difficult to compare with a uniform standard or motivate the development of a more appropriate and precise comparison tool. For example, the standards for happiness policies in Bhutan and United Kingdom cannot be identical. Defining the balanced point of happiness level and distribution in Bhutan based on western standards will restrict the autonomous implementation of happiness policies that are appropriate to the regional context. Recognizing this point, each country or province can establish the groundwork for pursuing a happiness policy that corresponds to their specific situation and sociocultural conditions.

3.3 Constructing Appropriate Social Conditions (Living Conditions)

Public happiness requires the establishment of an adequate level of social conditions or living conditions to support an individual's efforts to pursue happiness.

Happiness is not an emotional goal that can be achieved through passion or restraint. Therefore, there are limits to the suggestions of happiness-related books on ways to become happy (e.g., minimize desires), including positive psychology.[3] Happiness changes with emotional states, but is strongly related to objective items. Objective conditions have a significant effect on human happiness. With regard to this, a government should make efforts to establish the social conditions that support an individual's happiness efforts in order to increase public happiness. As mentioned before, social conditions include tangible conditions (social welfare, housing, public facilities, subsidies, etc.) and intangible conditions (social capital, institutions, culture, social ethics, etc.). Depending on how much of these social conditions need to be met, the social conditions will have a significant effect on

[3] Positive psychology was popularized by Martin Seligman (2002)'s "Authentic Happiness." The source of positive psychology is also seen as William James' healthy mindedness (1902). Most of the existing psychology research focuses on negative emotions such as depression, sadness, and addiction and conducts psychological research to alleviate them. However, Seligman advocated positive psychology as a wellbeing-oriented psychology, arguing that research on humans should focus on prosperity. He suggested that wellbeing is a key factor in PERMAS: positive emotions, engagement, relationships, meaning, and accomplishment.

happiness with individual capacity as a mediating factor. If such efforts are inadequate and the social conditions are not established in society, an individual's pursuit of happiness will be restricted and ultimately have a negative effect on public happiness.

Inferior social conditions do not stop at limiting members' activities to pursue happiness, but also increase the inequality of happiness. Why is that? If social conditions are at an inadequate level, an individual's happiness pursuit activities will be largely determined by the level of private resources. In this case, because of limited resources, the level of happiness one can achieve will be limited, and if there is an unequal distribution of resources among individuals, this will inhibit the equitable distribution of happiness. Considering this, we should make efforts to establish a basic level of social conditions, not only to raise the level of happiness but also to alleviate happiness inequality. In doing so, it is also necessary to pay attention to both the level and distribution of social conditions.

Social conditions affect individual happiness by themselves as well as supporting individuals' pursuit of happiness. For example, tangible resources like public transit systems or arts/cultural centers and intangible resources like political culture or social capital have a direct effect on individual happiness. We can say this is a direct effect because it does not have individual activities as a mediator. In contrast, the effect of social conditions on happiness that has individual activities as a mediator is indirect. Related, there will be a meaningful difference in policy design for public happiness depending on whether the direct or indirect effects of social conditions are emphasized.

If focusing on the direct effect, public policy does not assume a multiplier effect through the individual as mediator and thus needs to make it possible to achieve personal happiness with social conditions only. In this case, there is a limit to guaranteeing happiness effects with limited resources, and even if there were plenty of resources, there are limits to reflecting every individuals' preference. Furthermore, the individual is only the final consumer of social conditions, and this limits the participation of individuals in policymaking processes, which then also limits opportunities to improve civic attitudes through participation. This approach goes beyond establishing the basic frame of happiness to actually giving happiness to individuals and is closer to the approach of private happiness rather than public happiness. In contrast, if we focus on the indirect effect, public policy assumes a multiplier effect based on an individual's voluntary activities and does not assume that the establishment of social conditions will guarantee ultimate happiness for individuals. In this case, because of the multiplier effect of social conditions through individual activities, we can save the input of public resources and because we assume the voluntary participation of individuals, there is an incentive to reflect individual preferences in the public policy process or open participation in policy design. Moreover, there are opportunities to increase civic attitudes in the participation process.

Which effect do we focus on? A simple example of the direct and indirect effect above is similar to the one found in discussions of welfare policy—giving someone fish versus teaching someone how to fish. The former focuses on the direct effect, and the latter focuses on the indirect effect. In general, the latter is considered to be better for saving resources, protecting individual freedom, and having a sustainable impact. Similarly, in happiness policies, consideration of the multiplier effect of individual activities and related resource savings, incentives for policy participation, expectations for improving the distribution of happiness, gives more attention to the indirect effect of happiness policies rather than the direct effect.[4]

It is important to note that the establishment of social conditions is based on individuals' voluntary activities, thus, the policy direction for the establishment of social conditions should guarantee individual autonomy, and direct regulation on it should be restrained in principle. But there is an argument for strengthening active regulations on individual autonomy in order to promote happiness. For example, Layard (2005), who is exceptionally active in happiness policy recommendations, has suggested work–life balance through taxation, increased regulation of advertisement, income redistribution through a wealth tax, promotion of social capital through restrictions on migration, and enhancement of mental health through psychological diagnosis and treatment. Even when agreeing with the policy motivation, these suggestions may be criticized for their force and direct intervention that can infringe on individual freedoms excessively. Especially from a negative perspective on government intervention, these policies can interfere in the private sector with the excuse of increasing individual happiness (Kim et al., 2015; Sugden & Teng, 2016). The social conditions presented here do not require such forceful policies. Social conditions are based on the voluntary pursuit of happiness by each individual and aim to create the supporting conditions for these pursuits of happiness. Of course, some of the forceful suggestions of Layard can be included under the social enabling conditions, many policies have a regulatory characteristic, and thus, it can be difficult to distinguish the social conditions suggested here and Layard's happiness suggestions. Nevertheless, the criteria for distinguishing the two are clear. It is individual freedom. At its base, happiness is a voluntary emotion, and it is better to avoid a situation of artificially controlling this emotion from the outside. Thus, when promoting happiness policies, we should understand the tipping point between social conditions having an enhancing effect on individuals' pursuit of happiness and the infringement of individual freedom due to the establishment of social conditions and look for ways to maximize the former and minimize the latter.

3.4 Social Admissibility of Individual Happiness Values

Public happiness requires high social admissibility of individual happiness values. In a more neutral language, there should be a high level of consistency between individual and social values of happiness.

In order to enhance public happiness, high social admissibility of the happiness values (influencing factors and happiness factors) of constituents is necessary. First, the influencing factors of happiness should be socially admissible. Happiness

[4] The capability theory proposed by Sen (1999) is basically an argument that supports the indirect effect on happiness of the construction of basic social conditions as suggested here.

factors that are admissible to the individual will not always be socially admissible. To use an extreme example, illegal drugs can increase personal happiness. And it may also increase the level of public happiness and improve the distribution of happiness. However, there will be limits to accepting this as ideal from a public standpoint. Furthermore, the elements of happiness should also be socially admissible. In defining happiness, one view sees the hedonic components, while another sees eudaimonic components as happiness. This is a conceptual definition based on its elements, but is also a normative evaluation of what is happiness. In general, it is expected that the eudaimonic component will be more socially admissible than hedonic components. This is because the eudaimonic approach pursues meaning or fulfillment of life overall while emphasizing social approval and moral evaluation of different pleasures (Thin, 2012: 35).

Why is this social admissibility necessary? First, we need it for the increase of individual happiness. Basically, as a member of a community, humans pursue happiness while living in relationships with other individuals. However, individual happiness becomes more established when it is socially respected, whether this be pleasure or moral value. Related, Diener and Scollon (2003) indicated that the conditions for human happiness are provisional and they need social approval through conversations with others about their happiness.[5] However, if there is low social admissibility of an individual's happiness factor, achievement of happiness becomes unlikely as there is a disconnect between the individual aspect of happiness and the public aspect of happiness (and vice versa). Second, we need it for the sustainable development of society. The more community members pursue happiness of the community based on the interactive relationship among members, the more individual happiness factors and social happiness factors will become congruent. However, if one ignores the reciprocity among members and pursues their own happiness based on individualism and through unjust, illegal methods, then the conflict among members' will for happiness decrease happiness for society overall and will decrease the sustainable progress of society. Third, we need it for the smooth progress of happiness policies. If there is a big gap between individual happiness perceptions and social perceptions, this will negatively affect the policy implementation for increasing happiness. For example, in Utopia depicted by Thomas More, the hedonic components of happiness will have low social admissibility. In this case, public policies to boost the hedonic components for happiness are difficult to justify. In addition, the individual who values hedonic components is restricted in their efforts to pursue happiness by society's moral sentiments. Nevertheless, an individual that pursues a happiness factor that is in sharp contrast with social norms will inhibit the smooth implementation of happiness policies or will erode social norms. This adverse effect will become larger with the divide between an individual's happiness values and its social admissibility. Thus, for the increase of happiness through the connection of individual happiness

[5] This does not mean that people's subjective happiness can be judged externally and labeled as inauthentic. Happiness is subjective in nature, and it is not possible to clearly distinguish between authentic happiness and inauthentic happiness (Diener and Scollon 2003).

and public happiness, there should be more focus on increasing congruency between an individual's happiness factors and social norms.

In order to enhance the social admissibility of an individual's happiness values, it is important to make public efforts to increase the congruence between the individual's happiness values and the society's happiness values. However, this does not mean that uniform, top-down national involvement is desirable. Basically, the moral sentiment is a cultural phenomenon resulting from the history of a society and the average sentiment of the time, it is not appropriate for a government to control it with top-down authority, and there are limits to doing this artificially. Therefore, efforts to increase the congruence between individual and social moral sentiments on happiness should be bottom-up based on public debate and consensus, rather than top-down, authoritarian. For example, a forum for public deliberation in civil society, expansion of citizen participation in the public policy process, civic education, and information provision can be effective means. Of course, some may say that these efforts should be barred. However, this leaves the question of how to resolve the concern for decreasing happiness due to the incongruence of moral sentiments on happiness values. As long as individual autonomy is secured, there is no need to deny autonomous deliberation in civil society, active citizen participation, and civic education, as opposed to unilateral indoctrination and unilateral guidance. In the same context, Sugden and Teng (2016) suggest that instead of direct intervention, governments can give advice to individuals (personal message) or provide scientific evidence through social messages. At the same time, they criticize views like Layard (2005: 199) that argue for moral education as paternalistic. Moral education as a one-sided edification should be avoided, but civic education based on individual autonomy is necessary.

We should acknowledge that it is difficult to have a uniform and general criterion for the social admissibility or moral sentiments of happiness values due to regional and cultural differences. The acceptance of certain happiness values in one society does not guarantee the same acceptance in a different society. For example, if there is one society that values hedonistic happiness and another that values eudaimonic happiness, there will be limits to comparing the level and distribution of happiness with a uniform measure in these two different cultures. This is the reason for focusing on social, cultural differences in happiness debates, and the need for this applies to comparison both between countries and within countries.

Here, I summarize the principles of happiness presented above. First, individual happiness requires an active recognition of public responsibility. Second, the evaluation of happiness includes not only level, but also distribution. Third, happiness policies have a goal of establishing enabling conditions. Lastly, we should pay attention to the social admissibility of happiness values. From an attributes standpoint, the affirmation of public responsibility for public happiness is the ideology of public happiness; the level and distribution of happiness are the objects of happiness policies; the enabling conditions are the objective of happiness policies; and the social admissibility of happiness factors is related to happiness values. Also, the four principles are not items on the same level, but are in a means–ends relationship. That is, public responsibility is guaranteed through the practice of other items. The discussion of relationships among these is important because they provide basic direction for happiness policies and governance.

4 Research Toward Public Happiness

In this section, I provide an overview of current happiness research and evaluate it from the perspective of public happiness. Next, I present future directions of public happiness research.

4.1 Reflections on Current Research

In the previous section, four principles of public happiness were defined as follows: ① responsibility for public happiness, ② a balanced interest in the level and distribution of happiness, ③ efforts to establish social conditions, and ④ social admissibility of happiness values of members. Based on these demands of public happiness, the current research trend on happiness studies can be evaluated as follows.

Individuality bias
Most research is primarily interested in individual happiness. The majority of studies focus on individual happiness, and research on public happiness tends be the exception. For most studies, the individual is the unit of analysis since they are interested in individual happiness (Campbell et al. 1976; Pavot & Diener, 1993; Easterlin & Sawangfa, 2009; Shin, 2015; Park, 2003; Yoon & Kim, 2008, etc.). For example, Pavot and Diener (1993) and Easterlin and Sawangfa (2009) explain happiness as the emotional response of individuals and subconscious, physiological conditions. Shin (2015: 203) defines the influencing factors of happiness as an individual's age, income, occupation, and gender and explains that the most important causal factor in empirical analysis is the psychological element. These studies focusing on individual happiness do not consider the relationship with community members, the prosperity of the community, or other community-level variables. In this regard, Frawley (2015) indicated that previous studies adopted an individual perspective and remained within the frame of identifying influencing factors at the individual level. Even at the individual level, the influencing factors have been limited to income, employment, and marital status, which are individual traits.[6]

This research trend of focusing on individual happiness is understandable given that happiness is largely based on the subjective feeling or evaluation of an individual and is impossible to define absolutely. However, happiness is necessarily affected

[6] Frawley (2015) highlights five aspects—cultural bias, normativity, bad science, diminished subjectivity, individualization—as limitations of current happiness studies.

by social conditions, and thus, the current narrow focus on individual happiness needs to be corrected for the establishment and progress of public happiness studies. Furthermore, the practical interest of various countries and international organizations that are pursuing the promotion of public happiness is an important driver of the recent increase in happiness research and calls for expanding happiness research to a public happiness approach. Individual happiness-oriented research alone will limit the achievement of this macro-goal of promoting national happiness.

A few studies deal with happiness at the national or regional level (e.g., Bok, 2010; Bruni & Zamagni, 2007; Porta & Scazzieri, 2007; Thin, 2012; Zamagni, 2014).[7] However, even in such happiness studies, from a collective standpoint, the unit of analysis is mostly the individual, and there are few studies that focus on national or local public organizations as analytical units. Of course, this approach is not incorrect. It is because public happiness has a characteristic of collective happiness that is an extension of personal happiness. However, the sum of individual happiness is not the equivalent of public happiness. This is because the level of happiness, as well as the content of happiness, will change when connected with the community, not as an isolated individual. Therefore, when approaching public happiness, there seems to be a limit to adopting the individual as the unit of analysis. There is a need for more research on public happiness paying attention to the public dimension beyond the individual dimension.

Evaluation bias

Previous studies that evaluate happiness have focused on the average happiness level of citizens. Simply examining the average level of happiness is the same as seeing public happiness as the sum of individual happiness. However, for public happiness studies to become established, there needs to be an examination not only of the total level of happiness, but also the distribution. Public happiness is not just about individual happiness, but the relational happiness of community members and must look at overall happiness. Nevertheless, most studies are over-focused on the level of national happiness but not on the distribution. For example, the World Happiness Report (Helliwell et al., 2020) provides detailed rankings and ranking changes for each country for the level of happiness, whereas for the distribution of happiness, it only presents the happiness gap between urban and rural areas.

[7] Bruni and Zamagni (2007) offers a helpful review of the flow of public happiness discussions centered on Italian scholars in the Enlightenment period. Thin (2012) is notable for dealing with happiness issues at the level of mid-level social groups such as communities, families, and organizations beyond the individual level. However, it is not a macroscopic approach including the state. Bok (2010) is an exceptional study that has expressed direct interest in happiness at the national level. However, there is a limit to focusing on individual units in measuring happiness levels and identifying its factors. Several other studies (Easterlin 2013; Frey & Stutzer, 2012; Johns & Ormerod, 2007; Layard 2006; Kim, H., 2016; Kim, D.H., 2016; Koo et al., 2017, etc.) are related to public happiness research in the sense of discussing whether happiness can be applied as a policy goal. Most of the studies however still do not present an explicit discussion on the publicness of happiness, so supplementation is required.

Of course, it can be said that focusing only on the level of happiness is in part an important interest in public happiness. However, full-scale research on public happiness should go beyond a narrow attention to the average level of national happiness and include a balanced consideration of the two faces of public happiness, both the level and distribution.

Diagnosis bias

Interest in happiness studies has been reactivated in the twenty-first century, but this has not translated to practical interest in happiness policies and governance. At the risk of some over-generalization, most happiness studies focus on measuring happiness levels and identifying the influencing factors and thus have shown little interest in policy innovation for increasing happiness or changes in governance. Overall, there is a new approach to development goals, without efforts to adopt a new perspective on policies and policy implementation systems.

Some exceptional studies are focusing on happiness policies and are giving policy recommendations for each policy area. Di Tella et al. (2001) argue that happiness data should be used in shaping government policy, Veenhoven (2004a, b) maintains that government policies can create the conditions for increasing happiness, and thus happiness, rather than income maximization, should be a policy goal. Booth (2012: 56) asserts that government policy is necessary to increase happiness and that national policy that can override individual and local decisions is important. Some studies give specific policy recommendations. Also, Layard (2005) suggests that maximization of happiness, rather than income, should be a policy goal, and presents work-life balance through taxation, increased regulation of advertisement, income redistribution through a wealth tax, promotion of social capital through restrictions on migration, enhancement of mental health through psychological diagnosis and treatment as policy recommendations. Like Layard (2005), Frank (1999) assumes that relative welfare is important, and that in order to minimize income inequality, the adoption of a wealth tax on high-income earners is necessary. Graham and Haidt (2010). (2010) suggested that policies to encourage local festivals are important for increasing happiness.

However, these studies are still the exception. Most studies argue that happiness or wellbeing should be adopted as a developmental goal and stop short of giving fragmentary policy recommendations and do not expand to policy reorientation or the overall framework for happiness policies. There are tactics, but no strategies. Even though happiness studies have a prescriptive research topic, the relative lack and simplicity of prescriptive research has not produced meaningful prescriptions. Given that human happiness is affected by diverse factors, there needs to be an overall reorientation of policies for increasing happiness, and a prescription that only focuses on few policies cannot be a valid prescription. Furthermore, previous studies have shown little interest in the overall reorientation of policies and have been silent on the policy implementation structure of governance restructuring or renovation. Even if policy directions are reoriented, without an appropriate implementation system, policy implementation will be difficult.

In sum, current happiness studies are focused on the scientific measurement and identification of influencing factors (i.e., diagnosis) and in comparison show weak practical efforts to increase happiness or wellbeing through the innovation of governance and public policies. This lack of practical interest in happiness is due to the "beyond GDP" movement still being in its early stages, the lack of agreement on the validity of happiness as a goal, and the lack of serious consideration for the need to connect policy decision and governance to the transformation in national development goals. However, given that the recent motivation for happiness studies includes a practical one of increasing happiness, the lack of attention to governance or happiness policies in research is surprising. If there has been a major shift in national development goals, then of course, there should be a reflective reorientation of the overall policy system, and as such, there should be restructuring of governance as a policy implementation tool. Therefore, future happiness studies should go beyond measuring and identifying influencing factors of happiness and pay attention to the reorientation of policy direction and governance for the increase of public happiness.

In happiness policy and governance research, there should be an emphasis on combining happiness research and governance theories and an effort for diagnosis and prescription appropriate to each local context. Previous studies lacked discussion of appropriate theoretical foundations related to the change in policy and governance as per the change in development goals. Research that is led by theory can be generalized, and as such, there is a need for theory-driven research. Thus, the discussion of policy and governance change as related to the change in national development goals also requires a theory-based discussion. However, previous studies have lacked the theoretical interest in governance as an implementation system of development policies. This is a natural result of previous studies that did not actively connect happiness issues to policy or governance. Nevertheless, given that new paradigms, such as New Public Management, New Public Service, have replaced traditional management in previous policy or governance discussions, this theoretical indifference needs to be resolved. As long as happiness studies aims for public happiness, it has an inseparable relationship with governance.

Contextual bias

Happiness is related to an individual's feelings and is inevitably value-laden. As suggested above, in order to promote public happiness, it is required to increase social admissibility of individual happiness value, that is, to promote congruence between individual happiness value and social moral sentiments. However, the perception of the value of happiness varies according to regions and groups. That is, some regions may value hedonistic elements more, while others virtuous elements more, or some groups may emphasize group values over individual values, while some regions individual values over group values. Therefore, there is a limit to applying the uniform value standard for happiness across regions or groups. Nevertheless, many studies tend to ignore such differences. In particular, as Frawley (2015) indicated, happiness research has been developed in an atmosphere biased toward Western cultural and academic soils, and thus, consideration of the values of non-Western society is insufficient. This trend is easily observed in many comparative surveys of happiness between countries based on standard questionnaires. They attempt to compare happiness between countries based on standardized indicator systems, whether they are subjective or objective indicators, without careful consideration of differences between communities.[8] Of course, such attempts are not incorrect since there are not only differences between countries but also much in common, but the problem of sacrificing specific validity for generalization remains. It should be noted that even though standardization is inevitable for the purpose of comparison, there are limitations in attempting general evaluation based on limited standard (Cummins, 2013).

4.2 Directions for Public Happiness Research

The limitations of the current study of happiness are summarized in four aspects from the perspective of public happiness, but such limitations basically stem from the bias toward individual happiness. Most happiness studies so far have approached happiness from a private, individual perspective rather than a public aspect. And there has been limited attention to practical policy recommendations or governance for public happiness. Future studies should redirect their attention toward increasing the practical contributions of public happiness research.

If so, what approaches should public happiness research adopt? In comparison with individual happiness, public happiness research is subject to the following demands. As mentioned before, there are four biases in previous research, and they suggest the following future directions for research.

① Regarding the object of happiness: not only the happiness of private individual but also the happiness of public individual.

② Regarding the evaluation of happiness: not only the level of happiness but also the distribution of happiness is required.

③ Regarding the means of happiness instrument: not only diagnosis (measurement of happiness, finding factors) but also policy and governance as a means.

④ Regarding the context of happiness: research and acceptance of happiness values suitable for different groups and regions.

Table 2 summarizes the above compared with the current research with the tendency of individual happiness.

---

[8] OECD's Better Life Index tries to alleviate this problem by allowing users to arbitrarily apply weights to index items. However, the problem of the standardized index system has not been fundamentally solved, and while the randomness of the weights has been expanded, there seems to be a problem that the utilization is hampered due to the absence of reference standards for weight application.

Table 2 Future direction for research on public happiness: compared with research tendency on individual happiness

	Individual happiness research	Public happiness research
Object	Happiness of private individual	Happiness of public individuals
Evaluation	Level of happiness	Level and distribution of happiness
Instrument	Policy fragmented/diagnosis (measurement, identifying conditions)	Policy comprehensive/ governance
Context	Value-neutral approach	Social admissibility of happiness values (value-laden approach)

References

Alesina, A., Di Tella, R., & MacCulloch, R. (2004). Inequality and happiness: Are Europeans and Americans different? *Journal of Public Economics, 88*(9–10), 2009–2042.

Allin, P., & Hand, D. J. (2014). *The well-being of nations: Meaning, motive and measurement*. John Wiley & Sons.

Bartolini, S., Bilancini, E., Bruni, L., & Porta, P. L. (Eds.). (2016). *Policies for happiness*. Oxford University Press.

Bjørnskov, C., Dreher, A., & Fischer, J. A. (2007). The bigger the better? Evidence of the effect of government size on life satisfaction around the world. *Public Choice, 130*(3), 267–292.

Bok, D. (2010). *The politics of happiness: What government can learn from the new research on well-being*. Princeton University Press.

Booth, P. (Ed.). (2012). *... And the pursuit of happiness-well-being and the role of government*. Institute of Economic Affairs.

Boyce, C. J., Brown, G. D., & Moore, S. C. (2010). Money and happiness: Rank of income, not income, affects life satisfaction. *Psychological Science, 21*(4), 471–475.

Brooks, A. C. (2008). *Gross national happiness: Why happiness matters for America and how we can get more of it*. Basic Books.

Bruni, L., & Zamagni, S. (2007). *Civil economy: Efficiency, equity, public happiness*. Peter Lang.

Campbell, A., Converse, P. E., & Rodgers, W. L. (1976). *The quality of American life: Perceptions, evaluations, and satisfactions*. Russell Sage Foundation.

Canadian Index of Wellbeing. (2012). https://uwaterloo.ca/canadian-index-wellbeing/. Accessed May 7, 2012.

Carson, R. (2002). *Silent spring*. Houghton Mifflin Harcourt.

Cho, Y. (2013). A study on paradigm transfer problems from export-oriented policy to domestic demand based policy for economic growth. *The Journal of Korean Public Policy, 15*(4), 213–238. (Korean).

Clark, A. E. (2016). Adaptation and the Easterlin paradox. In T. Tachibanaki (Ed.), *Advances in happiness research* (pp. 75–94). Springer.

Clark, A. E., & Oswald, A. J. (1996). Satisfaction and comparison income. *Journal of Public Economics, 61*(3), 359–381.

Coggburn, J. D., & Schneider, S. K. (2003). The relationship between state government performance and state quality of life. *International Journal of Public Administration, 26*(12), 1337–1354.

Crum, A. J., & Salovey, P. (2013). Emotionally intelligent happiness. In S. A. David, I. Boniwell, & A. Conley Ayers (Eds.), *Oxford handbook of happiness* (pp. 73–87). Oxford: Oxford University Press.

Cummins, R. A. (2013). Measuring happiness and subjective well-being. In S. A. David, I. Boniwell, & A. Conley Ayers (Eds.), *Oxford handbook of happiness* (pp. 185–200). Oxford University Press.

Diener, E. (Ed.). (2009). *Assessing well-being: The collected works of Ed Diener*. Springer.
Di Tella, R., & MacCulloch, R. (2005). Partisan social happiness. *The Review of Economic Studies, 72*(2), 367–393.
Di Tella, R., MacCulloch, R., & Oswald, A. (2001). Preferences over inflation and unemployment: Evidence from surveys of happiness. *The American Economic Review, 91*(1), 335–341.
Diener, E., & Scollon, C. (2003). Subjective well-being is desirable, but not the summum bonum. *Paper to be delivered at the University of Minnesota Interdisciplinary Workshop on Well-Being*, Minneapolis.
Diener, E. (2000). Subjective well-being: The science of happiness and a proposal for a national index. *American Psychologist, 55*(1), 34–43.
Dreher, A., & Öhler, H. (2011). Does government ideology affect personal happiness? A Test. *Economics Letters, 111*(2), 161–165.
Duncan, G. (2005). What do we mean by "happiness"? The relevance of subjective wellbeing to social policy. *Social Policy Journal of New Zealand, 25*, 16–31.
Duncan, G. (2010). Should happiness-maximization be the goal of government? *Journal of Happiness Studies, 11*(2), 163–178.
Durand, M. (2018). Countries' experiences with well-being and happiness metrics. Global Happiness. In J. Sachs, R. Layard, & J. F. Helliwell (Eds.), *Global happiness policy report 2018* (201–227). Sustainable Development Solutions Network.
Dutt, A. K., & Radcliff, B. (Eds.). (2009). *Happiness, economics and politics: Towards a multi-disciplinary approach*. Edward Elgar Publishing.
Easterlin, R. A., & Angelescu, L. (2009). Happiness and growth the world over: Time series evidence on the happiness-income paradox. *IZA discussion papers No. 4060*. Institute for the Study of Labor.
Easterlin, R. A. (1974). Does economic growth improve the human lot? Some empirical evidence. In P. A. David & M. W. Reder (Eds.), *Nations and households in economic growth* (pp. 89–125). Academic Press.
Easterlin, R. A. (2013). Happiness, growth, and public policy. *Economic Inquiry, 51*(1), 1–15.
Easterlin, R. A., McVey, L. A., Switek, M., Sawangfa, O., & Zweig, J. S. (2010). The happiness–income paradox revisited. *Proceedings of the National Academy of Sciences, 107*(52), 22463–22468.
Easterlin, R. A., & Sawangfa, O. (2009). Happiness and domain satisfaction: New directions for the economics of happiness. In A. K. Dutt & B. Radcliff (Eds.), *Happiness, economics and politics* (pp. 70–94). Edward Elgar Publishing.
Eiji, Y. (2009). The Influence of government size on economic growth and life satisfaction: A case study from Japan. Resource document. *Munich Personal RePEc Archive MPRA Paper No. 17879*. https://mpra.ub.uni-muenchen.de/18439/. Accessed May 2, 2020.
Eren, K. A., & Aşıcı, A. A. (2016). The determinants of happiness in Turkey: Evidence from city-level data. *Journal of Happiness Studies, 17*, 1–23.
Frank, R. H. (1999). *Luxury fever: Why money fails to satisfy in an era of excess*. Free Press.
Frawley, A. (2015). Happiness research: A review of critiques. *Sociology Compass, 9*(1), 62–77.
Frey, B. S. (2008). *Happiness: A revolution in economics*. MIT press.
Frey, B. S., Benz, M., & Stutzer, A. (2004). Introducing procedural utility: Not only what, but also how matters. *Journal of Institutional and Theoretical Economics (JITE)/Zeitschrift für die gesamte Staatswissenschaft, 160*(3), 377–401.
Frey, B. S., & Stutzer, A. (2012). The use of happiness research for public policy. *Social Choice and Welfare, 38*(4), 659–674.
Graham, C. (2011). *The pursuit of happiness: An economy of well-being*. Brookings Institution Press.
Graham, J., & Haidt, J. (2010). Beyond beliefs: Religions bind individuals into moral communities. *Personality and Social Psychology Review, 14*(1), 140–150.
Gulati, R., Mayo, A., & Nohria, N. (2017). *Management: An integrated approach*. Cengage Learning.

Halpern, D. (2010). *The hidden wealth of nations*. Polity.
Helliwell, J. F. (2006). Well-being, social capital and public policy: What's new? *The Economic Journal, 116*(510), C34–C45.
Helliwell, J. F., Layard, R., & Sachs, J. (Eds.). (2020). *World happiness report 2020*. Sustainable Development Solutions Network.
Helliwell, J. F., & Putnam, R. D. (2004). The social context of well-being. *Philosophical Transactions of the Royal Society of London Series B Biological Sciences, 359*(1449), 1435–1446.
Herzberg, F., Mauser, B., & Snyderman, B. (1959). *The motivation to work*. John Wiley & Sons.
Hirsch, F. (2005). *Social limits to growth*. Routledge.
Holden, M., & Phillips, R. (2010). Best research from the Community Indicators Consortium 2009: Introduction to the special issue. *Applied Research in Quality of Life, 5*(4), 261–272.
Inglehart, R., Foa, R., Peterson, C., & Welzel, C. (2008). Development, freedom, and rising happiness: A global perspective (1981–2007). *Perspectives on Psychological Science, 3*(4), 264–285.
Johns, H., & Ormerod, P. (2007). *Happiness, economics and public policy*. Institute of Economic Affairs.
Kacapyr, E. (2008). Cross-country determinants of satisfaction with life. *International Journal of Social Economics, 35*(6), 400–416.
Kahneman, D., & Deaton, A. (2010). High income improves evaluation of life but not emotional well-being. *Proceedings of the National Academy of Sciences, 107*(38), 16489–16493.
Kelly, A. (2012, December 1). Gross national happiness in Bhutan: The big idea from a tiny state that could change the world. *The Guardian*.
Kim, E. (2011). Local good governance: A research framework. *Journal of Korean Politics, 20*(2), 209–234. (Korean).
Kim, D. G. (2013). Study on policy direction of people's happiness enhancement of Park Geun-hye government at the level of regional development. *Korean Balanced Development Studies, 4*(2), 39–63. (Korean).
Kim, B., Kang, H., & Kim, H. (2015). A Study on the Moderating Effect of Quality of Life on the Relationship between Public Service Satisfaction and Citizens Happiness. *Korean Journal of Public Administration, 53*(3), 29–56. (Korean).
Kim. D. H. (2016). Developing a happiness measure and its application for Japanese localities. *Korean Policy Studies Review, 25*(3), 133–177. (Korean).
Kim, H. (2016). Exploring the influence of perceived income inequality on happiness: Focusing on the moderating effect of perceived upward social mobility. *Korean Policy Studies Review, 25*(2), 559–587. (Korean).
Kim, S., & Kim, D. (2012). Does government make people happy? Exploring new research directions for government's roles in happiness. *Journal of Happiness Studies, 13*(5), 875–899.
Koo, K., Lim, J., & Choi, S. (2017). *What makes us happy?* Seoul: Jipmoondang. (Korean).
Kroll, C. (2008). *Social capital and the happiness of nations: The importance of trust and networks for life satisfaction in a cross-national perspective*. Peter Lang.
Lane, R. E. (1994). Quality of life and quality of persons: A new role for government? *Political Theory, 22*(2), 219–252.
Lapinski, J. S., Riemann, C. R., Shapiro, R. Y., Stevens, M. F., & Jacobs, L. R. (1998). Welfare state regimes and subjective well-being: A cross-national study. *International Journal of Public Opinion Research, 10*(1), 2–24.
Large, J. (2010, April 22). The new pursuit of happiness. *The Seattle Times*.
Layard, P. R. G., & Layard, R. (2011). *Happiness: Lessons from a new science*. Penguin UK.
Layard, R. (1980). Human satisfactions and public policy. *The Economic Journal, 90*(360), 737–750.
Layard, R. (2005). *Happiness: Lessons from a new science*. Penguin Books/Penguin Group.
Layard, R. (2006). Happiness and public policy: A challenge to the profession. *The Economic Journal, 116*(510), C24–C33.

Lee, K. (2019). A study of the development and establishment of the history of public administration: Focusing on the Interrelationship between Public Administration Science, Public Administration Philosophy, and Humanism. *Korean Public Administration Review, 53*(3), 211–242. (Korean).
Luttmer, E. F. (2004). Neighbors as negatives: Relative earnings and well-being. *National Bureau of Economic Research*. https://doi.org/10.3386/w10667
Mizobuchi, H. (2017). Measuring socio-economic factors and sensitivity of happiness. *Journal of Happiness Studies, 18*(2), 463–504.
Musikanski, L. (2014). Happiness in public policy. *Journal of Social Change, 6*(1), 5.
Musikanski, L., & Polley, C. (2016). Life, liberty, and the pursuit of happiness: Measuring what matters. *Journal of Social Change, 8*(1), 5.
Nettle, D. (2006). *Happiness: The science behind your smile*. Oxford University Press.
Ng, Y. K., & Ho, L. S. (Eds.). (2006). *Happiness and public policy*. Palgrave Macmillan.
O'Donnell, G., Deaton, A., Durand, M., Halpern, D., & Layard, R. (2014). *Well-being and policy*. Legatum Institute.
OECD. (2013). *OECD guidelines on measuring subjective well-being*. OECD Publishing.
Oshio, T. (2017). Which is more relevant for perceived happiness, individual-level or area-level social capital? A multilevel mediation analysis. *Journal of Happiness Studies, 18*(3), 765–783.
Ott, J. (2005). Level and inequality of happiness in nations: Does greater happiness of a greater number imply greater inequality in happiness? *Journal of Happiness Studies, 6*(4), 397–420.
Ott, J. (2011). Government and happiness in 130 nations: Good governance fosters higher level and more equality of happiness. *Social Indicators Research, 102*(1), 3–22.
Ott, J. (2013). Greater happiness for a greater number: Some non-controversial options for governments. In A. Delle Fave (Ed.), *The Exploration of Happiness* (pp. 321–340). Springer.
Park, S. (2003). The concept and comparison method of quality of life. *Korean Policy Science Review, 7*(3), 57–80. (Korean).
Park, H. (2008). *Strategic planning for public organizations*. Goyang: Daeyoung Publishing. (Korean).
Pavot, W., & Diener, E. (1993). Review of the satisfaction with life scale. *Psychological Assessment, 5*(2), 164–172.
Pellerin, C. (2016, February 16). Constitutional considerations of happiness. *Columbia Undergraduate Law Review*.
Pfeiffer, D., & Cloutier, S. (2016). Planning for happy neighborhoods. *Journal of the American Planning Association, 82*(3), 267–279.
Porta, P. L., & Scazzieri, R. (2007). Public happiness and civil society. In L. Bruni & P. L. Porta (Eds.), *Handbook on the Economics of Happiness* (pp. 95–109). Edward Elgar Publishing.
Prycker, V. (2010). Happiness on the political agenda? Pros and Cons. *Journal of Happiness Studies, 11*(5), 585–603.
Pugno, M. (2009). The Easterlin paradox and the decline of social capital: An integrated explanation. *The Journal of Socio-Economics, 38*(4), 590–600.
Radcliff, B. (2001). Politics, markets, and life satisfaction: *The political economy of human happiness. American Political Science Review, 95*(4), 939–952.
Ram, R. (2010). Social capital and happiness: Additional cross-country evidence. *Journal of Happiness Studies, 11*(4), 409–418.
Raz, J. (1994). *Ethics in the public domain: Essays in the morality of law and politics*. Oxford University Press.
Rodrik, D. (1999). Where did all the growth go? External shocks, social conflict, and growth collapses. *Journal of Economic Growth, 4*(4), 385–412.
Sacks, D. W., Stevenson, B., & Wolfers, J. (2010). Subjective well-being, income, economic development and growth. *National Bureau of Economic Research*. https://doi.org/10.3386/w16441
Sacks, D. W., Stevenson, B., & Wolfers, J. (2012). The new stylized facts about income and subjective well-being. *Emotion, 12*(6), 1181.

Salichs, M. A., & Malfaz, M. (2006). Using emotions on autonomous agents. the role of happiness, sadness and fear. *Integrative Approaches to Machine Consciousness, Part of AISB, 6*, 157–164.

Schumacher, E. F. (1973). *Small is beautiful: Economics as if people really mattered*. Blond and Briggs.

Scitovsky, T. (1976). *The joyless economy: An inquiry into human satisfaction and consumer dissatisfaction*. Oxford University Press.

Seligman, M. E. P. (2002). *Authentic happiness: Using the new positive psychology to realize your potential for lasting fulfillment*. Free Press.

Sen, A. (1999). *Development as freedom*. Anchor Books.

Sheldon, K. M., & Houser-Marko, L. (2001). Self-concordance, goal attainment, and the pursuit of happiness: Can there be an upward spiral? *Journal of Personality and Social Psychology, 80*(1), 152–165.

Shin, S. (2015). The analysis on the determinants of happiness in Korea. *Kookmin Social Science Review 41*(2), 183–208. (Korean).

Stevenson, B., & Wolfers, J. (2008). Economic growth and subjective well-being: Reassessing the Easterlin paradox. *National Bureau of Economic Research*. https://doi.org/10.3386/w14282

Stiglitz, J. E., Sen, A., & Fitoussi, J. P. (2009a). Report by the commission on the measurement of economic performance and social progress. Resource document. Commission on the Measurement of Economic Performance and Social Progress. http://www.stiglitzsen-fitoussi.fr/documents/rapport_anglais.pdf. Accessed June 15, 2020.

Stiglitz, J., Sen, A., & Fitoussi, J. P. (2009b). The measurement of economic performance and social progress revisited. Reflections and overview. Resource document. Commission on the Measurement of Economic Performance and Social Progress. https://hal-sciencespo.archives-ouvertes.fr/hal-01069384/document. Accessed June 15, 2020.

Stiglitz, J. E., Sen, A., & Fitoussi, J. P. (2010). *Mismeasuring our lives: Why GDP doesn't add up*. The New Press.

Sugden, R., & Teng, J. C. Y. (2016). Is happiness a matter for governments? In S. Bartolini, E. Bilancini, L. Bruni, & P. L. Porta (Eds.), *Policies for happiness* (pp. 36–57). Oxford University Press.

Thin, N. (2012). *Social happiness: Theory into policy and practice*. Policy Press.

United Nations General Assembly. (2011). Happiness: Towards a holistic approach to development (Resolution 65/309). 64th session: 109th plenary meeting. http://www.un.org/ga/search/view_doc.asp?symbol=A/RES/65/309. Accessed May 25, 2012.

United Kingdom Office for National Statistics. (2012). https://www.ons.gov.uk/. Accessed June 15, 2015.

Veenhoven, R. (2004a). Happiness as an aim in public policy: The greatest happiness principle. In P. A. Linley & S. Joseph (Eds.), *Positive psychology in practice* (pp. 658–678). Wiley.

Veenhoven, R. (2004b). Happy life years: A measure of gross national happiness. In K. Ura, & K. Galay (Eds.), *Gross national happiness and development, Proceedings of the First International Seminar on Operationalization of Gross National Happiness* (pp. 287–318). Thimphu: Centre for Bhutan Studies.

Veenhoven, R. (2005). Inequality of happiness in nations. *Journal of Happiness Studies, 6*(4), 351–355.

Veenhoven, R. (2010). Greater happiness for a greater number. *Journal of Happiness Studies, 11*(5), 605–629.

Weimann, J., Knabe, A., & Schöb, R. (2015). *Measuring happiness: The economics of well-being*. MIT press.

Welsch, H. (2009). Implications of happiness research for environmental economics. *Ecological Economics, 68*(11), 2735–2742.

Woo, C. (2013). Possibilities and Limitations of Public Policies in the Pursuit of Happiness. *Korean Journal of Public Administration, 51*(2), 283–318. (Korean).

Woo, C. (2014a). Exploring an alternative approach to the global development: Theoretical foundation and policy implications of happiness approach in the context of global development. *Korean Society and Public Administration, 24*(4), 411–434. (Korean).

Woo, C. (2014b). The effect of good governance on happiness of the people: Does technical quality precedes democracy? *Korean Journal of Public Administration, 52*(1), 219–246. (Korean).

Yoon, I., & Kim, S. (2008). The impact of socioeconomic status and subjective class identification on life satisfaction-with a focus on mediating effects of high-class leisure activity. *Journal of the Korean Urban Management Association, 21*(2), 153–185. (Korean).

Zak, P. J., & Knack, S. (2001). Trust and growth. *The Economic Journal, 111*(470), 295–321.

Zamagni, S. (2014). Public happiness in today's economics. *International Review of Economics, 61*(2), 191–196.

Zorondo-Rodríguez, F., Gómez-Baggethun, E., Demps, K., Ariza-Montobbio, P., García, C., & Reyes-García, V. (2014). What defines quality of life? The gap between public policies and locally defined indicators among residents of Kodagu, Karnataka (India). *Social Indicators Research, 115*(1), 441–456.

Chapter 4
Measurement of Public Happiness

1 Significance of Measurement

Measurement of happiness is important for the progress of happiness research or the implementation of happiness policies. This is because scientific discussion of happiness research is difficult without measuring happiness. But measuring happiness is not easy. This is because the concept of happiness is multifaceted and has subjective properties. Nevertheless, measuring happiness is not impossible. Anand (2016: viii) is one of the researchers who believe that happiness can be measured. In response to some criticism that happiness is neither empirical nor measurable, he asserts that factors for happiness exist in a certain pattern:

> (W)e have been interested in measuring human flourishing and using the resulting data to understand how wellbeing is produced and distributed. The field attracts its fair share of work on the technicalities of index design and our own research has included some such activity but here I want to focus on some more basic but equally important issues, namely what are the dimensions in which human wellbeing resides, what are the drivers or causes of wellbeing, and how do all of these change over the human life course? There have been those who thought that science should focus on things that are 'hard' and measurable and that happiness was neither, but the perspective no longer feels like the majority view it might once have been. At a population level, there are clearly some common patterns that tell us about the kinds of things that help life go well (or otherwise).

If, as Anand argues, there is a certain pattern related to happiness, it raises expectations for measuring happiness. In fact, many researchers have attempted to measure happiness in this light and, as a result, have accumulated substantial results. The main method applied to the measurement of happiness is based on individual self-assessment, and at center-stage is a survey targeting a large number of individuals. Other methods are also used. For example, experience-sampling methodology (ESM) is used to measure an individual's objective happiness in real time. The Day Reconstruction Method (DRM) is used to measure the holistic view of the respondents' experience through diary records. It is also possible to indirectly measure the happiness of a target individual through the evaluation of those who have close interactions with the target individual, such as family members, neighbors, and friends. Clinical

S. J. Lee, *Public Happiness*, Community Quality-of-Life and Well-Being,
https://doi.org/10.1007/978-3-030-89643-0_4

interviews, record content analysis, and so on are also available options (Ludwigs, 2018: 8; Pavot & Diener, 2013). Nevertheless, the method based on the response of the respondents in terms of frequency of use is overwhelming. The reason why the questioning method is so highly employed is that it is very difficult to draw implications about psychological states like happiness from overt behavior. Therefore, most evaluation of psychological states rely on questionnaires. Of course, these self-reports have issues of validity and reliability.

A survey or interview is basically a question-based measurement method, and Veenhoven (1991a, b) summarizes the limitations and possibilities of such methods as follows. First, there is an issue of whether happiness can be measured through external observation. Basically, it is difficult to objectively measure life satisfaction through observations of overt behavior. Like other attitudes, happiness is only partially reflected in social behaviors. Not only happy people but also unfortunate people act as active, outgoing, or friendly. In fact, the correlation between external evaluation of happiness and one's own evaluation is not high. It should be recognized that even the causes of suicide are reported to have cultural and personal variation.

Second, there is an issue of whether people can measure their thoughts through questions. If it is difficult to evaluate happiness through external observation of behavior and questions through interviews or surveys are an alternative. However, there is a lot of skepticism about the validity of self-assessment for happiness. First of all, there is a criticism that responses to questions reflect other factors because people do not have opinions or interests about their satisfaction in life. In fact, some people do not have specific opinions about happiness, so they are significantly affected by situational factors. Even those who have a definite opinion on happiness may also have a global opinion on happiness, so the specific response value for a subdivided scale may change. There may also be uncertainty in reproducing opinions about happiness. But those concerns should not be exaggerated. According to several surveys, most people actively think about life satisfaction, and thus, the answer to the question of happiness is prompt, stable, and no-response is low. On the other hand, there are criticisms that respondents tend to exaggerate their happiness due to the ego-defensive or social desirability effect. However, the evidence to support such criticism is uncertain. Although there is evidence that responses to questions about happiness are related to various situational influences such as interview location, interviewee, weather, and mood, such situational influences are random errors that disappear by repeated measurements. As other contextual factors, the influence of wording of questions, answer formats, sequence of questions, context of the interview, etc. induces more systematic errors, but not enough to nullify the efforts to measure happiness.

Fortunately, the response to happiness is found to be quite stable. For example, Cummins (2018: 12) in claiming homeostasis of happiness observes that happiness or subjective wellbeing shows a normal distribution between about 70–90 points on the 0–100-point scale based on the results of existing studies.[1] The specific results he presented are follows: Hartman's (1934, recited from Cummins, 2018) study shows

[1] He regards subjective wellbeing as emotion-stripping mood happiness and sees such happiness as maintaining homeostasis around set points.

the reliability of the test–retest of happiness measurement was 0.7. When Cummins (2018: 18) reviewed the results of 16 population surveys on happiness, the average score was 75 points and the standard deviation was 2.5. The results of 31 surveys conducted by the Australian Unity Wellbeing Index project until 2014 reported that the average score was 75.3 and the standard deviation was 0.72 (Cummins, 2018: 19). Anglim et al. (2015) in their measurements of happiness reported that the average score was 75 points, the standard deviation was 6.60, and the test–retest reliability was 0.76.

As such not only has research shown that the questioning method has considerable stability, but also in situations where it is difficult to find a viable alternative to the questioning method, surveys and interviews are being used as practical tools for measuring happiness. Among the two, surveys occupy the position of a more important measurement tool as a method for targeting an anonymous majority at low cost, compared to interviews where the scope of the target is relatively limited due to the cost and constraints of the implementation environment. In this context, national surveys conducted in various countries become an important basis for happiness research and policy development through the measurement and collection of extensive data on happiness.

Considering the property that happiness is basically a self-assessment of individuals' lives, despite some limitations, the questioning method for respondents is not only necessary but also reasonable as a key instrument for measuring happiness. In fact, despite the advantage of objectivity, the measurement based on observations of respondents' behaviors may be biased in the process of external observers evaluating respondents from an omniscient point of view. Nevertheless, there still remain problems with the questioning method. Because of the ambiguity or multidimensionality of the concept of happiness, there is a lack of consensus on what specific questions are appropriate to ask. Also, confusion arises in questions when mixing wellbeing and happiness or measuring both the condition of happiness and happiness per se. As a result, a wide variety of measurement tools are mixed in question content and scale. This is why continuous research and supplementation are needed in using the question method for measuring happiness in the future (Cummins, 2018: 22).

Meanwhile, many measurement tools not only ask subjective questions but also include objective indicators in the survey at the same time. Basically, the objects to be measured are the same, so the results of both must match. However, measurement errors are inevitable, and it is difficult for both to be identical. Also, the relationship between the two is not uniform. It is not only difficult to secure validity due to the data collection limit of objective indicators, but also because, as Veenhoven (1991a, b) pointed out, there is inherent uncertainty in the external expression of respondents' opinions in subjective indicators. Therefore, rather than resolving the disagreement between the two, it is necessary to make efforts to improve the indicator system while paying attention to the advantages and limitations of each indicator. In this regard, it is also necessary to pay attention to intersubjective indicators, especially those that can complement subjective indicators, as described later.

2 Happiness Research

2.1 *Major Surveys*

As happiness is reappearing as an important development goal, there is heightened academic and practical interest in happiness, but it is still in its early stages and remains in the stage of developing happiness measurement indicators rather than the development of practical policies. Measurement of happiness is often done through various social surveys or calculating a happiness index. Exemplary social surveys related to happiness include the following: The Better Life Index of OECD, the Human Development Index of UNDP (United Nations Development Program), the wellbeing section in the Gallup World Poll, the World Value Survey of World Value Survey Association, and the Gross National Happiness Survey of Bhutan, etc. For reference, Table 1 briefly summarizes the basic composition and indicators of relatively well-known surveys including these.

2.2 *Evaluation of Current Measures*

We briefly introduced some of the well-known happiness-related measurement surveys. Overall, most surveys are comprehensive, complex, and tend to mix subjective and objective indicators. Here, with the questionnaires in mind, the composition of the indicators is discussed.

Inclusiveness of Measures

Despite the fact that the recent widespread survey of happiness is due to an upsurge of new interest in happiness, it is difficult to find a survey focusing on happiness. Most surveys list indicators of happiness and related factors (influencing and resultant) together in a metric dashboard (Global Council for Happiness and Wellbeing, 2019: 11). For example, the OECD (2013) includes quality of life and material conditions under the wellbeing domain, and includes happiness (subjective wellbeing) as a lower domain of quality of life. Such categorization has limitations. Such an approach has the problem of hindering the original umbrella role of happiness by treating happiness not as a central concept associated with the good life but as one of several sub-elements associated with the good life. This does not correctly reflect the recent growing demand for happiness and is an incorrect measurement rather than just measurement bias. A survey that does not put happiness at the center, whatever its name, actually has the character of a general survey on the "good life" in general. The good life is not a new concept. Several social welfare-related surveys in the past have been conducted with the good life in mind. That is, while the vast majority of current happiness-related surveys conceptually include happiness, the actual surveys are not significantly different from previous welfare surveys. Welfare surveys existed long before the start of happiness research, and if they are the same, there is no reason to

Table 1 Exemplary surveys related to happiness: structure and measures

Name	Measure types	Domain/indicators	Number of indicators	Components of happiness	Presentations	Data sources
World values survey (WVS)	Subjective	11 (happiness, health, control over life, life satisfaction, financial situation, food, safety, medical aid, income, shelter, standard of living)	Multi-indicators	Experience, evaluation	Listing	Survey
Human development index (UNDP)	Objective	3 (long and health life, knowledge, a decent standard of living)	**Multi-indicators**	–	**Summary index**	Hard data
Gallup world poll (GWP)	Subjective	13 (anger, sadness, stress, worry, enjoyment, learning, life evaluation, life past, life today, negative experience, positive experience, smile or laugh, respectful treatment)	**Multi-indicators**	**Experience, evaluation, eudaimonia**	**Listing**	Survey
WHOQOL (WHO)	Subjective	7 (physical, psychological, independence, social relations, environment, religious/personal beliefs, overall quality of life)	**Multidomains and multi-indicators**	**Experience, evaluation, Eudaimonia**	**Listing**	Average of individual responses and national level measures

(continued)

Table 1 (continued)

Name	Measure types	Domain/indicators	Number of indicators	Components of happiness	Presentations	Data sources
Better life index (OECD)	Mixed	11 (income and wealth, job and wage, housing, work–life balance, health status, education and capacity, social relations, citizen participation and governance, quality of environment, personal safety, subjective wellbeing)	**Multidomains and multi-indicators**	**Evaluation**	**Summary index**	Average of individual responses and national level measures
Happy planet index (HPI)	Mixed	4 (life expectancy, experienced wellbeing, inequality of outcomes, ecological footprint)	**Multi-indicators**	**Experience, evaluation**	**Summary index**	Average of individual responses and national level measures
World happiness index (UN)	Mixed	7 (happiness, GDP per capita, social support, healthy life expectancy, freedom to life choices, generosity, corruption)	**Multidomains and multi-indicators**	**Experience, evaluation**	**Representative index**	Average of individual responses and national level measures

(continued)

Table 1 (continued)

Name	Measure types	Domain/indicators	Number of indicators	Components of happiness	Presentations	Data sources
Canadian indicators of Wellbeing[a] (Canada)	Mixed	8 (living conditions, health, sustainable environment, viable community, education, work–life balance, democratic participation, leisure and cultural activity)	**Multidomains and multi-indicators**	**Evaluation**	**Summary index**	Average of individual responses and national level measures
New wealth indicators France)	Mixed	10 (employment rate, research effort, debt, life Expectancy, life satisfaction, income inequality, poverty, early exit from school, carbon footprint, soil artificialization)	**Multidomains and multi-indicators**	**Evaluation**	**Listing**	Average of individual responses and national level measures
Indicators of children's wellbeing (US)	Mixed	7 (family and social, Economic, health care, physical environment, behavior, education, health)	**Multidomains and multi-indicators**	**Experience**	**Listing**	Average of individual responses and national level measures

(continued)

Table 1 (continued)

Name	Measure types	Domain/indicators	Number of indicators	Components of happiness	Presentations	Data sources
Measuring national wellbeing (UK)	Mixed	10 (personal wellbeing, relationships, health, daily life living conditions, financial conditions, economy, education and skills, governance, environment)	**Multidomains and multi-indicators**	**Experience, evaluation, eudaimonia**	**Listing**	Average of individual responses and national level measures
Measuring Australia's progress [a] (Australia)	Mixed	4 society, economy, environment, governance)	**Multidomains and multi-indicators**	[b]	**Representative index**	Average of individual responses and national level measures
Gross national happiness (Bhutan)	Mixed	9 emotional wellbeing, health, time use, education, cultural diversity and resilience, good governance, vital community, ecological diversity and resilience, quality of life)	**Multidomains and multi-indicators**	**Experience, evaluation,**	**Summary index**	Average of individual responses and national level measures
Wellbeing indicators (Japan)	Mixed	5 (subjective wellbeing, socioeconomic conditions, health, relatedness, sustainability)	**Multidomains and multi-indicators**	**Experience**	**Listing**	Average of individual responses and national level measures

(continued)

Table 1 (continued)

Name	Measure types	Domain/indicators	Number of indicators	Components of happiness	Presentations	Data sources
Wellbeing in Germany Index (Germany)	Mixed	12 (health, work, education, time, income, security, areas, family and society, economy, nature, law, global responsibility)	**Multidomains and multi-indicators**	**Evaluation**	**Listing**	Average of individual responses and national level measures
Life Quality Indicators (Spain)	Mixed	9 (material conditions, work, health, education, social relation, security, governance, environment, subjective sell-being)	**Multidomains and multi-indicators**	**Evaluation**	**Representative index**	Average of individual responses and national level measures
Community Wellbeing index (Korea)	Subjective/intersubjective	6 (human development, economy, environment, infra, social, governance) and happiness	**Multidomains and multi-indicators**	**Experience, evaluation, Eudaimonia**	**Summary index**	Survey

[a]There is no usable data for some indicators
[b]No indicator for subjective wellbeing (happiness)

add more surveys under the name of happiness research. This will only create more confusion by introducing a new word.

Various surveys list many indicators for a good life in an all-inclusive manner for economic reasons to measure not only happiness but also various related factors through one survey, but also because interest in happiness policy is not yet firm and an integrated understanding of the concept of happiness has not been established. Of course, these all-inclusive indicator systems are not completely wrong. Initially, it may be desirable to save financial resources to include not only happiness but also several factors related to happiness in one survey. In addition, it may have the benefit of leading to discoveries of trade-offs and synergies across each indicator domain, and it may be advantageous for the division of roles and evaluations among public agencies per domain (Global Council for Happiness and Wellbeing, 2019: 11).

Nonetheless, an all-inclusive measurement system that combines happiness and related factors into the sub-factors of quality of life or good life without a clear purpose, neglects the uniqueness and usefulness of happiness variables. It interferes with helping to promote a consistent happiness policy by dispersing interest in happiness factors or treating them as secondary factors, not to mention the aforementioned possibility of confusion between happiness research and other similar research of quality of life, wellbeing, progress, etc. In order to alleviate such a problem, it is necessary to conduct a survey with a clear emphasis on happiness by which various analyses on the relationship between happiness and related factors can be performed. In this regard, for example, the approach of Ludwigs (2018) seems fair. He clearly mentions that in the introduction his research is about subjective wellbeing among various wellbeing concepts like wellbeing, objective wellbeing, and subjective wellbeing and suggests appropriate measurement tools for subjective wellbeing.

Diversity of Measurement Indicators

Various indicators and methods for measuring happiness have been developed and applied, and there is not an agreement among nations to use a single indicator like GDP in measuring economic performance, or a set of indicators like Sustainable Development Goals (SDGs) indicators proposed by the United Nations (Iriarte & Musikanski, 2019). In the current situation wherein various indicator systems are mixed, it is difficult to carry out not only comparative research but a stable policy because consistent information on the state of happiness cannot be provided. Thus, although the study of happiness is abundant on the outside, there is a concern that it will remain in a poor state in practice.

As aforementioned, most surveys measure not only happiness but also various factors related to wellbeing, so they include indicators in various areas. As shown in Table 1, the number of measurement domains varies from 3 to 12 depending on the survey. This may be natural because wellbeing is a complex concept including various factors. But this increase in the measurement area is also due to the inclusion of factors related to the good life in the measurement items rather than focusing on happiness and related factors. On the other hand, most surveys apply multiple indicators by domain to increase the validity of measurements, thus taking the form of multidomains and multi-indicators. A problem is that the composition of measurement indicators becomes more complex and numerous, which not only reduces the possibility of integrating indicators and increases the cost of collecting indicators, but also increases the burden on respondents, thereby reducing the expectation of policy utilization of measurement results.

Mixing of Subjective and Objective Indicators

Most surveys apply objective and subjective indicators in parallel in measuring the factors related to a good life (Table 2). In other words, it is simultaneously collecting statistical data on objective conditions and conducting a survey on subjective emotions and evaluation. Thus, the Human Development Index using only objective indicators or the WHOQOL or World Value Survey using only subjective indicators are the exception. It is interesting to look at when these indicators were first developed. HDI, WHOQOL, and World Value Survey (1981) developed in 1990, 1994, and 1981 respectively, precede most wellbeing surveys including the Better Life Index (2011) of the OECD and World Happiness Index (2012) of the United Nations. We can see here that relatively later developed indicators are more comprehensive. This phenomenon can be interpreted as a result of the more widespread interest in happiness or wellbeing in the 2000s, and the increased discussions of happiness and wellbeing-related factors, which has changed in a more complex way. This is because the increase in complexity causes problems such as an increase in cost, difficulty in comparative analysis of measurement results, and restrictions on the application of policies, despite the possibility of improving measurement validity as an effort to develop indicators.

For objective indicators, various indicators in the physical, economic, social, environmental, and political fields are used as a whole. The indicators that are particularly emphasized in various surveys include health and life expectancy (physical domain), income and economic status (economic domain), education level and safety (social domain), democratization, political rights, individual freedom, and government capacity (political domain), etc. Recently, more environmental and ecological conditions have been included. The application of objective indicators is basically

Table 2 Thin (2012)'s framework for analyzing happiness

	Hedonic tone: good versus bad feelings	Life evaluation: satisfaction versus disappointments	Existential interpretation: meaning making versus doubt and alienation
Future (anticipation)	Optimism versus fear	High versus low expectations	Life story imagined as coherent/purposeful or not
Present (current experience)	Enjoyment versus suffering	Belief that current life is good/bad	Sense of current fulfilment or purpose
Past (memory and synthesis)	Happy versus unhappy memories	Degree of satisfaction with achievements	Making sense of the past or not

under the implicit assumption that happiness will be high if these factors are in good condition. Therefore, objective conditions have the characteristics of factors that influence happiness. However, data collection on objective indicators does not necessarily take place in relation to happiness. In addition, these objective indicators are composed of indicators that can be measured in a specific and familiar way about life conditions and have the advantage of being quantified, enabling verification and comparative analysis. However, there is a problem that, along with the limitations of data collection, the measurement of material conditions alone is not enough to accurately understand the quality of life (Cummins, 2018: 3).

With the exception of the UNDP (1990)'s Human Development Index (HDI), which focuses entirely on objective indicators such as life expectancy, literacy, and national income, objective indicators are generally applied together with subjective indicators. Subjective indicators are also not without problems. This is because subjective indicators have limitations in reliability due to individual subjective evaluations of respondents, despite the advantage that more comprehensive data can be obtained compared to objective indicators. Basically, objective indicators and subjective indicators both have possibilities and limitations, respectively. In this regard, attention should be paid to the "intersubjective indicators" to be introduced later as an additional supplementary effort along with efforts to improve both indicators.

Subjective indicators related to happiness generally include three factors: positive or negative emotions of an individual, satisfaction with life, and evaluation of the meaning of life. These broadly encompass the elements presented by two approaches to happiness, the hedonic and eudaimonic approach. The hedonistic approach sees happiness as including both positive and negative affects and life satisfaction. These elements were suggested by Diener (1984), who has contributed to the scientification of happiness research by overcoming the conceptual ambiguity of happiness by introducing the concept of subjective wellbeing. Since then, many surveys centered on psychology have followed this method (Koo et al., 2015: 19). Individuals' affect is measured by dividing affect into positive affect and negative affect, and the evaluation of an individual's emotion is based on the gap between the two factors. The measurement of life satisfaction includes a method of asking overall satisfaction for life as a whole and a method of asking satisfaction for each specific life domain (domain satisfaction). The domains of each domain satisfaction overlap with the domains (components) of the objective indicator, but there is a difference in that it obtains information from individuals' subjective responses. For example, in terms of "income" of economic conditions, measuring the actual income level becomes an objective condition indicator for the income domain, and measuring satisfaction with the income level becomes a subjective satisfaction index for the income domain. In this regard, some scholars have suggested that objective conditions and subjective measurement results are quite consistent (Pfeiffer & Cloutier, 2016).

Surveys not only include hedonistic components such as affects (positive and negative) and life satisfaction, but also eudaimonic components centered on the meaning and values of life. Eudaimonia is an ancient Greek concept in which humans achieve happiness through experiences such as life purpose, challenges, and growth, and flourishing is commonly used as an English expression for this (National Research

Council, 2013). Purpose, meaning or values of life, social relationship, engagement, caring others, competence, self-appraisal, social trust, religiosity or spirituality, optimism about future, respectful life, and accomplishment are frequently used as indicators for measuring this (Diener & Biswas-Diener, 2008: 240; Huppert et al., 2013).

Specifically, which factors of happiness are included in the measurement items vary depending on the survey. For example, in Table 2, the WHO's WHOQOL and the UK's MNWs include experience (affect), evaluation, and eudaimonic measures, while other surveys do not include eudaimonic components. For hedonic components, WHI and GNH include experience (affect) and life evaluation together, but other surveys include only a few of them as indicators. Even when subjective indicators are included, some indicators of subjective wellbeing (happiness, life satisfaction, etc.) are not included, as in the case of Australian MAP. Overall, hedonistic components are included in the index at least partially, whereas the index for eudaimonic components is included in the survey almost only as an exception. The reason for this is that the development of indicators for eudaimonic aspects is relatively delayed, in addition to the tendency to understand happiness as subjective wellbeing, as presented by Diener. However, from an integrated perspective that sees happiness as including both hedonistic and eudaimonic components, including only hedonistic components in a question has limitations as a partial measurement to happiness. Fortunately, in recent years, there is a growing tendency to include three factors in the indicator from an integrated perspective (Diener & Biswas-Diener, 2008; National Research Council, 2013).

3 Measurement Strategies

3.1 Establishing the Direction of Happiness Measurement

In surveys related to the good life, two complementary perceptions are needed. First, it is necessary to increase the number of surveys conducted with measuring happiness as the survey objective. In other words, there should be more surveys that approach happiness as a central concept. Considering that the reason for the emphasis on happiness in the twenty-first century is the increased interest in happiness, which has been neglected in policy goals, future surveys on the good life will go beyond the conventional welfare-related research that focused on objective life conditions. Nevertheless, as mentioned earlier, most current surveys show little distinction from conventional welfare-focused surveys by presenting happiness in an expanded inventory format along with various related factors of a good life without a clear focus on happiness. The problem is that, despite the possibility of providing measurement results for various factors, the survey method that treats happiness as a peripheral factor has limitations in terms of grasping the concept of a good life and of helping to implement a happiness policy, due to the limitations of happiness-related questions and the lack of prior consideration of the relationship between happiness and related factors. On the other hand, a survey focused on measuring happiness is expected to contribute more to understanding happiness and the establishment of more effective happiness policies by enabling more diverse questions to be employed and more dynamic hypothesis testing on the relationship between happiness and related factors.

Second, in the survey design, a conceptual distinction between happiness and conditions of happiness should be made (Feldman, 2010: 9). Most of the current surveys present both happiness and happiness conditions, causing confusion. Of course, it does not mean that happiness and happiness-related factors must be presented separately on the questionnaire, or that only the question of happiness itself should be included in the questionnaire while removing the happiness-related factors. In fact, it is not necessary to inform respondents of the structure of the questionnaire. However, in designing the survey questionnaires, the survey designer should have prior recognition of the distinction between happiness and happiness conditions, and the hypothetical relationship between happiness and related factors, and reflect this in the survey design. Enumerating various questions related to a good life without serious prior consideration of the structure of the question is not desirable since it limits the systematic nature of the analysis or the utilization of the results.

3.2 Measurement Models of Happiness

In order to measure happiness, a model for measuring happiness must first be established. Assuming that the components of happiness include hedonistic components (affect and life evaluation) and eudaimonic components, it is desirable to adopt an integrated approach that includes all the factors suggested by both perspectives as a measurement model for happiness. This is because there is a limit to grasping the complex reality of happiness by a partial approach, and even when an integrated model is adopted as a basis, the range of measurement factors can be adjusted according to needs and conditions.

As a model for measuring happiness suggested from an integrated perspective, the survey guideline proposed by the OECD (2013: 29) is well known. The OECD emphasized that the characteristics and scope of the concept should be clarified before measuring happiness (subjective wellbeing) and synthesized the existing discussions and suggested three measures of happiness: affect, life evaluation, and eudaimonia. Affect is defined as the momentary emotion and feeling of experiencing an event at a specific point in time. It is expressed as a positive or negative feeling. Life evaluation is defined as a reflective, cognitive assessment on a person's life as a whole or a part of it, and is determined based on an individual's overall judgment rather than a momentary emotional state.

On the other hand, eudaimonia is a concept that focuses on individual capability as much as the ultimate goal of life and includes autonomy or meaning and purpose (OECD, 2013). In addition, the OECD proposes 6 modules such as ① overall happiness and life satisfaction, ② life evolution, ③ affects, ④ eudaimonia, ⑤ domain evaluations, and ⑥ experience for practical application. Ludwigs (2018: 8) confirms its standard character by referring to the OECD guideline as a golden standard for measuring subjective wellbeing.

Thin (2012: 36) proposes a more sophisticated happiness measurement model by overlaying the three elements of happiness with the time points of future, present, and past (Table 2). In the table, the three components of happiness correspond to existing happiness factors. Such a model can be said to be a step forward considering that most surveys, including the OECD guideline presented above, did not pay special attention to time dimensions. By applying such a measurement model, it is possible to hold more in-depth information on the dynamic changes between happiness and conditions of happiness, which is expected to contribute more to the promotion of effective happiness policies along with the progress of happiness research.

As previously discussed, a measure of happiness based on an integrated perspective is not just about happiness but includes measurements of objective conditions (impact factors or outcomes) related to happiness. This is because it is possible to capture the correlation between the two by measuring conditions related to happiness along with happiness, and based on this, it will be possible to implement policies for the promotion of happiness or to measure the social effects of happiness. As long as happiness is in a causal relationship with external conditions, measuring only the state of happiness irrespective of such objective conditions is reducing the meaning by half. In view of this need, an integrated measurement model that encompasses the conditions of happiness and happiness in relation to a good life is presented in

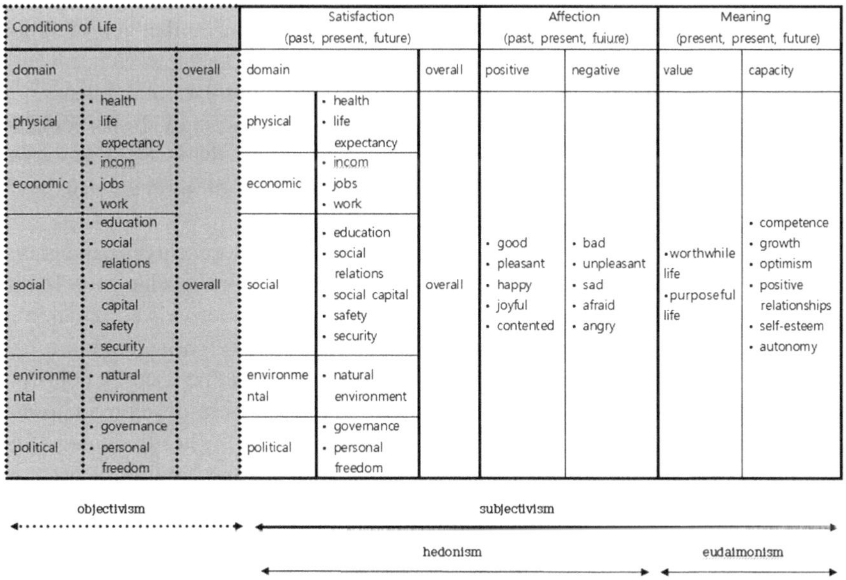

Fig. 1 Integrated measurement model of happiness and condition

Fig. 1.[2] Satisfaction, affection, and meaning are the components of happiness, and the measurement of happiness targets these three areas. Measurements in these areas basically employ subjective indicators based on respondents' evaluations. Satisfaction and affection are areas corresponding to the hedonistic approach, and meaning corresponds to the eudaimonic approach. The indicators of each domain can be subdivided in the temporal dimension of the past, present, and future. As an objective factor that affects or is affected by happiness, the conditions of life or quality of life can be approached from a holistic point of view or from a domain level such as physical, economic, social, environmental, and political domains. These measurements may be approached based on objective data but may also be measured based on the respondent's subjective assessment of life conditions. That is, the measurement method for life conditions is not fixed, and objective and subjective indicators can be used alone or in combination. In the table, the measurement areas of condition of life and satisfaction are marked equally to indicate this.

Regarding the establishment of a measurement model for happiness, one thing to keep in mind is that there will be a limit to the application of uniform indicators because there are cultural differences between countries and regions. Therefore, it is necessary to develop and apply indicators in consideration of cultural differences. Of course, if a certain measurement model aims to be applied only in the region, it will not be appropriate to point out cultural differences. However, if any measurement model is applied across the region, it is necessary to consider cultural differences. Regarding the problem of cultural differences in measurement, Cummins (2018: 32–38) stated that there are differences in language interpretation of respondents in subjective wellbeing surveys, differences in factors affecting happiness, and systematic differences in respondents' self-expression methods. It is emphasized that consideration of cultural differences is necessary because they will exist. Despite such needs, it is problematic that indicators are developed and applied with universal application in mind rather than paying attention to cultural differences until now. In particular, a more cautious approach is needed to compare and measure the level of happiness of each country in cross-sectional data based on the result of applying a uniform indicator system without considering cultural differences.

There may be two ways to supplement this. One is the development of an integrated model that reflects cultural differences while maintaining universal elements. To this end, while appropriately modifying the measurement items, it will be possible to give flexibility to appropriately adjust the index items or weight according to the region. For example, the Better Life Index allows margins to be used by adjusting the weights of measurement items by country. The other is to develop additional measurement models suitable for specific cultures. That is, instead of integrating the models, establishing a new alternative model and analyzing differences between multiple measurement models to enhance the adequacy of each model. In any case, cross-cultural communication between Western and non-Western regions along with the spread of interest in non-Western regions is essential. The current situation is due to the fact that major measurement models were developed in the West and inevitably became more suitable for Western culture.

[2] The preparation of this graph was assisted by Lee Yeon-kyung.

The integrated measurement model for happiness and related factors presented here is for the measurement domain and is not intended to limit the measurement method. Of course, surveys and interviews are generally used to measure subjective happiness, and to measure objective conditions, much effort to collect statistical data along with surveys are exerted. But these are not all of the application methods. In this regard, Thin (2012: 104) indicated that relying excessively on surveys based on standardized questions as in the present is problematic, and more humane, holistic, interesting, participatory, cheap, and simple social learning methods (such as story-telling, focus groups, role-play, appreciative enquiry) need more attention. As he suggested, in measuring happiness in the future, it would be desirable to adopt more diverse alternative methods depending on the purpose. However, there will be a limit to the practical application of such criticism. This is because the establishment of a happiness policy requires national attention and effort, and for this purpose, a method such as a survey targeting the majority can be more economical and more effective in arousing policy interest.

3.3 Conciseness of Indicators

Currently, many surveys have too many areas to measure or too many indicators, which increases the measurement cost as well as lowering the reliability of the measurement results, hindering the intuitive understanding of measurement results and policy utilization. In addition, complex or excessive indicators will inevitably cause a problem of mass-producing data that will not be consumed. Thin (2012: 102) referred to this problem as the data grave yard problem and proposed to limit unnecessary surveys and make them as concise and economical as possible. Surveys based on concise indicators will have an expected effect of not only controlling the mass production of unnecessary data, but also increasing the efficiency and reliability of surveys and increasing the policy utilization of measurement results.

A good example of a concise indicator is the GDP, a representative economic indicator. Despite the criticism that GDP does not properly reflect the country's development status or production activities, the reason why it has maintained its position as a prominent representative indicator so far is its simplicity. Another example of simplifying a complex indicator system is the WHOQOL. The full version of WHO's WHOQOL initially included 100 indicators, but the limitations of measuring all 100 indicators in the field were revealed, and the WHOQOL-BREF was developed, which reduced the number of indicators. It is evaluated as an effort to increase the efficiency and reliability of indicators by simplifying them.

A study by Cummins (2018) is noteworthy regarding the need for simplicity in the measure of happiness. The summary of his research is as follows. He compares three subjective wellbeing measures: Global Life Satisfaction (GLS) as a short list measure, Satisfaction with Life Scale (SWLS) as an intermediate measure, and Personal Wellbeing Index (PWI) as a long list measure. GLS (Andrews & Withey, 1976) employs a single question asking global wellbeing as a measurement item.

Specifically, the response to the question "How do you feel about your life as a whole?" is measured with a seven-choice response scale. SWLS, suggested by Diener et al. (1985), measures subjective wellbeing through a total of five questions. The five questions of SWLS also use a seven-choice response scale and are as follows: ① In most ways, my life is close to my ideal. ② The conditions of my life are excellent. ③ I am satisfied with my life. ④ So far I have gotten the important things I want in life. ⑤ If I could live my life over, I would change almost nothing. PWI suggested by the International Wellbeing Group (2013) measures responses to questions about satisfaction in seven core domains on an 11-point scale. The specific question is as follows: How satisfied are you with: ① your standard of living? ② your health? ③ what you are achieving in life? ④ your personal relationships? ⑤ how safe you feel? ⑥ feeling part of your community? ⑦ your spirituality or religion(optional)? SWLS measures a single domain of GLS through multiple questions, while PWI is a model that extends the measurement range from a single domain to multiple separate domains.

Based on the number of indicators, GLS, SWLS, and PWI each correspond to short list measures that contain only a minimum number of indicators, intermediate measures that use multiple questions for one domain, and extended measures that use multiple questions for multiple domains. Each indicator system has its strengths and weaknesses in measuring subjective wellbeing. Short list measures such as GLS are concise and have the advantage of not having a large difference in response according to the composition method of the scale, but it is impossible to evaluate each components of happiness, react sensitively to situational factors such as mood and cultural heterogeneity. Intermediate measures such as SWLS can obtain a relatively high level of measurement reliability compared to minimum indicators but have the disadvantage that the validity of the indicators can be compromised if the respondent does not clearly understand them. While extended indicators such as PWI can secure high levels of measurement reliability, distinguish between the contribution of each domain to happiness, and have the advantage of being less affected by situational factors, they may not have interdomain consistency and independent explanatory power for GLS (Cummins, 2018).

It is worth noting that according to the empirical study of Cummins (2018: 32), the correlation between the measurement results is quite high for the three indicator types despite their differences as shown below (recited):

GLS versus SWLS: 0.77 (Anglim et al., 2015), 0.66 (van Beuningen, 2012).

GLS versus PWI: 0.78 (Anglim et al., 2015), 0.60 (Casas et al., 2009).

PWI versus SWLS: 0.75 (Anglim et al., 2015), 0.78 (Renn et al., 2009).

Such results provide meaningful implications for the demand for concise happiness measurements. In other words, if the correlation between the three types of indicators crosses each other and the correlation between them is high in the measurement results, the relative weight should be placed on the indicator types that are advantageous in terms of ease of measurement and cost. In this regard, Cummins (2019), who reported that the measure of the single indicator of happiness (GLS) is fairly stable and reliable, with a score of 70–80% on the 100% scale, further supported the call for a simplified happiness indicator. Based on these results, Cummins (2018:

61) explicitly suggests that the method of measuring subjective wellbeing should be through more simple items, fewer in numbers, and reliable measures as much as possible. Of course, since the strengths and weaknesses of the three indicator types are not of a single dimension but of different properties, there is a limit to using only conciseness as a criterion for selection of indicators. However, if there are no conditions that are in conflict with conciseness in particular, more consideration of conciseness is needed. Basically, in order to secure an agreed happiness indicator that has the same status as GDP, a simple indicator should be developed and agreed upon as much as possible. Currently, the reason why different researchers and countries use different indicator systems is that they are basically adopting an extended indicator system. As such, it is difficult to reach consensus in a situation where there are multiple indicators. The simpler the indicator, the easier it is to agree.

3.4 Employing Intersubjective Measures

Necessities

Indicators for measuring happiness are classified into objective indicators and subjective indicators. Objective indicators are indicators that do not reflect the opinions of the subject of investigation and can be identified consistently to anyone from the point of view of a third party according to their objective status. For example, objective conditions such as income, employment rate, housing conditions, and social overhead capital are objective indicators that can measure their frequency or quantity in a standardized way. GDP, which has traditionally been used as a measure of national development, is a representative objective indicator. Among wellbeing indicators, the Human Development Index, which consists of life expectancy, training period, and GNI per person, is a representative objective indicator. Objective indicators have an advantage in measuring and comparing tangible factors, but there is a problem that it is difficult to measure subjective dimensions such as happiness as well as partial measurement problems due to limitations in data availability. This is because it is difficult to obtain objective data on subjective emotions. Although there has been an attempt to evaluate happiness based on externally revealed behavior (Kahneman, 1999), support for such an attempt is weak, and in general, the measurement of happiness is based on subjective indicators that depend on the subjective evaluation of respondents. For example, the UN's WHI and the OECD's BLI are measuring how happy respondents feel in terms of subjective wellbeing. Subjective indicators are used not only in domains such as one's mood or satisfaction, but also for evaluating satisfaction with the environment in which the person is located. For example, an indicator such as WHO's WHOQOL measures an individual's satisfaction with material conditions such as his or her surrounding environment (natural environment, living environment, etc.) or traffic conditions. Subjective indicators also have limitations. Subjective indicators mainly measure responses to questions, so if respondents do not have a common background or value, the validity of the results can be questioned. This problem can be particularly serious in when measuring respondents with cultural heterogeneity. In this regard, Cummins (2018) pointed out that if subjective wellbeing is well defined and theoretically robust, it would be possible to properly measure subjective wellbeing in different cultures, but this process is very difficult in reality.

Overall, objective indicators have a problem of limiting the measurement range due to the limitation of data acquisition, despite ensuring the objectivity of measurement, and the subjective indicators have limitations in securing objectivity of measurement, despite the relative ease of data acquisition and high flexibility in the measurement range. If so, are there any alternative indicators that can overcome the limitations while taking advantages of both? This document proposes intersubjective measures as a useful alternative with such a possibility.

What are Intersubjective Measures?

As mentioned in Chap. 2, the Community Wellbeing Project in Korea has adopted and developed wellbeing measures at the collective level beyond the individual level. As Weeranakin and Promphakping (2018) and Thin (2018) have properly pointed out, most wellbeing-related studies have shown limitations in measuring the sum of individual wellbeing rather than directly measuring wellbeing at the community level. This research project established a unique measurement model for community wellbeing as an effort to supplement the limitations of this trend and introduced an intersubjective measure in the process of its application.

A brief summary of the project's community wellbeing measurement model is as follows (Kee et al., 2014; Kim & Lee, 2014). This model measures community level wellbeing based on the perspective of capital. Specific measurement indicators include a total of 41 indicators, 17 dimensions across six capitals: human development (education, health, welfare), economy (employment, regional economy), environment (physical and ecological environments), infrastructure (housing, ICT, transportation, safety), society (community relations, citizenship, trust, culture). In addition, a general indicator for each dimension is included to allow choice between the specific indicators and general indicator for each dimension in parallel or selectively. Each indicator asks respondents to make both an intersubjective and a subjective assessment of the living conditions of their community by using the question, "How would you evaluate your local community, and to what extent are you personally satisfied with the area you live in?" All responses are measured on a 10-point scale.

Intersubjective measures go beyond subjective and objective indicators to measure wellbeing based on "intersubjectivity." In general, intersubjectivity can be defined as "the diverse relationships among the various perspectives of individual, group, and traditions" and is considered a key element for understanding the social behaviors of humans (Gillespie & Cornish, 2010). The perspective of emphasizing intersubjectivity does not agree with the argument that values or perceptions can only be experienced at an individual level and argues that people have a collective understanding of "how the community that they belong to appears" which ultimately affects people's collective and individual sense of worth (White, 2010). Thus, a specific and objective definition is not always necessary when measuring an abstract concept like values and intersubjective indicators can be a good alternative when group constituents have a shared consciousness under a specific context (Burford et al., 2013). In short, intersubjectivity is understood to mean that an individual has the cognitive ability to make certain judgments or evaluations at the collective level beyond the individual level. If so, subjectivity can be interconnected with objectivity, and in this context, intersubjectivity can be understood as meaning a subjective evaluation of an objective state. Although intersubjectivity is still subjective in the sense of individual evaluation, it can be said to be objective in that the direction of the evaluation is not tied to oneself and aims to cover the evaluation of the objective state.

Table 3 compares measures according to the characteristics of wellbeing concepts. Of course, the intersubjective measure is not a measure that applies only to wellbeing, but comparing the measurement indicators of various wellbeing concepts will help us understand the properties of the intersubjective measure. In Chap. 2, the concepts related to wellbeing were summarized into five categories: objective IWB, subjective IWB, objective CWB, subjective CWB, and intersubjective CWB (see Fig. 3 in Chap. 2). For the measurement of objective wellbeing, both objective indicators and subjective indicators can be used for both individual and collective dimensions. In measuring subjective wellbeing, subjective indicators will be used at both the individual and collective levels. In contrast, for the measurement of an objective evaluation of community wellbeing, an intersubjective measure can be applied. Here, the intersubjective measure is related to the collective level at the individual-aggregate dimension and has the characteristic of an indicator that pursues both objectivity and subjectivity in relation to the subjective–objective dimension.

Intersubjective indicators are based on individual responses to questions in their measurement method and are therefore similar in appearance to subjective indicators. However, intersubjective indicators differ from subjective indicators in that it is asking respondents to evaluate the community (collective) level rather than the individual level satisfaction. For example, the subjective indicator tries to measure the individual level of satisfaction of respondents through questions such as "Are you satisfied with the wellbeing level of your community?" In comparison, the intersubjective indicator purports to measure the individual "evaluation" of the community level rather than the "satisfaction" of the individual respondent, through questions such as "How do you evaluate the wellbeing level of your community?" In other words, the intersubjective indicator goes through a subjective form but aims for objectivity beyond subjectivity. Of course, to such an attempt, a question may be raised whether it is possible to simultaneously ask and respond to the same respondents' own satisfaction (subjective evaluation) and third-party evaluation (subjective evaluation) for community wellbeing. In other words, it is a question of whether there is a significant difference between subjective evaluation and intersubjective evaluation in the question result for the same respondent. In this regard, Choi & Lee (2020) found that respondents differentiated between subjective questions about satisfaction at the individual level and intersubjective questions about community. Specifically, in order to measure the wellbeing level of 27 Korean communities, this study collected objective statistical data, subjective satisfaction data, and intersubjective evaluation data, and performed a comparative analysis based on applying

Table 3 Comparing wellbeing-related measures

	Objective (individual) wellbeing	Subjective (individual) wellbeing	Objective community wellbeing	Subjective community wellbeing	Intersubjective community wellbeing
Object	Individual status (income, education, education, health), condition (living area)	Subjective satisfaction of individual status and conditions	Community service(sanitation), condition (population density)	Subjective satisfaction of community service, conditions	Objective evaluation of community service, conditions
Key words	Status, condition	Satisfaction	Status, condition	Satisfaction	Evaluation
Method of measurement	Hard data, survey	Survey	Hard data, survey	Survey	Survey
Exemplary question	What is your income?	How satisfied are you with your income?	How often is garbage collection in your community?	How satisfied are you with the garbage collection service in your community?	How would you evaluate your community's garbage collection service?
Happiness component	Individual happiness conditions	Individual happiness	Public happiness conditions	Public happiness domain	Public happiness domain
Service aspect	Supply	Demand	Supply	Close to supply	Demand

distance analysis, mean comparison, and correlational analysis. It showed that there was a significant difference between the intersubjective indicator and subjective or objective indicators in their analytical results. This confirms the unique usefulness of the intersubjective indicator in measuring wellbeing at the community or collective level.

The Usefulness of Intersubjective Indicators

Intersubjective indicators are useful measurement instruments that can complement the shortcomings of objective indicators and subjective indicators. In particular, it will be more useful when there is a lack of objective data at the collective level related to public happiness. The usefulness of the intersubjective indicator is as follows.

① Proxy measures of objective indicators: When collection of objective data at the collective level is difficult or impossible, we can use intersubjective indicators as proxies. Such an advantage is greater especially for small communities in which data availability is a problem most of the time. Intersubjective indicators are not merely proxies of objective data. If intersubjective data is perceived as low quality, then there is a high probability that intersubjective data will always become second choice to objective data when they exist. The existence of objective data does not guarantee accurate measurement of objective conditions. Existing data is necessarily partial and thus in many cases, they do not objectively reflect the conditions of a community. They are partial by nature. Intersubjective evaluation has the benefit of trying to evaluate from a more comprehensive perspective. For example, there will be a limit to measuring the level of cultural services in the community with only the number of libraries, an objective indicator. In this case, the evaluation of cultural services in the entire region can be obtained through intersubjective questions, not limited to some services. Thus, intersubjective indicators may in fact be better and not inferior to objective indicators.

② Complementing the subjective indicators: When conducting a survey to acquire subjective data, it is necessary to allocate more than a certain number of samples for each community, but it is often difficult to cover the cost required for such a survey. In addition, in evaluating the community status, there is a limit to matching the average of individual responses with the community status. For example, when the average value of individual satisfaction for public services of a community is not the same as the level of public services of the community, there is a limit to accept the latter as equivalent to the former. In this regard, the intersubjective indicator asks respondents to evaluate the status of the community from a third party's standpoint, not from a view of individual preference. There is a possibility to secure a reliability level close to or exceeding the subjective satisfaction survey even with a relatively small number of respondents. If so, the cost associated with the survey can also be reduced.

③ Indicator of policy performance: When public policy is implemented in units of regions or groups, evaluation at the community (or collective) level has important implications for effective implementation. It is fair that such evaluation is made by the consumer, not the supplier. This is because public policy is not implemented for the government but is implemented for the wellbeing of citizens who are the consumers. Therefore, no matter how well the government implements public policy, it is difficult to determine such a policy as a good policy unless the citizens acknowledge it as such. This is especially true for happiness policies for which subjective evaluation of citizens is important. The intersubjective indicator can be useful for community level evaluations. This is true even when an objective indicator exists. This is because objective indicators are data prior to evaluation and intersubjective indicators are data that reflect the evaluation of consumers. Of course, one may ask about subjective satisfaction instead of the intersubjective evaluation, because subjective satisfaction is also the evaluation of consumers. However, if you put emphasis on objectivity, one will be more interested in the intersubjective indicator than the subjective indicator, because subjective satisfaction is a subjective evaluation at the individual level, whereas the intersubjective s evaluation is an objective evaluation at the community level.

④ Civic education effect: Intersubjective indicators have a secondary effect of civic education. Intersubjective indicators have the effect of expanding civic attitudes by encouraging people to consider the community aspect above and beyond the individual. That is, the intersubjective indicator has the effect of broadening the horizon of respondents by inducing them to consider the community (region, group) level beyond the individual level in the questioning process. When considering an issue, thinking about how it relates to me and thinking about how it relates to the community have clear differences in the scope and level of cognition. Of course, surveys are not tools of civic education, but if the scope and level of civic attitudes are expanded through a survey then that in itself will change wellbeing perceptions and can have an indirect effect on wellbeing policies. In this regard, Thin (2012: 103) suggested that we should not only pursue hypothetical instrumental values in measuring happiness but should pay attention to the education of respondents. In other words, he argued for the necessity of providing learning opportunities for happiness in the measurement process, beyond interest in acquiring and using information, so that civic interest in happiness and value change can take place. Beyond the educational effect on happiness, the intersubjective indicator is expected to have the effect of universal civic education that strengthens the scope and level of individual cognition from the individual level to the community level. In addition, this learning effect is thought to have an aspect that contributes to the overall happiness policy by improving the attitudes of not only the respondents but also the policymakers who are exposed to these survey results.

⑤ Utilization as a public perspective survey tool: An intersubjective survey using intersubjective indicators is based on public opinion formed from a public perspective. Unlike the standard survey that is commonly used, it is more suitable for use as evidence for policymaking. The existing standard survey has two limitations. First, standard surveys require respondents to improvise with a superficial knowledge or lack of understanding of the question. Of course, many surveys try to reduce responses when they are not suitable for responding by allowing respondents to choose the option of "I don't know," but superficial response issues still remain. Also, respondents who are not actually familiar with the content of the question may not choose the option of "I don't know." Second, most existing surveys do not seek the opinions of respondents from a public perspective but ask for opinions (e.g., satisfaction) from the perspective of individual (private) interests. For example, when asking about the educational conditions of a community, instead of asking whether the conditions are appropriate from a public perspective, they ask individual satisfaction with the educational conditions. Although such a survey can measure individual satisfaction, it has limitations in determining whether it is appropriate at the collective level. This is because individual responses reflect the respondent's individual interests. Even if individual responses are combined, these basic attributes do not change. This is because the total or average of individual interests may represent the population of respondents, but not the public interest. Therefore, although such a survey method is frequently called "public" opinion survey, the meaning of "public" means the majority or collectivity of people, but not publicness. A more precise term would be "individual" or "collective" opinion survey. This is because the basic attribute of such surveys is an individual opinion survey that measures personal preference or satisfaction.

The deliberative public opinion survey has been proposed as a complementary effort to address the limitations of standard surveys based on respondents' superficial and spontaneous responses (Dryzek, 1990; Fishkin, 1991). The deliberative public opinion survey is a method designed to collect informed responses based on deliberation rather than superficial opinions, by asking respondents to go through a deliberation process in addition to the standard investigation. The standard method of the deliberative public opinion survey is comprised of a general opinion survey, followed by deliberation (often with involvement of experts), and finally another general opinion survey and an attempt to measure changes in participant opinions before and after deliberation. It is considered an alternative that can alleviate or overcome the problems of the spontaneity or superficiality of standard surveys. However, such methods are time-consuming and expensive, the procedure is complicated, the influence of experts can be large, and the sample size is limited. Opinions that have changed after the deliberation process (although there are disagreements about the possibility and degree of the change) still have the limit of being individual opinions on personal preference or satisfaction from a private perspective. Of course, as they gain deeper knowledge and understanding of issues in the deliberation process, there is a possibility that respondents will approach the issues from a more public perspective. This is because the deliberation process not only expands knowledge about the issue but also discusses the need to look at the issue from a public perspective. However, this does not fundamentally change the perspective that operates when responding to a question unless the nature of the question fundamentally changes, and therefore, the response in deliberative public opinion surveys basically maintains the characteristics of the individual opinion presented in terms of private interests.

In sum, deliberative public opinion surveys can be a good way to overcome the improvisation and self-interest bias, but it is not a practical alternative to the other limit.

The intersubjective survey presented here, unlike the traditional survey or deliberative survey which has the nature of an opinion survey based on the perspective of private interest, has the characteristic of an opinion survey from a *public* perspective. This is because the intersubjective survey is a method that asks respondents for public evaluation based on personal reflection on the public dimension, not personal preference or satisfaction. These differences have important implications in relation to the public use of survey results. The results of the two existing surveys are "private" or "collective" opinions, which aggregate individual preferences or satisfactions, and have limitations as information to be used in the process of public policy decisions which aim for public interest. In contrast, the result of the intersubjective survey is more of a "public opinion" based on the evaluative opinions formed from the public perspective, and accordingly, it is more suitable as information to be used in the policymaking process pursuing the public interest. In addition, as the method of intersubjective survey gets settled, the views of respondent citizens will evolve into more civilized citizens who have a higher interest in the public dimension; thus, the utilization of the intersubjective survey results can be increased. In this regard, one could say that the perspective that works for respondents is still a private perspective, as in the deliberative survey where the private view dominates the respondents even after deliberation. However, the attribute of the intersubjective question itself is different from the questions of the other two opinion surveys. Accordingly, the perspective that dominates respondents in the intersubjective survey will be public at its basis.

The intersubjective survey is also useful as an alternative that can overcome much of the spontaneity of standard surveys. Respondents in the intersubjective survey will undergo psychological reflection internally in order to respond to a question from the public perspective. Such reflection process is a process of expanding the innate private perspective to the public perspective, and it corresponds to the effects of deliberation that respondents go through in the deliberative survey. There is a difference, however, that deliberation in the intersubjective survey is an individual and internal reflection, while deliberation in the deliberative survey is collective and external. Notwithstanding such differences, the individual and internal reflection in the intersubjective survey is expected to have the effect of alleviating spontaneous responses as in the collective and external deliberation process. In sum, the intersubjective survey suggested here is a survey method that collects public opinion based on a public perspective, overcomes the limitations of the standard survey and the deliberative survey, and has the potential for policy utilization. The discussion so far is summarized in Table 4.

Limitations

Despite the usefulness of the intersubjective survey, there is a concern that respondents may have difficulty distinguishing between personal satisfaction and public evaluation in responding to the actual survey. Naturally, it may be a difficult problem

Table 4 Comparison of standard survey, public opinion survey, and regarded official survey

	Standard survey	Deliberative survey	Intersubjective survey
Characteristic of questions	Spontaneous, superficial	Collective deliberation	Individual deliberation (reflection)
Perspectives of responses	Individual preferences (private satisfaction)	Individual preferences (private satisfaction)	Public evaluation (public satisfaction)
Usefulness for public policy	Low	Middle	High

for the same respondent to distinguish between the degree of "satisfaction" in terms of their interests and the degree of "evaluation" from a public point of view for the same question item. Fortunately, respondents can make a distinction between the two. In the aforementioned Community Wellbeing Project, respondents were asked to evaluate individual subjective satisfaction and regard for the same question item (e.g., community safety) simultaneously. The analysis results showed that there was a significant difference between the subjective satisfaction of the respondents and the subjective evaluation, which confirms that there is not much concern about confusion between the subjective satisfaction and the subjective evaluation (Choi & Lee, 2020).

3.5 *Presentation of Measurement Results*

After measurement using indicators, how to present the results is also an important issue. Since the ultimate purpose of making happiness indicators is to promote citizen happiness through the use of these indicators, it is important to communicate well the content of the indicators to the users including policy makers, policy analysts, and also the general public (Eurostat, 2014). Relatedly, Shim and Lee (2016) explain that the ways to present quality of life indexes can be broadly divided into the format of suite of indicators and creating a composite index. The suite of indicators format does not calculate a summary index but simply lists the level (or change) of all indicators in order and the UK's Measuring National Wellbeing is an example. The composite index format uses weights to summarize the indicators into one number and Canada's Canadian Index of Wellbeing is an example. The suite of indicators format has the strength of allowing users to choose and use the indicators that they are interested in but when there are too many indicators, it can be difficult to have an intuitive understanding of the whole picture. In contrast, the summary index format can be easily understood because it provides one number, but there can be issues with the fairness or political neutrality in terms of the weights used for each indicator. Because the pros and cons of each method are clear, there have been efforts to supplement them. A notable example is OECD's Better Life Index (OECD BLI) that does not predetermine the weights of measurement items but allows users to assign weights and calculate a summary index. Other examples include Australia's Measures of Australia's Progress that select headline progress indicators with other indicators in the category for each theme. For another method, as in the Korean Community Wellbeing Project, a comprehensive or selective method of calculating the measurement results may be taken by separately presenting the overall indicators together with the detailed indicators.

4 Measuring Happiness

4.1 The Components of Happiness

As discussed before, happiness can be categorized into hedonic and eudaimonic, depending on perspective. The former explains happiness with temporary and direct feelings such as "pleasure (feeling)" and "satisfaction" while the latter is about sustainable conditions such as the purpose of life and self-realization. The hedonic and eudaimonic perspective of happiness can be summarized into the three aspects of affect, life satisfaction, and eudaimonia, or the four aspects ofpositive affect, negative affect, life satisfaction, and eudaimonia (Diener & Biswas-Diener, 2008: 249; OECD, 2013: 29).

Lee and Lee (2016) conducted a factor analysis to see whether this theoretical concept categorization matches empirical data. For the analysis, data from the Survey Research Center, Graduate School of Public Administration, Seoul National University's "2014 National Survey of the Civic Perceptions on the Role of Government and Quality of Life." This survey aimed to explore the scope and process of government tasks and how to improve them and Korean citizens' perception of quality of life and the role of government to provide basic data for policymaking. The survey was conducted from October 2, 2014–November 24, 2014, (54 days) with effective sample of 5940 adults age 19 and older nationwide. The sampling method was stratified sampling. The questionnaire used 10-point scale answers and the specific survey items used in the factor analysis for happiness components were as follows. First, regarding feelings, the following ten questions were asked including both positive and negative feelings: (1) How joyful did you feel? (2) How peaceful did you feel?, (3) How much did you worry?, (4) How sad were you?, (5) How happy were you?, (6) How depressed were you?, (7) How angry were you?, (8) How stressed were you?, (9) How tired were you?, (10) How much did you smile or laugh?." Second, for satisfaction, respondents were asked to evaluate the two following items: (1) My life conditions are satisfactory, (2) I am satisfied with my life." Third, for life meaning, respondents were asked to assess the following three items: (1) I have a choice about how to live my life, (2) I believe my work is meaningful, (3) overall, I feel a sense of accomplishment about what I have done."

A factor analysis of happiness components produced four factors as shown in Table 5. The first factor "negative emotions" includes worry, sadness, depression,

Table 5 Factor analysis of the components of happiness

Measurement items	Happiness			
	Negative feeling	Positive feeling	Life meaning	Life satisfaction
How much did you worry?	0.755	−0.105	−0.037	−0.019
How sad were you?	0.787	−0.177	−0.178	0.132
How depressed were you?	0.793	−0.221	−0.160	0.050
How angry were you?	0.837	−0.108	−0.089	−0.018
How stressed were you?	0.794	−0.037	0.091	−0.215
How tired were you?	0.639	0.144	0.194	−0.385
How joyful did you feel?	−0.147	0.800	0.163	0.308
How peaceful did you feel?	−0.155	0.805	0.179	0.245
How happy were you?	−0.147	0.795	0.218	0.179
How much did you smile or laugh?	−0.022	0.766	0.259	0.009
I have a choice about how to live my life	−0.076	0.213	0.798	−0.004
I believe my work is meaningful	−0.061	0.201	0.845	0.206
Overall, I feel a sense of accomplishment about what I have done	−0.046	0.246	0.783	0.268
My life conditions are satisfactory	−0.018	0.303	0.210	0.805
I am satisfied with my life	−0.042	0.356	0.275	0.743
Eigen value	5.4006	3.0249	1.2521	1.0422
Variance	0.2426	0.1997	0.1579	0.1145
Cumulative	0.2426	0.4423	0.6002	0.7147

angry, stress, and tiredness, and the second factor "positive emotions" includes joy, peace, happy, laugh, or smile. The third factor "life meaning" includes choice over life, meaningful work, sense of accomplishment. Lastly, the fourth factor "life satisfaction" includes satisfaction with life conditions, and satisfaction with my life. These results show that the happiness component includes the factors suggested by both the hedonic approach and the eudaimonic approach, and the feeling factor can be divided into negative and positive factors.

4.2 Level and Distribution of Happiness

Public happiness must be measured and pursued at the collective level beyond the individual level. This is because public happiness cannot be maintained in a private dimension isolated from the public community by nature and can only be secured in a close relationship with constituents of the community. As well expressed by Bhutan's King Khesar (2013), who advocated for Gross National Happiness, "Happiness feeds on community and fraternity." In situations where the constituents of the community are not happy together, individual happiness is difficult to exist, and even if it exists, it cannot be sustained. Public happiness is based on this perspective. Therefore, discussions on public happiness should be made with equal interest not only in the level of happiness but also in the distribution of happiness in a community whether big or small. Nevertheless, most of the interests and discussions about happiness are excessively focused on the level of happiness. Of course, the level of happiness should be an important concern because the primary concern of an individual is to increase their level of happiness. However, from the perspective of the community, it is not justified to pay attention only to the level of happiness whether of individual or of community. Basically, the level of happiness apart from the distribution of happiness may be a necessary condition for public happiness but not a sufficient condition. That is, public happiness demands both the improvement of the level of happiness and the balance of the distribution of happiness in the community.

Then what does it mean to measure happiness levels? This means measuring the mean value of each individual or group happiness. The mean value is a key indicator that is used to evaluate, compare, and analyze certain phenomena in various areas. However, there are some problems with examining happiness with a mean value only. Above all, there is an excessive generalization error. This does not take outliers into consideration and thus a mean value only shows the characteristics of the midpoint in the sample but does not show any location information of how the data are spread out. There is a limit to not knowing whether the mean value is high because one person's happiness is significantly greater than other constituents' happiness or because every constituent of a society has a similarly high level of happiness. Furthermore, excessive concentration on the mean happiness value causes side effects that hinder positive change in society. In particular, it does not help to derive policy implications for the improvement of an unfair society. This is because it discourages efforts to identify conflicting factors that increase the level of happiness but decrease the equality of happiness. Therefore, in order to construct a happy community together, it is necessary to measure and analyze the level and distribution of happiness, and factors related to them, buttressed by the balanced interest between the level and distribution of happiness.

As a response to this need, Seung Jong Lee et al. (2020) analyzed the relationship between the level and distribution of happiness at the national level by aggregating the time series data of the World Happiness Report from 2008 to 2018. First, Fig. 2 schematically shows how the mean value of the level and distribution of happiness in the 150 countries changed during the analysis period. In the figure, the *X*-axis

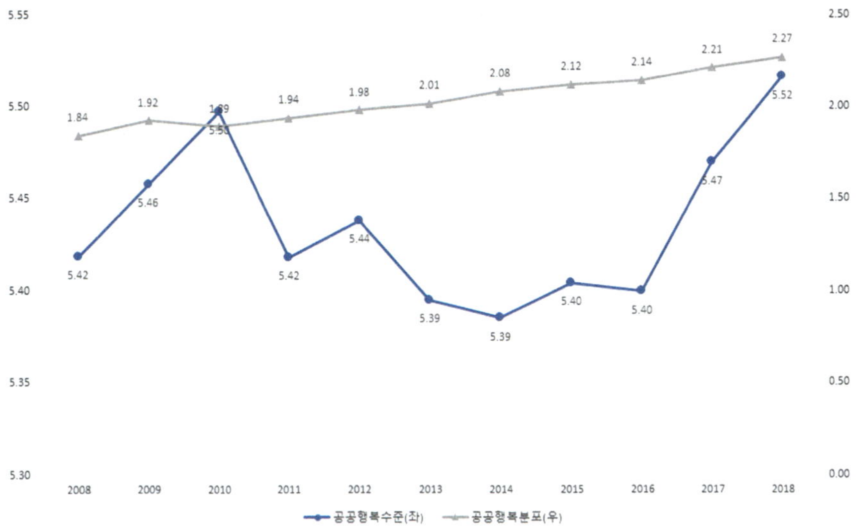

Fig. 2 Trend of public happiness level and distribution inequality (2008–2018). *Source* Lee et al. (2020)

represents the level of happiness by country, and the *Y*-axis represents the distribution (the degree of inequality) of happiness by country. As shown in the figure, the level of happiness in each country increased rapidly from 2008 to 2010 and then declined until 2016. This recession is interpreted to reflect problems such as the global economic recession, worsening unemployment rate, and social polarization since 2011. After some period of this recession, happiness levels rebound from 2017 to 2018. Thus, while the level of happiness has ups and downs, the distribution of happiness, that is, the degree of inequality, shows a continuous increasing trend over the entire period of analysis. As such, it has been found that there is some gap between the level of happiness and the distribution, which makes it difficult to secure public happiness only with interest in the level or distribution of happiness.

Fortunately, the level and distribution of happiness are not entirely moving in the opposite direction. Figure 2 shows that there is a discrepancy between the level and distribution of happiness, but the degree is not so serious. Specifically, the distribution of happiness is stable, whereas the level of happiness is curved, but overall, the progression of happiness level is not significantly different from the progression of happiness distribution. This assessment becomes more evident from Fig. 3. The figure shows the aggregation of all happiness levels and distributions during the period analyzed by country. When observed by country, happiness levels and distribution do not necessarily coincide but are generally found to have a positive correlation ($r = 0.44$). Although the correlation is not high, it can be said that countries with a high level of happiness tend to have low happiness inequality. This may be a positive basis for alleviating concerns about the trade-off between policies aiming at

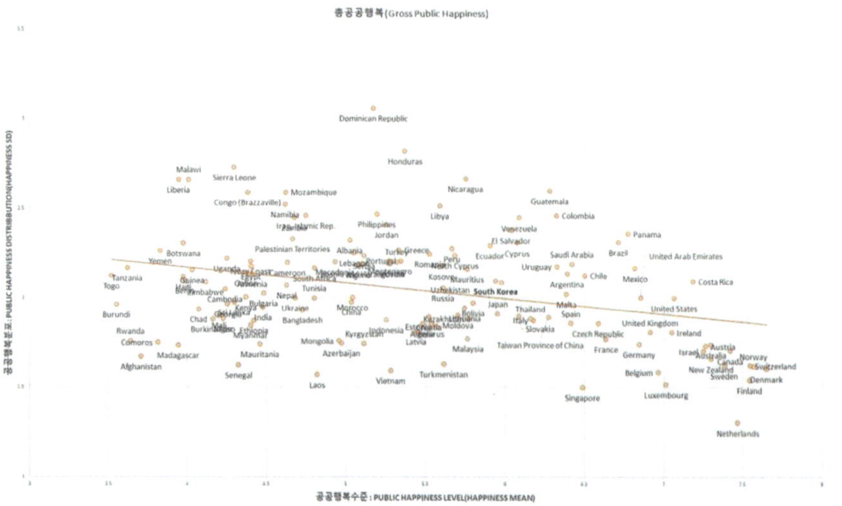

Fig. 3 State of public happiness by Country: level and distribution (2008–2018). *Source* Lee et al. (2020)

increasing happiness and policies aiming at improving the distribution of happiness (cf. Ott, 2005).

The implications of Figs. 2 and 3 together are clear. Since there is only a weak correlation between the level of happiness and its distribution, policy interest focused on only one of the level and distribution of happiness is not desirable in terms of the promotion of public happiness, and therefore, it is necessary to pursue both in a balanced manner. At the same time, such efforts can be supported by a synergy effect between the two, since there is some positive, though not strong, relationship between the level and distribution of happiness.

References

Anand, P. (2016). *Happiness explained: What human flourishing is and what we can do to promote it*. Oxford University Press.

Andrews, F. M., & Withey, S. B. (1976). *Social indicators of well-being: Americans' perceptions of life quality*. Plenum Press.

Anglim, J., Weinberg, M. K., & Cummins, R. A. (2015). Bayesian hierarchical modeling of the temporal dynamics of subjective well-being: A 10 year longitudinal analysis. *Journal of Research in Personality, 59*, 1–14.

Burford, G., Hoover, E., Velasco, I., Janoušková, S., Jimenez, A., Piggot, G., Podger, D., & Harder, M. K. (2013). Bringing the "missing pillar" into sustainable development goals: Towards intersubjective values-based indicators. *Sustainability, 5*(7), 3035-3059.

Casas, F. et al. (2009). Satisfaction with spirituality, satisfaction with religion and personal well-being among Spanish adolescents and young university students. *Applied Research in Quality of Life, 4*, 23–45.

Choi, N., & Lee, S. J. (2020). The usefulness of intersubjective community wellbeing as a community development indicator: Evidence from comparing three approaches to measuring community wellbeing. *International Journal of Community Well-Being, 3*(2), 173–192.

Cummins, R. A. (2018). *Measuring and interpreting subjective wellbeing in different cultural contexts: A review and way forward*. Cambridge University Press.

Cummins, R. A. (2019). *ACQol Bulletin Vol 3/21: 230519. Resource document. Australian centre on quality of life bulletin archive*. http://www.acqol.com.au/publications. Accessed May 17, 2020.

Diener, E. (1984). Subjective well-being. *Psychological Bulletin, 95*(3), 542–575.

Diener, E., & Biswas-Diener, R. (2008). *Happiness: Unlocking the mysteries of psychological wealth*. Oxford: Wiley-Blackwell.

Diener, E., Emmons, R. A., Larsen, R. J., & Griffin, S. (1985). The Satisfaction with Life Scale. *Journal of Personality Assessment, 49*(1), 71–75.

Dryzek, J. S. (1990). *Discursive democracy: Politics, policy, and political science*. Cambridge University Press.

Eurostat. (2014). *Getting messages across using indicators: A handbook based on experiences from assessing Sustainable Development Indicators*. Publications Office of the European Union.

Feldman, F. (2010). *What is this thing called happiness?* Oxford University Press.

Fishkin, J. S. (1991). *Democracy and deliberation: New directions for democratic reform*. Yale University Press.

Gillespie, A., & Cornish, F. (2010). Intersubjectivity: Towards a dialogical analysis. *Journal for the Theory of Social Behaviour, 40*(1), 19–46.

Global Council for Happiness and Wellbeing. (2019). *Global happiness and wellbeing policy report 2019*. Sustainable Development Solutions Network.

Hartmann, G. W. (1934). Personality traits associated with variations in happiness. *The Journal of Abnormal and Social Psychology, 29*(2), 202–212.

Huppert, F. A., & So, T. T. (2013). Flourishing across Europe: Application of a new conceptual framework for defining well-being. *Social Indicators Research, 110*(3), 837–861.

International Wellbeing Group. (2013). *Personal wellbeing index: 5th Edition*. http://www.acqol.com.au/instruments#measures. Accessed June 25, 2019.

Iriarte, L., & Musikanski, L. (2019). Bridging the Gap between the sustainable development goals and happiness metrics. *International Journal of Community Wellbeing, 1*(2), 115–135.

Kahneman, D. (1999). Objective happiness. In D. Kahneman, E. Diener, & N. Schwarz (Eds.), *Well-being: The foundations of hedonic psychology* (pp. 3–25). Russell Sage Foundation.

Kee, Y., Kim, Y., & Philips, R. (2014). *Community well-being: Learning in communities*. Springer Briefs Series, forthcoming.

Khesar, J. (2013). Happiness experienced: The science of subjective well-being. In S. A. David, I. Boniwell, & A. Conley Ayers (Eds.), *Oxford handbook of happiness*. (pp. 7–9). Oxford: Oxford University Press.

Kim, Y., & Lee, S. J. (2014). The development and application of a community wellbeing index in Korean metropolitan cities. *Social Indicators Research, 119*(2), 533–558.

Koo, K., Lim, J., & Choi, S. (2015). A synoptic review of the research on happiness. *Journal of Governmental Studies. 21*(2), 95–130. (Korean).

Lee, S. J., & Lee, J. E. (2016). Differential effects of prospective and retrospective government performance on trust in government. *A paper presented at the conference held by Lehman College*. New York, USA.

Lee, S. J., Lee, S., & Jo, C. (2020). A study on the differential factors that affect public happiness level and distribution. *Korean Public Administration Review, 54*(1), 171–197. (Korean)

Ludwigs, K. (2018). *The happiness analyzer: A new technique for measuring subjective well-being*. Erasmus University Rotterdam.

National Research Council. (2013). *Subjective well-being: Measuring happiness, suffering, and other dimensions of experience*. National Academy Press.
OECD. (2013). *OECD guidelines on measuring subjective well-being*. OECD Publishing.
Pavot, W., & Diener, E. (2013). Happiness experienced: The science of subjective well-being. In S. A. David, I. Boniwell, & A. Conley Ayers (Eds.), *Oxford handbook of happiness* (pp. 134–151). Oxford: Oxford University Press.
Pfeiffer, D., & Cloutier, S. (2016). Planning for happy neighborhoods. *Journal of the American Planning Association, 82*(3), 267–279.
Renn, D. et al. (2009). International well-being index: the Australian version. *Social Indicators Research, 90*, 243–256.
Shim, S., & Lee, H. (2016). Measuring quality of life: The international trends and the response by Korean National statistical office. *Survey Research, 17*(2), 185–205. (Korean).
Thin, N. (2012). *Social happiness: Theory into policy and practice*. Policy Press.
Thin, N. (2018). Qualitative approaches to culture and well-being. In E. Diener, S. Oishi, & L. Tay (Eds.), *Handbook of well-being* (pp. 108–127). DEF Publishers.
UNDP. (1990). *Human development report 1990: Concept and measurement of human development*. United Nations Development Programme.
van Beuningen (2012) *The satisfaction with life scale examining construct validity*. Discussion paper. Statistics Netherlands.
Veenhoven, R. (1991a). Questions on happiness: Classical topics, modern answers, blind spots. In F. Strack, M. Argyle, & N. Schwarz (Eds.), *Subjective well-being: An interdisciplinary perspective* (pp. 7–26). Pergamon Press.
Veenhoven, R. (1991b). Is happiness relative? *Social Indicators Research, 24*, 1–34.
Weeranakin, P., & Promphakping, B. (2018). Local meanings of well-being and the construction of well-being indicators. *Social Indicators Research, 138*(2), 689–703.
White, S. C. (2010). Analysing well-being: A framework for development practice. *Development in Practice, 20*(2), 158–172.

Chapter 5
Determinants of Happiness

1 Explanatory Models of Happiness

There are various explanatory models for factors influencing happiness. Broadly speaking, there are two theoretical models: adaptation theory which emphasizes individual personality traits and reactivity theory which emphasizes objective external circumstances (Sirgy, 2001). Adaptation theory is primarily a psychologist's approach, with individual personality traits such as extraversion, agreeableness, conscientiousness, emotional stability, and openness rather than objective conditions as key influencing variables (Maggino, 2015; Yeh et al., 2015). This theory posits that satisfaction with life experiences or public services affects happiness through a filtering process by pre-determined personality traits, and improvement of objective conditions or increasing positive experiences does not increase happiness. Rather, personality traits influence the emotions and evaluations of various objective situations. In contrast, reactivity theory is the main approach of various social scientists including economics and sociology and posits that objective external conditions at individual and social levels such as income, age, gender, marriage, occupation, family, region, and government. Conditions and so on are linked to happiness. In the process, individual experiences and evaluations are determined by passive reactions to objective conditions, so objective conditions become an important influencing variable of happiness (Diener, 1984; Ko, 2013).

Adaptation and response theories are each called by various names. Adaptation theory, which focuses on internal traits of individuals, is also referred to as personal trait or disposition theory, internal factor theory, set point theory, top-down spillover theory, etc. Reactivity theory, which focuses on objective external conditions, is also called in various ways such as situation theory, external factor theory, needs satisfaction theory, and bottom-up spillover theory. Among these various names, some additional explanation is needed for the distinction between the top-down spillover approach and the bottom-up spillover approach. Both approaches focus on the spillover process of happiness. A spillover is a phenomenon in which satisfaction in one domain of life affects satisfaction in another domain and can be divided into

S. J. Lee, *Public Happiness*, Community Quality-of-Life and Well-Being,
https://doi.org/10.1007/978-3-030-89643-0_5

vertical diffusion and horizontal diffusion. Vertical diffusion assumes that there is a hierarchy in the domain of life. The domain of overall life such as life satisfaction, happiness, or subjective wellbeing is the highest domain, and the major domains of life such as such as family, leisure, health, or income are sub-domains. Vertical diffusion is about the mutual influence between the upper and lower areas of life, while horizontal diffusion is about the mutual influence between the life domains at the same level (Sirgy et al., 2001). Both the top-down approach and the bottom-up approach explain vertical diffusion, that is, the relationship between happiness (or quality of life) and the subdomains of life, that is, the diffusion process. The former describes a process in which happiness, which is determined according to an individual's disposition, diffuses downward to satisfaction in the lower domains of life, while the latter describes the process in which satisfaction by sub-domain of life is upwardly diffused to happiness, which is the upper domain of life. The distinction between the two has the advantage of being an instrument to simultaneously identify the direction of the diffusion of happiness, along with discussions on whether individual factors are important or environmental factors are important in determining happiness. However, these approaches do not explain the horizontal diffusion between domains of life at the same level.

Classifying the approach model as such based on psychological and objective factors has important implications with regard to public policies for promoting happiness. The former implies that individual propensities are more important than the environment in determining happiness, thus diluting the significance of policy efforts to improve the environment. The latter implies that the environment is more important than an individual's propensity in determining happiness, thus underscoring the importance of policy efforts to improve the environment. As each approach has its limitations, there is a good reason to embrace both from an integrated standpoint. It is a model that simultaneously considers adaptation based on individual propensity and reaction to external objective conditions. Each model is discussed below.

1.1 Adaptation Theory

Adaptation theory argues that the individual's personality trait or disposition is an important factor in determining happiness, not living conditions. It assumes that there is a preliminary process that broadly influences an individual's assessment of overall life to have a certain tendency. Such tendencies are due to individual personality traits (Costa & McCrae, 1980), genetic factors (Bok, 2010), and chronic cognitive process (Diener & Biswas-Diener, 2008), and are stable. Of course, everyday experiences bring temporary effects, but an individual's evaluations eventually return to their original set points due to stable personal disposition (Headey, 2008; Lance et al., 1995; Maggino, 2015; Pavot & Diener 1993; Sugden & Teng, 2016).

Adaptation theory has been the name of a theoretical paradigm that has dominated empirical research on happiness or subjective wellbeing since the 1970s, but recently, it is commonly called set point theory (Headey, 2008). The central argument of adaptation theory or set point theory is that adults have a stable level of happiness. Brickman and Campbell (1971), one of the classic works of adaptation theory, argued that people are destined to experience a stable level of wellbeing through adaptation, even for the most extreme positive or negative life experiences. Of course, depending on the event, fluctuations centered on a set point occur, but such fluctuations are limited to a short period of time and the level of happiness returns to the previous level. This is because an individual's adaptability is very strong and stable (Lykken & Tellegen, 1996), and the individual's adaptability works in the same way for both positive and negative events. Even when a good event occurs, individual happiness is not significantly improved. This is because aspiration rises, offsetting the increase in the utility of favorable events. Even when negative events occur, individual happiness is not significantly degraded. This is because it compensates the decrease in utility caused by negative events through adaptation to the new situation. Adaptation and aspiration can work in the same way for situations as well as events. Graham (2009: 151)'s "paradox of happy peasant and miserable millionaires," which refers to the fact that poor farmers can be happier than the rich ones, explains this well. The paradox is explained by the downward adaptation of the poor farmer and the upward aspiration of the wealthy millionaire. As such, the set point effect is characterized as a repetitive process as aspirations are generated by the individual's desire and adaptation occurs at a certain level (Binswanger, 2006: 367). And at this time, the adaptability of an individual depends on the individual's personality traits or genetic factors and is regarded as a universal trait that everyone has.

Adaptation theory is frequently compared to a treadmill in which the foot moves in the opposite direction of the ground and no matter how long one runs the person stays in the same spot. There are two types of treadmill effects: the hedonic treadmill and the aspiration treadmill (Bruni & Zamagni, 2007: 235). The hedonic treadmill refers to the return of happiness to a previous level due to psychological adaptation to a new situation. For example, when an individual increases his income and owns a better car, his comfort level increases, but soon his happiness level returns to a similar level as before through psychological adaptation to his new condition. What is secured already is no longer new and eventually turns into boredom. What affects happiness is novelty, not comfort, which eventually becomes boredom (Scitovsky, 1976 cited in Bruni & Zamagni, 2007: 235). The aspiration treadmill focuses on the level of aspiration that demarcates satisfying results from unsatisfying results. When aspirations increase, happiness cannot increase even if situations improve. This is because even more situational improvement is required to maintain the same satisfaction level. For example, when an individual has a better car due to an increased income, the new car increases the individual's objective wellbeing, but if the aspiration for a nice car is higher than before as income increases, the increase in objective wellbeing does not increase subjective happiness.

The analogy of these two kinds of treadmills explains the process by which individual happiness is maintained at a certain level despite changing circumstances. However, there seems to be no need to approach psychological adaptation and aspiration change separately. The two are not independent, but rather inextricably related phenomena. In the previous example, when a new car is purchased with an increase in income, the adaptation to the new car and the increase in the desire for a better car occur simultaneously. Adaptation to a new car is the familiarization of a new situation, and new aspirations increase in proportion to the familiarization. In other words, familiarization is an increase in aspiration, and an increase in aspiration is an increase in familiarity. Therefore, the two treadmills above only have a difference in which aspect is emphasized in the adaptation process and are not actually different models.

A substantial number of studies support the set point or treadmill effect. Easterlin (2001) and Larsen (2000) explained that even if objective living conditions change, humans soon adapt to them, which creates new aspirations and eventually does not have a significant impact on the level of happiness as if happiness were spinning around. Lykken and Tellegen (1996) developed subjective wellbeing's set point theory through a study, "Happiness is a stochastic phenomenon." They developed the Multidimensional Personality Questionnaire to measure the wellbeing of twins and published a research result that found that the association between individual emotional stability, life events, and subjective wellbeing was more dependent on genetics than socioeconomic status, income, and educational attainment. Pagán-Rodríguez (2010) reported in an analysis of time series data on disabled people that they adapt well to new situations 5 years after the occurrence of disability, recovering the overall satisfaction level before the accident despite the need for personal assistance or care. In addition, various related theories have been developed to support or supplement the set point theory including adaptation level theory (Brickman & Campbell, 1971), SWB personality theory (Costa & McCrae, 1980), dynamic equilibrium theory (Headey & Wearing, 1989, 1992), multiple discrepancies theory (Michalos, 1985), homeostatic theory (Cummins, 2005), etc.

There are also studies that are critical of the set point theory. Lucas et al. (2003) analyzed the effect of marital transition (positive transition such as marriage and negative transition like widowhood) on life satisfaction based on data from the German Socio-Economic Panel Study (GSOEP). Analytical results showed that individuals on average reacted to events and then adapted back toward baseline levels. Specifically, individuals who initially reacted strongly were still far apart from the baseline level years later, and many people exhibited trajectories that were in the opposite direction to that predicted by adaptation theory. They concluded that marital transitions could be associated with long-lasting changes in satisfaction. And, they added that this effect is easy to overlook when looking only at average trends. Using the same panel data, Lucas et al. (2004) analyzed the relationship between unemployment and life satisfaction. The results were similar. They conclude: "In accordance with set point theories, individuals reacted strongly to unemployment and then shifted back toward their baseline levels of life satisfaction. On average, however, individuals did not completely return to their previous levels of satisfaction, even after they became reemployed." The results were the same for those who had already experienced unemployment in the past. These research results basically indicate that the magnitude of adaptation is exaggerated.

Cummins et al., (2014: 24) acknowledge that most empirical studies on the set point effect reported a phenomenon of reverting back to baseline after a certain period of adaptation after a life event occurred. However, they pointed out that there is a limit to analyzing the effect of adaptation only over time and argue that it is necessary to recognize that adaptation occurs by a balance of two factors. They argue: "One component is the strength and persistence of the psychological challenge provided by the event, and the other is the material and psychological resources of individuals to recover homeostatic control. Therefore, recovery time through adaptation is highly idiosyncratic and may never occur if the balance of challenge versus resources remains strongly unfavorable." This research strongly suggests the need for theoretical modification of adaptation. In this regard, Diener et al., (2009: 103) propose five modifications to the adaptation theory based on recent research results: "First, individuals' set points are not hedonically neutral. Second, people have different set points, which are partly dependent on their temperaments. Third, a single person may have multiple happiness set points: Different components of wellbeing such as pleasant emotions, unpleasant emotions, and life satisfaction can move in different directions. Fourth, wellbeing set points can change under some conditions. Finally, individuals differ in their adaptation to events, with some individuals changing their set point and others not changing in reaction to some external event." They add that "These revisions offer hope for psychologists and policymakers who aim to decrease human misery and increase happiness."

From a practical perspective, the implications of adaptation theory are twofold. On the one hand, by diluting expectations for the impact of environmental conditions on happiness, it undermines the importance of policy efforts to improve social conditions for happiness improvement, and on the other hand, it functions as a rationale to save public resources required for such policy efforts.

From a theoretical perspective, adaptation theory has the power of logic that encompasses theories related to the paradox of happiness. Given that the paradox of happiness is a question of the proportional relationship between the consumption of income and goods and happiness which has traditionally been valued, adaptation, the core logic of the set point effect, is the same as asserting the paradox in that it negates the association between external conditions and happiness. The versatility of this theory is particularly notable in relation to the argument that the magnitude and sustainability of happiness individuals get will differ depending on the type of consumption. For example, in conspicuous consumption (Veblen, 1899) or comparative consumption (Duesenberry, 1949), it is argued that the comparative advantage determines happiness, not the objective level of consumption. In this way, in consumption behaviors pursuing a relative position, the paradox arises that comparative value, not the size of objective benefits, determines happiness (Easterlin, 1973; Solnick & Hemenway, 1998: 375; Sugden & Teng, 2016). In addition, the argument that the consumption of relational goods consumed within reciprocity with others is important for the promotion of happiness is also related to the paradox of happiness in that material consumption has a limit to affect happiness (Bruni & Zamagni, 2007: 239). Therefore, the adaptive theory, which denies the direct relationship between external conditions and happiness, has the potential to be applied broadly to theories related to not only convenience goods but also comparative goods or relational goods. Of course, there may be variations in the level or direction of adaptation depending on the type of consumption. In this regard, Bruni and Zamagni (2007: 239) indicated that "adaptations and aspirations act less intensively in the consumptions of the familial, affectional, or civic relations which are of non-economic realms. The treadmill syndrome is not total, and a rich familial and relational life makes everybody, on average, happier." However, despite the differences according to consumption types, the existence of adaptation is not completely denied, and the general applicability of adaptation theory is accepted to that extent.

Basically, adaptability theory maintains that adaptability is due to personality traits of an individual and that it is stable and universal across individuals. Of course, everyone goes through short-term fluctuations, but in the end, they will adapt to the same level and direction. Two questions need to be addressed in order for such an argument to be sustained: First, are the individual personality traits stable? Second, is the mode of adaptation universal regardless of individual personality trait differences?

① Stability of personal orientation: Substantial number of studies support the stability of personal orientation. Brickman and Campbell (1971), for example, supports the stability of personal orientation by arguing that humans, like all other organisms, tend to try to maintain homeostasis and therefore adapt to good luck or misfortune. Pagán-Rodríguez (2010, 2012) supports the robustness of personal disposition by reporting that people's global satisfaction levels recover even when they need personal assistance or care.

Cummins (2018) also provide strong support for the stability of personal orientation through the homeostatically protected mood theory.[1] Homeostasis can be defined as the management of an essential variable to a set point, representing an optimal level for the operation of an individual (Cummins, 2018: 12). According to him, "SWB is not dominantly evaluative and more affective, and the main source of the affective component is source from "mood" which is chronic and trait-like affect not from emotion which is acute affect." He argues that mood has a genetic base and provides a set point for individuals. The mood is reported to be fairly stable regardless of the measurement method. The normal range of set points was reported as 70–90 points on the 0–100-point scale (Cummins, 2010: 18), 73.8–76.7 points (Cummins et al., 2014). Anglim et al. (2015, cited from Cummins, 2018: 18) reported that the average happiness level was 75.0 points and the standard deviation was 6.60 points. The results of empirical studies on the set point appear quite robust.

As such, Cummins argues that the source of stability of the happiness level was the stability of HP mood, but also explains that the HP mood is not robust but fragile. There are two cases when the mood is not stable and fragile. One is the mood is genetically unstable, and the other is when life experiences lead to loss of emotional stability (e.g., experience of assault). Excluding exceptional cases, such a HP mood theory, is an important support for adaptation theory. However, the theory's support is somewhat limited in scope. The HP mood theory is presented by focusing on affect, especially the stable mood, among the many elements of happiness, because mood is presumed as the dominant factor for SWB. However, if SWB is composed of moods

[1] Homeostasis is defined as the management of an essential variable to a set point, representing an optimal level for the operation for an individual (Cummins 2018: 12).

acting in short period (moods) and disposition acting in longer period as argued by Kozma et al. (1990), then the HP mood theory's support for the adaptation theory based on individual orientation is weakened to that extent.

② Universality of personal orientation: Adaptation theory assumes that everyone adapts to environmental conditions at the same level and direction. However, the assumption that despite the differences in personal disposition, responses to the external environment are identical is too simple. People with different personalities react differently to the same situation. That is, even in the same situation, individuals with a positive orientation respond more positively, and individuals with a negative orientation respond more negatively. The well-known precept that, looking at half a glass of juice, positive individuals say "half full" and negative individuals say "half empty" show us that differences in personal disposition are important in response to external circumstances. Moreover, as aforementioned, there is a possibility that the level of adaptation of an individual differs depending on the positive and negative situations. Nevertheless, the adaptation theory narrowly focuses on the adaptation result and thus does not pay proper attention to the adaptation process, i.e., the dynamic relation between individual propensity and adaptation experience. While emphasizing the stability of personality trait, it does not pay attention to individual differences in disposition. Accordingly, it does not clearly explain whether the set point effect is a result of the same adaptation mode deriving from the same personality trait or a result of the same adaptation mode despite the difference in personality trait.

There are two complementary approaches to overcome this limitation. One is an approach that explains the difference in adaptation mode by focusing on the difference in external conditions that the adaptive theory pays little attention to. For example, Lucas (2007) and Lucas and Diener (2009) argue that traumatic events such as divorce, death of a spouse, unemployment, and disability lead to long-term changes in SWB, contrary to the expectations of adaptation theory. They also argue that there are individual differences in adaptation and that adaptation does not always occur either. The reason individual adaptation does not work equally for positive events or negative events is explained by a general tendency to give more weight to perceived losses than gains (Schwarz & Strack, 1999). In response to this trend, Kahneman and Tversky (1979) stated that the value function for losses is steeper than the value function for gains, and the differential sensitivity to losses and gains is loss aversion. Nevertheless, it seems that these arguments partially support adaptation rather than entirely denying adaptation. This is because they indicate that in shocking situations a reaction occurs rather than an adaptation, and in general situations adaptation occurs rather than a reaction. In addition, Bruni and Porta (2005: 45) and Easterlin (2003) argued that adaptation occurs in areas of life related to material living conditions, but adaptation in family or health domains occurs at a much lower level. Weick (2015) reported that adaptation is difficult because basic human needs are not met for those who require personal assistance and care due to illness, disability, or age. These examples highlight differences in adaptation according to differences in external conditions.

A second approach is to explain the differences in adaptation according to the type of personality. For example, Boyce and Wood (2011) reported that in a survey of 307 disabled persons over a 4-year period, life satisfaction depends on personality trait. They argued that although becoming disabled has a severe impact on life satisfaction, this effect is significantly moderated by pre-disability personality. Specifically, agreeable individuals adapt more quickly and completely to disability, while disagreeable individuals may need additional support to adapt. Similarly, Bruni and Zamagni (2007: 239) stated that altruistic people are on average happier than egocentric people and that those who regularly volunteer consider themselves to be happy and are also considered happy by others. Of course, an argument that there is a difference in adaptation according to personality trait is not the same as the argument against the stability of personality. According to the difference in personality type, the direction and degree of adaptation will differ, and there will be a difference in the level of happiness accordingly, but the level of happiness can be within a certain limit regardless of the personality type. In other words, the discussion of personality types does not entirely deny the stability of adaptation, which is the core basis of the set point theory. However, unlike the simple set point theory, this suggests that the degree of adaptation will differ depending on individual personality types. If the difference in adaptation depending on personality types is not large, the set point theory will remain valid and vice versa. This is a matter of empirical investigation. Nevertheless, as long as there are still diverse personality types, the stability of the adaptive theory becomes unstable to a certain degree.

1.2 Reactivity Theory

Reactivity theory posits that an individual's level of happiness is determined by external conditions. Rather than the individual's adaptation to the external environment, how much the external objective condition satisfies the individual's needs becomes a significant influencing factor of happiness. In other words, individual happiness is determined by the individual's reactivity to the environment in various areas of life. Therefore, when the environment changes positively or negatively, the individual's level of happiness changes positively or negatively accordingly. Individuals are receptive but not active in their reactions to the external environment. In other words, the individual is an independent variable in adaptive theory, whereas in response theory, the independent variable is not an individual, but an external environmental condition. Therefore, as the set point theory argues, the level of happiness after an event does not return to the level before the event. This is because the changed life conditions are reflected in the individual life. If so, the set point theory is incorrect or exaggerated.

A representative model of reactivity theory is the needs satisfaction theory, which assumes that happiness is promoted when needs are satisfied. Representative theories include Maslow's hierarchy of needs (1943), Existence needs, Relatedness needs, Growth needs (ERG) theory by Alderfer (1972), Herzberg et al.'s (1959) motivation-hygiene theory or two-factor theory, trichotomy of needs theory by McClelland (1961), and the fundamental human needs theory of Max-Neef (1991), etc. These theories are similar in that they regard human needs as a major factor influencing happiness.

The most well-known needs satisfaction theory is Maslow's hierarchy of needs. Maslow (1943) argued that humans have basic needs to lead a life in the study of "A Theory of human Motivation." Basic needs are a set of goals that motivate humans. Human needs are composed of five levels of needs: physiological needs, safety needs, love and belonging needs, esteem needs, and self-actualization. Maslow divided these five levels of needs into the basic and being needs. Self-actualization corresponds to being needs, while the other four needs correspond to basic needs (see Fig. 1). When a need is fairly well satisfied, the next higher need emerges. And, the higher the level of needs, the greater the level of satisfaction. Satisfaction of one level of needs is replaced by the next higher level, and the needs that have already been satisfied lose their function of motivation. In the end, the most prominent goal will monopolize consciousness. Maslow's basic needs theory has important meaning as a leading research that indicates that need is an important factor in human wellbeing. However, there are criticisms against the argument that there are different stages of need.

Alderfer (1969) and McClelland (1961) made efforts to complement the limitations of Maslow's hierarchy of needs. First, McClelland explained in "Trichotomy of needs theory" that the needs for achievement, power, and affiliation are the motivations that make people act. These three needs are evaluated as a condensed integration of Maslow's needs stages, transcending characteristics such as race and gender. Alderfer (1969, 1972)'s ERG theory encompasses Maslow's five stages of needs, into three areas: existence needs (physiological and physical safety needs), relatedness needs (social relationships and external esteem), and growth needs (self-esteem and self-actualization). These needs classify domains of needs into the existence, relatedness, and growth, respectively, in terms of the object of needs. ERG theory is based on Maslow's theory, but it assumes that human needs are not hierarchical,

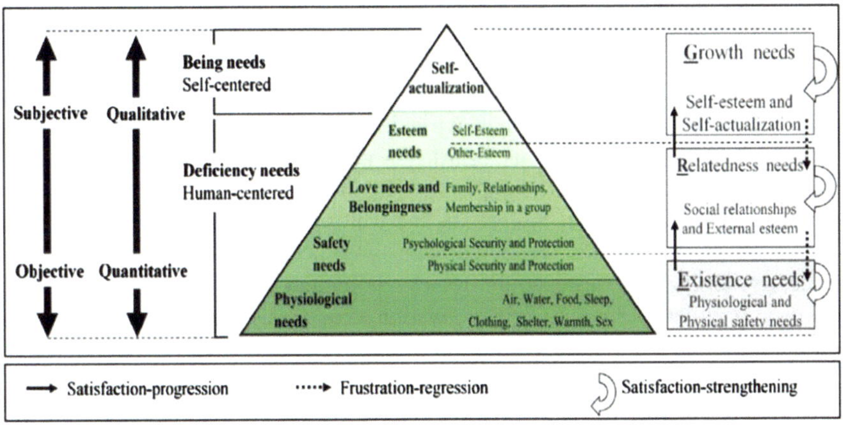

Fig. 1 Maslow's hierarchy of needs and Alderfer's ERG theory. *Source* Estaji (2014: 27)

and thus, they may all emerge at one time. Instead of Maslow's hierarchical logic, there are three mechanisms between the three categories: satisfaction progression, frustration regression and satisfaction- strengthening. Figure 1 shows a comparison between Aldermen's model and Maslow's model (Estaji, 2014: 27). As shown in the figure, the domain of the need stage theory and the domain of ERG do not exactly match. For example, Alderfer's existence needs include some of the safety needs (physical security and protection) along with the physiological needs in the need stage theory. Such overlapping is the same for other domains. Furthermore, the figure shows how each needs domain corresponds to the subjective-qualitative domain and the objective-quantitative domain.

The two-factor theory or motivation-hygiene theory of Herzberg et al. (1959) divides human needs into a motivator that leads to motivation and a hygiene factor that only leads to prevention of dissatisfaction rather than motivation. This differs from the assumptions of previous research that the satisfaction of all needs is linked to motivation regardless of the type of needs. Motivation factors include achievement, recognition, work itself, responsibility, advancement, growth, etc., which generally corresponds to Maslow's needs for recognition and self-actualization. Hygiene factors include organizational policy, supervision, relation with superiors, work conditions, salary, relationship with peers, etc., which generally correspond to Maslow's physiological, safety, and belongingness needs. While Maslow's vertical motivational theory or Alderfer's horizontal motivational theory focused on the relational properties between needs domains, Herzberg broadened the horizons of needs theory to the dimension of motivation beyond the analysis of needs. According to this theory, it is expected that the qualitative difference of motivation will occur depending on the nature of the external conditions, and accordingly, the form of achievement of happiness will change. That is, since satisfaction and dissatisfaction are not of the same dimension but of an independent dimension, efforts to create external conditions for motivation need to be made differently.

Self-determination theory of Ryan and Deci (2000) garnered attention by suggesting that individual autonomous motivation is important for human growth or psychological wellbeing, and the manifestation of that motivation is influenced by external conditions. In general, self-determination theory (SDT) is a psychological theory about human motivation that posits that intrinsic motivation (e.g., a sense of achievement) is more important than extrinsic motivation (e.g., promotion) in determining individual behavior. In this regard, they propose three intrinsic needs involved in self-motivation: the need for competence, autonomy, and relatedness, which when satisfied yield enhanced self-motivation and wellbeing and when thwarted leads to diminished motivation and wellbeing. The three needs are considered universal, innate, psychological, and essential for psychological wellbeing of an individual. However, in order for this intrinsic motivation to be manifested, the existence of an appropriate external environment is important.

They argue that various human behaviors are more than a function of dispositional differences or biological endowments, but a wide range of reactions to social environments. More specifically, social contexts catalyze both within- and between-person differences in motivation and personal growth, resulting in people being more self-motivated, energized, and integrated in some situations, domains, and cultures than in others. In short, the external environment fosters or undermines the manifestation of human motivation, and accordingly, the psychological wellbeing of humans is varied. Their self-determination theory is different in that they have expanded their interest in revealing social conditions that influence the manifestation of human motivations beyond the existing motivational studies that focused on extricating the structure of human motivations.

The fundamental human needs theory of Max-Neef (1991: 8–33) is a need theory that advocates human scale development as a counter model for developmentalism focused on economic growth. Max-Neef distinguishes between needs and satisfiers of needs, criticizing the theoretical limitations that past studies have focused only on needs. He also argues that unlike "wants" (hope) which are infinite and insatiable, fundamental human needs are finite, classifiable, and the same across all cultures and historical periods. Such satisfiers of needs may include forms of organization, political structures, social practices, values and norms, spaces, types of behavior and attitudes. That is, satisfiers are considered to encompass not only external objective conditions but also internal factors. He classifies needs into existential needs and axiological needs.

Existential needs include four components: being (attributes), having (institutions, norms etc.), doing (actions), interacting (location, milieus), and axiological needs include nine components: subsistence, protection, affection, understanding, participation, idleness, creation, identity, and freedom. Intersecting these components results in 36 categories of satisfiers. With this classification, Max-Neef presents specific satisfiers for each category. The satisfiers presented are indeterministic and large in number, and thus, instead of listing all suggested satisfiers, I only present one category of satisfiers here as an example: being-subsistence satisfier category includes satisfiers like physical health, mental health, equilibrium, sense of humor, and adaptability. Overall, including this example, satisfiers encompass objective external conditions such as social setting and internal propensity factors such as adaptability. As such, the satisfiers suggested by the fundamental human needs theory are notable as suggesting the need or possibility to dilute the boundary between the internal and external factors in relation to the existing approaches that distinguish between the two factors as factors influencing happiness.

1.3 Integration Theory

Adaptation theory and reaction theory contribute to expanding understandings of the effect of individual disposition and external environment on happiness, respectively, but the adaptive model shows a limit that neglects the situation and the reactivity model neglects personality. However, both circumstances and dispositions are factors of happiness that are difficult to ignore. Therefore, there is a need for an integrated model linking both models. In fact, existing studies have been developed in the direction of confirming that both factors are effective in influencing happiness.

This is confirmed by the fact that the modification or criticism of the adaptation theory has been connected to the acceptance of external environmental factors, and the modification or criticism of the reaction theory has been connected to the acceptance of internal propensity factors. That is, unless adhering to the typical prototype of each theoretical model, both theories have followed the direction of linkage or integration. We find this possibility in Lucas and Diener (2009), well-known happiness researchers. They acknowledged the stability of personality, the basis of adaptation theory, but also showed a reservation for it. They stated that personality is stable over time, but can change over time. In addition, they stated that personality is important for determining the level of happiness, thus forming a set point, while situations and life circumstances can in some cases have considerable influence as well. Accordingly, they conclude that set point theory is "moderately supported not definitely" from the standpoint of acknowledging the influence of the environment while acknowledging personality-based adaptation. Although not explicitly mentioned, the same logic could have been applied to the reaction theory. Similarly, several studies support an integrated approach of simultaneously accepting personal disposition and external environment as explanatory factors of happiness (Brief et al., 1993; Lance et al., 1995; Maggino, 2015; Sirgy, 2001 etc.). Such a possibility has been suggested in the aforementioned study by Max-Neef (1991).

Figure 2 is an integrated model for the decision of subjective wellbeing proposed by Brief et al. (1993: 648), which shows that personality trait and external circumstances are simultaneously linked to happiness. Their framework posits that both objective life circumstances and global personality indirectly affect SWB through their effects on the interpretation of life circumstances. It was tested both cross-sectionally and longitudinally with a sample of approximately 375 men and women. Personality was operationalized in terms of the dispositional trait negative affectivity

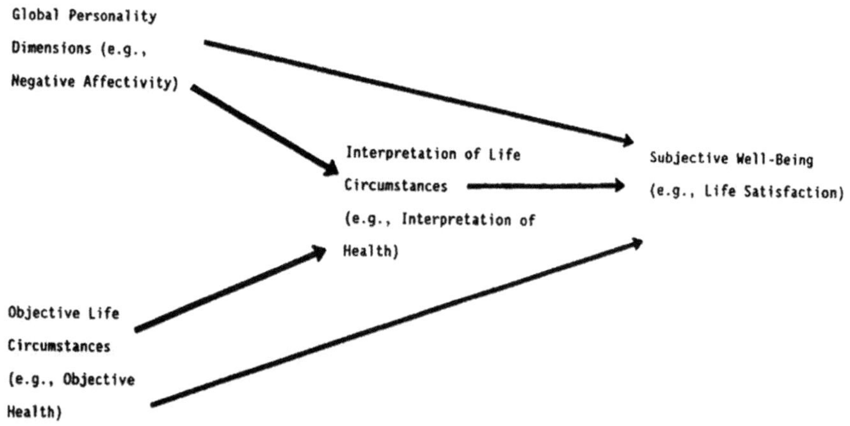

Fig. 2 Integrating adaptation (downward diffusion) and reactivity (upward diffusion) models (Brief et al., 1993: 648)

Table 1 Direction of happiness level according to personality and environment characteristics

		Personality types		
		Aspiration escalating	Aspiration restraining	Aspiration adapting
Environment change (events)	Positive	Little change in happiness	Increase in happiness	Little change in happiness
	Negative	Decrease in happiness	Little change in happiness	Little change in happiness

(NA), and the measure of life circumstance investigated was health. The analytical result strongly supported the model. However, there still remains an uncertain aspect about the interaction between the environment and personal preferences in the decision-making process. To confirm this, it may be worthwhile to verify a revised model in which an individual's propensity acts as a moderating variable in the relationship of the influence of the environment on happiness, or another model in which the environment acts as a moderating variable in the relationship of an impact of personal propensity on happiness.

Along with the identification of the paths between environment, personality trait, and happiness, another important issue is how happiness varies according to the difference in environmental factors and personality. In this regard, I would like to present a hypothesis on the direction of change in happiness according to environmental characteristics and personality types (see Table 1). This is meaningful as an attempt to take into account the differential effect of environmental characteristics and individual personality on happiness as an effort to integrate the two factors of happiness.

To put it simply, reactivity theory has a tendency to presume uniformly that a positive environment has a positive effect on happiness and a negative environment has a negative effect. This assumption comes from disregarding the effect of personality on happiness. The adaptation theory has also exhibited a similar pattern. In other words, it has focused on the assumption that individual personality neutralizes environmental impact and has not paid much attention to the fact that adaptation patterns can change depending on individual personality traits, and accordingly, the impact on happiness may vary. It goes without saying that the effect of the environment on happiness was neglected. However, the individual's reaction to the environment becomes varied in its influence on happiness when it intersects with the personality traits of the individual, and the individual's adaptation to the environment also becomes varied in its influence on happiness when it intersects with the environmental characteristics. That is, when considering environmental characteristics and personality traits at the same time, the effects of adaptation and reaction on happiness that the existing adaptation theory or reactivity theory assumes, respectively, are not uniform and become more variable. How does it change then?

To answer the question, it is necessary to categorize the environment and personality traits. First, environments are simply classified into a positive environment and a negative environment. Personality types of individuals are categorized into an aspiration escalating type (unsatisfying personality type), an aspiration restraining type (or ascetic personality type), and an aspiration adapting type (or satisfaction personality type) based on the characteristic of individual aspirations. By crossing the environmental factors and personality factors, as shown in Table 1, the direction of happiness changes according to personality traits and environmental characteristics can be projected. For convenience, I will explain how personality traits affect happiness when combined with environmental traits.

First, aspiration escalating or unsatisfying personality is a type that seeks a higher level of satisfaction without being satisfied with the current state. Living in a society and forming relationships with others, individuals often compare their own condition with the condition of others. The question is the form of comparison. In comparing, the aspiration escalating personality pursues an upward comparison, a comparison with a higher level than their own, which is a negative factor for happiness (Schwarz & Strack, 1999). For this type of personality, a positive change in environment will not change the level of happiness due to the increase of aspirations that offset the increase in utility from the environment change. However, a negative change in environment will decrease the level of happiness due to the combining effect of the decrease in utility resulting from the environment change and personal frustration. In other words, for this type of personality, positive environmental changes have little effect, and negative environmental changes have amplified effects on happiness.

Second, the aspiration restraining or ascetic personality suppresses the aspiration itself and tolerates a lower level of desire than others. In comparing, there will be a downward comparison, which is a positive factor of happiness (Schwarz & Strack, 1999). For this type of personality, a positive change in environment will increase the level of happiness by suppressing aspirations along with the utility increase from the environment change. However, a negative change in environment will not change the level of happiness due to the effect of suppressing personal aspirations which offsets the utility decrease from the environment change.

Third, the aspiration adapting or satisfaction personality is a type that adapts to reality and is close to the personality type assumed by the set point theory. It is a personality type found in the "sour grapes and foxes" in Aesop's fables. This type is passive in comparing one's current condition with the condition of others, and therefore, there is little increase or decrease in happiness according to the comparison. For this personality type, a positive change in environment will not change the level of happiness due to increased aspiration that offsets the increased utility from the environment change. A negative change in environment will also have little effect on happiness levels due to the effect of personal adaptation that offsets the reduced utility from the environment change.

Thus far, we have discussed the explanatory models for determining happiness. Evaluation of the necessity of public policies for promoting happiness varies depending on which approach you take. There will be limitations in setting the role of the government based on the adaptation theory or the downward theory, and if the reaction theory or the upward theory is accepted, policy efforts to improve the external environment for the promotion of happiness will be supported (Ko, 2013: 8; Veenhoven 1991a, 1991b). According to an integrated perspective, the support and direction of happiness policy will differ depending on the relative importance between the two factors, adaptation and reactivity, or the linkage between the two. It should be noted that most of the discussion of adaptation theory, reactivity theory, or integrated model focuses on affect or satisfaction, but little on eudaimonia. However, since happiness includes the eudaimonic aspect, not just affect or satisfaction, it will be necessary to expand this interest. Although existing studies did not explicitly cover the components of happiness in searching for the factors influencing happiness, the core hypothesis of each theory can be applied to all components of happiness in principle.

2 Factors Influencing Happiness

A discussion of factors influencing happiness is important for promoting happiness. This is like having a diagnosis before treating a patient. Diagnosis requires an understanding of the patient's current state and analyzing the cause of the disease. Likewise, the measurement of the actual state of happiness and the identification of factors influencing happiness become a basic requirement for happiness promotion. This knowledge is particularly important to policymakers.

This is because if they do not have knowledge about the actual state of happiness and the influencing factors, they not only waste resources, but also harm happiness through wrong policies. The discussion on the explanatory models of happiness presented above is actually about the relative importance between external conditions and individual personality as factors influencing happiness. However, even if external conditions are more important, internal factors cannot be ignored, and vice versa. Despite the differences in relative importance, both have been discussed as important factors influencing happiness. The integrated perspective is based on this understanding. Nonetheless, in the happiness policy process, the influencing factor that is of primary interest should be the external environmental condition rather than the individual personality. The reason for this is as follows.

First, the purpose of public policy is basically to pursue changes in external conditions. Happiness policy is also basically a government activity that attempts to influence happiness through changes in external conditions. Of course, it is not that internal personality cannot be a policy object. However, in general, public policy focuses on changes in external conditions. Second, efforts to change personality through public policy are both normatively and practically limited. If a policy that pursues a change in personality exceeds a certain threshold, there is a risk of infringing too much on individual autonomy, and even if it does not, it is unlikely that personality can change significantly by policy, considering the basic argument of the adaptation theory. Third, compared to the progress of discussions on the relationship between personal disposition and happiness so far, evidence for a causal relationship between external conditions and happiness is insufficient. If this situation persists, it will result in the waste of resources and efforts put into policy. Therefore, even if there is some trial and error in the early stage, it is necessary to stabilize the effectiveness of happiness policy based on the accumulation of practical knowledge between external conditions and happiness in the policy process. Based on this recognition, the next section discusses which factors have meaningful influences on happiness, focusing on external environmental conditions.

In the 2000s, research on factors influencing happiness increased significantly (e.g., Diener et al., 1993; Dorn et al., 2007; Easterlin, 2001; Eren & Aşıcı, 2016; Frey & Stutzer, 2000, 2010; Hartog & Oosterbeek 1998; Kahneman & Krueger, 2006; Mizobuchi, 2017; Oshio, 2017; Ott, 2011; Rode, 2013 etc.). Regarding external conditions, the classification criteria adopted by various studies are the nature of factors such as politics, economy, social, culture, and demographic factors (Jang, 2011; Kim, 2016), income versus non-income factors (Lim et al., 2016), individual, regional, or national level (Eren & Aşıcı, 2016; Oshio, 2017; Thin, 2012). Here, influencing factors of happiness will be discussed by dividing them into individual-level and collective-level factors.

2.1 *Influencing Factors at the Individual Level*

Besides personality, influencing factors of happiness at the individual level include a variety of external factors such as marriage, family and friendships, social relationships, community services, charity, employment, perceived health, religion, volunteering, and political (Bok, 2010: 17). The first factor to be mentioned is individual personality. As we have seen in the discussion on the theory of adaptation in the previous chapter, personal disposition is a significant factor affecting happiness. The core argument of the adaptation theory is that an individual's personality is an important factor that determines happiness rather than external conditions. Such an approach has accumulated considerable theoretical and practical discussions centered on psychologists (e.g., Cummins, 2018; Diener, 1984; Kahneman, 1999; Vittersø, 2013, etc.).

At the individual level, the external condition most often referred to as an influencing factor for happiness is income. As for the effect of individual income on happiness, the argument for substantial effectiveness and the argument for limited effectiveness are in opposition. The substantial effect approach considers that income is a significant influencing factor for happiness. Income gives people opportunities to do what they want, enables them to obtain the goods and services they need, and permits them to enjoy a higher socioeconomic status. In this way, income, an important means of satisfying needs, is widely recognized as a significant influencing factor of happiness. Also, this perception is empirically supported in several studies. Frey and Stutzer (2002a, 2002b) found a strong correlation between income and happiness in both periods in a panel data survey of Americans, 1972–1974 and 1994–1996: In the lowest decile of income, the mean happiness scores were 1.92 (for 1972–74) and 1.94 (for 1994–96), for the fifth decile the score was 2.19, and for the tenth and highest decile, it was 2.36. Di Tella et al. (1999)'s analysis of the data for Europe from the Eurobarometer Survey Series (1975–91) reported a similar result: In the upper quartile of the income bracket, 88% of persons rated themselves to be "fairly satisfied" or "very satisfied," while in the lowest income percentile, only 66% of those rated likewise. Veenhoven (1991a, 1991b) argued that the claim that happiness is relative is untrue, and poor living conditions such as war or isolation, including poverty, are a direct cause of deterioration of happiness. Of course, income is included in such conditions.

On the other hand, there is a position that income is not a significant influencer of happiness. Easterlin (2001: 465) conducted an empirical study to find out whether individual income can bring greater happiness. He proved that happiness temporarily increases with expectations for the future at the beginning of income growth, but aspirations increase with income over the life cycle, reducing the effect of income on happiness. Diener et al. (1993) reported that, in an analysis of the effect of individual income level on wellbeing, income change in poor areas has some effect on wellbeing, but the connection between income change and subjective wellbeing is not supported overall. Kahneman et al. (2006) argue as follows based on the results of a survey: "The belief that high income is associated with good mood is widespread but mostly illusory. People with above-average income are relatively satisfied with their lives but are barely happier than others in moment-to-moment experience. Moreover, the effect of income on life satisfaction seems to be transient. …[P]eople exaggerate the effect of income to happiness because they tend to focus on conventional achievements when evaluating life." In addition, several studies such as Inglehart et al. (2008), Layard (2005), and Luttmer (2004) also argue that the effect of increasing happiness on income is limited. This argument corresponds to the adaptation theory or set point theory.

Despite the debate over the happiness effect of income, whether it is large or small, stable or unstable, it is certain that income is a positive influencing factor for happiness. In empirical studies, the correlation between income and happiness was small to moderate (around 0.2, Diener & Oishi, 2000; Diener et al., 1999). The strength of correlations is not high, but it is difficult to find a negative evidence. However, as the low correlation indicates, income is not a variable that sufficiently predicts the level of happiness. Income is an important factor, but may not be the most important factor.

Another factor that is being actively studied in relation to determinants of happiness at the individual level is education (Eren & Aşıcı, 2016; Hartog & Oosterbeek 1998; Kahneman & Krueger, 2006; Koo et al., 2014; Mizobuchi, 2017; Michalos, 2008; Subramanian et al., 2005). Education, along with health and income, is a key item of UNDP's "Human Development Index (HDI)." Many studies support education as a positive influencer of happiness. For example, Hartog and Oosterbeek (1998) analyzed the effects of wealth, education, and health on happiness for the Dutch, and the analytical results showed that education, along with health, is a strong influencing factor of happiness. A study by Subramanian et al. (2005) found that the higher the level of education, the more likely respondents perceived that they were healthier and happier. On the other hand, there is also a study showing limited effects of education on happiness. Michalos (2008) argues that overall support for the impact of education on happiness is not great. He points out that despite many studies that support the positive effects of education, in general, evidence for the effectiveness of education in terms of happiness is not strong. In this regard, he points out that Witter et al. (1984), based on a review of 90 American studies, concluded that educational attainment accounts for between 1 and 3% of the variance in adult subjective wellbeing. Also, he cites as an example Layard (2005: 62)'s statement that "education has only a small direct effect on happiness, though of course it raises happiness by raising a person's income.'' Instead, Michalos argues that if happiness is understood in the robust eudaimonist sense of overall human wellbeing, then education evidently has an enormous impact. He also suggests that related studies will be able to more appropriately evaluate the effects of education on happiness by paying more attention to indirect effects as well as direct effects of education.

Unemployment is an important factor that hinders happiness. Clark and Oswald (1994) reported that unemployment was a more serious detrimental factor than divorce or separation in an analysis of the British Household Panel Study. However, there was a difference in the degree of the impact, and it was found that young people, local workers with a high unemployment rate, and long-term unemployment were relatively less unhappy. Winkelmann and Winkelmann (1998) argued that because unemployment has a large negative impact on life satisfaction, income must be increased by 7 times to offset this.

In addition to the variables discussed above, demographic factors such as health, family and social relations, marriage, religion, sex, and age are also included as variables affecting happiness at the individual level (Blanchflower & Oswald, 2005; Eren & Aşıcı, 2016; Kahneman & Krueger, 2006; Rode, 2013; Shin, 2015, etc.). In general, rather than focusing on only one variable, most studies combine and analyze all the factors that may affect happiness. For example, Kahneman and Krueger (2006) presents recent environmental changes as a list of factors that influence happiness such as smiling frequency, eye smile, the level of happiness evaluated by friends, the frequency of the verbal expression of positive emotions, sociability and extraversion, sleep quality, friends' evaluation of the happiness level, self-evaluation of the happiness level, wages within the reference group, socioeconomic status, active involvement in religion, marriage, income growth and so on. Mizobuchi (2017) presents the factors of happiness in 11 socioeconomic dimensions, including sensitivity, housing, income, occupation, community, education, environment, civic participation, health, safety, and work–life balance. Eren and Aşıcı (2016) present the following 14 items as factors influencing happiness: sex, level of education, marital status and marriage satisfaction, employment and satisfaction. and employment satisfaction, materialism, degree of hope, household income, household income satisfaction, satisfaction from housing, satisfaction from friends' network, self-reported health, perception of safety, comparisons to 5 years before, expectations from 5 years later.

2.2 Influencing Factors at the Collective (National) Level

Influencing factors of happiness at the collective level include political, economic, and social factors. That is, the structural factors of the community affect the happiness of individual members.

Political Factors

There is less research on political factors related to happiness than studies on economic factors or psychological factors. Among them, the main items presented as political factors affecting happiness at the collective level include democracy, rule of law, freedom of politics, efficiency of government, and transparency of government, corruption, etc. (Bennett & Nikolaev, 2016; Dorn et al., 2007; Frey & Stutzer, 2000; Helliwell & Huang, 2008; Inglehart & Klingemann, 2000; Ott, 2001; Veenhoven, 1990, etc.). The object of most interest is how democracy is related to happiness, and several studies report that countries with developed democracy have a high level of national happiness. For example, Inglehart and Klingemann (2000: 179–180) found that in an analysis of World Happiness Survey (WVS) data, flourishing of democratic institutions is closely related to happiness ($r = 0.78$). Frey and Stutzer (2002a, 2002b: 143) reported the more democracy and the more decentralization, the happier people tend to be in a study of Cantons in Switzerland. According to them, there was an 11% difference in happiness level between residents living in regions with the highest democracy index and those in the regions with lowest index, and a difference of 3.2% between residents in areas with a high degree of devolution and those in areas with a low degree of devolution. In addition to these, Dorn et al. (2007), Inglehart and Welzel (2005), Inglehart et al. (2008), Haller and Hadler (2006), Ott (2001), Rode (2013), Veenhoven (2000), Welsch (2003), report that democracy is an important factor for promoting the happiness of people.

Other political factors have been suggested as important factors influencing happiness. Such factors include government efficiency, government transparency, government regulation, and corruption control (Bennett & Nikolaev, 2016; Dorn et al., 2007; Frey & Stutzer, 2000; Helliwell & Huang, 2008; Ott, 2001, 2005), and political freedom (Bennett, 2016; Inglehart et al., 2008; Kalmijn et al., 2005; Veenhoven, 2000), political stability, rule of law, and civic participation (Kaufmann et al. 2007).

There are also discussions on how government policy relates to happiness. Layard (2005) is a leading scholar on the positivity of happiness policy. He proposes various policies such as wealth redistribution through higher taxation, work–life balance, controlling advertisement, employment protection, promotion of social capital, caring mental health to promote national happiness, etc. Similarly, Bok (2010) suggests happiness policies for child care, education, marriage and family, leisure, employment, health care, retirement income, urban commuting, etc. Halpern (2010), under the premise that a smooth relationship between citizens is more important than economic growth as a cause of happiness, proposes various policies for promoting happiness polices such as promoting parenting and care skills, supporting complementary currencies, supply of information to and from citizen consumers, responses to local and global environmental threats, fighting drug and sex pathologies, devolution and democratic innovation, etc. There are also empirical studies examining the relationship between government policy and happiness. Most of these studies are characterized by a focus on government spending. Pacek and Radcliff (2008) find, in a comparative analysis of 18 industrial democracies from 1981 to 2000, that welfare state generosity exerts a positive and significant impact on life satisfaction and happiness (see also Radcliff, 2001). Rothstein (2010) argues that the universal welfare state has a positive relationship with happiness, by increasing economic and social equality, promoting common values among people, and generating procedural fairness. Bjørnskov et al. (2007) and Kacapyr (2008) found that fiscal decentralization has a positive relationship with happiness, and Ram (2009) reported that in a comparative study of 140 countries, government expenditure was not significant, but had a positive relationship with the level of happiness.

There is also skepticism. Veenhoven (2000) performed a comparative study of 41 nations from 1980 to 1990 and found that welfare expenditures (measured by social security expenditures) is not related to the wellbeing of citizens (measured by the degree to which they lead healthy and happy lives) or equality in wellbeing among citizens. However, he does not deny the policy effect on happiness. Veenhoven (2004a, 2004b) found that social policies that promote the rule of law and civil rights, economic freedom, and tolerance of minorities are positively correlated with popular happiness. He adopts the position that an appropriate happiness policy is useful. Kacapyr (2008) found no significant association between the size of government spending and life satisfaction. Bjørnskov et al. (2007) reported that life satisfaction is negatively related to government consumption in a cross-sectional analysis of 74 countries. Yamamura (2011) reported negative correlation between government expenditure and life satisfaction when government size impedes economic growth.

Some studies report that the relationship between government policy and happiness is not uniformly positive or negative, but rather appears differently depending on the situation or policy types. For example, Ott (2011) reported that the relation between the size of government and national happiness depends heavily on the quality of government in a comparative study of 130 countries. Specifically, the good-big government was positively related to happiness, but the bad-big government was not. Based on this result, he suggested that the quality of the government is more important than the simple size of the government (measured by consumption and expenditures), and that, for the quality of government, technical quality (such as government effectiveness, regulatory quality, rule of law, and corruption control) is more important than the democratic quality of the government (such as voice and accountability, and political stability). Gao and Meng (2015), in an analysis of five rounds of surveys on Chinese elders across 22 provinces between 1998 and 2008, reported that the size of the government had a negative effect on the satisfaction of the elderly in general, but the effect was different depending on regional characteristics. In more developed regions, negative effects of government size were found, and positive effects were stronger in less developed regions. Kim et al. (2015) found that public services of local governments in Korea have a positive effect on the happiness of residents, but the magnitude of the influence was different depending on the quality of life of the target group. Bjørnskov (2005), in an analysis of the results of a three-year survey (1973, 1982, 2002) of nine European countries, found that democracy or welfare expenditures had no significant relationship with happiness, but that policies for growth, trade, business, or revenue reduction were associated with happiness. This shows that the effect of happiness can be different depending on the type of policy.

Overall, public policy is an important influence variable related to happiness, but unequivocal conclusions have not been reached on the direction and mode of its effect. With the accumulation of additional research in the future, a clearer demonstration of the policy effect will be needed. It should be indicated that there are different opinions on the necessity of the happiness policy per se. For example, Thin (2012: 84–89) criticizes that even if we concede the legitimacy of the purpose for such active happiness policies as Layard proposes, it is excessively interventionistic and undesirable for the government to actively pursue such policies. He also points out that it is difficult to find substantial evidence to support the assumptions about the relationship between happiness and the policies proposed by the active proponents of happiness policy. He then argues that between ignoring happiness, and seizing it as the sole objective, there is a wide range of government options and responsibilities. Of course, excessive government intervention has the danger of violating privacy, freedom, and autonomy. If, however, government policy does not have to promote happiness as the sole goal, these concerns need not be considered as a total denial of the happiness policy. It is understood that Thin also expresses the necessity of approaching the happiness policy from a balanced standpoint rather than completely denying the necessity of government's policy. The question is at what level and what type of happiness policy should be pursued? To help make this decision, more research on the causal relationship between policy and happiness is needed. Although the happiness policy encompasses policies in various fields, most of the related studies have been centered on government expenditures, and the verification of the relationship between various policy proposals and happiness is still in dearth.

In exploring the relationship between public policy and happiness, it should be recognized that policy itself is an element of social conditions and at the same time constructs other social conditions. For example, environmental policy is itself a social condition and at the same time a factor influencing environmental conditions. In other words, the effects of government policies on happiness include direct effects on happiness and indirect effects through construction of other external conditions. Nevertheless, if attention is focused only on the direct effect in the analysis of the relationship between policy and happiness, the total effect of public policy on happiness cannot be adequately captured. This point suggests that on the one hand, a more detailed understanding of the path through which government policy affects happiness is required and, on the other hand, prematurely ignoring the usefulness of government policy be restrained.

Basically, the questions raised about the happiness policy are related to the policy objective and the effect of the happiness policy. In response to this, the next chapter discusses the necessity of a happiness policy in more detail.

Economic Factors

Among the economic variables discussed as a factor influencing happiness at the collective level, the key variable is national income (GDP). If national income increases, does the level of happiness increase? Until the recent rise of interest in happiness research, it was considered common sense that if the country's income level is high, people's level of happiness would also be high. Of course, this common sense has not been proved in a situation where comparative studies of happiness between countries rarely exist, but it is implicitly supported by the fact that most happiness studies have reported that richer people in individual countries enjoy higher levels of happiness. However, this common sense faces a critical challenge. Richard Easterlin (1974) in his seminal work "Does Economic Growth Improve the Human Lot? Some Empirical Evidence" discovered that countries with higher average incomes do not show higher levels of happiness. This is the well-known Easterlin paradox, and as a result of this study, follow-up studies focusing on the relationship between wealth and happiness have been actively progressing to support or supplement Easterlin's hypothesis (e.g., Choudhary et al., 2012; Clark, 2016; Eren & Aşıcı, 2016; Graham, 2011; Pugno, 2009; Sacks et al., 2012 etc.).

Nevertheless, there is still strong support for the relationship between national income and the level of happiness of the people. For example, Di Tella et al. (2003) argue that GDP is an important variable for a country's level of happiness. Hagerty and Veenhoven (2003) reported that there was a positive relationship between income growth and national happiness through a time series analysis of 21 countries from 1958 to 1996. Veenhoven and Vergunst (2014) demonstrated that income growth and national happiness had a positive relationship based on the analytical results of 67 countries over a period of 40 years. In addition, a study by Howell and Howell (2008) empirically revealed that the positive relationship between income and happiness was strong in countries with low national income. Stevenson and Wolfers (2013) argued that income is a significant influencer of happiness regardless of space and time, based on the analytical results of long-term data. More specifically, they reported that each country's GDP per capita had a "clear positive link" with subjective well-being, and there was no evidence of a satiation point beyond which wealthier countries have no further increases in subjective wellbeing. They also reported that the relationship between income and subjective wellbeing across countries was similar to the relationship within countries, which was similar to the time series relationship, the happiness of countries at different points in time as they became richer or poorer. Such results emphasize the importance of absolute income rather than relative comparison with respect to happiness and at the same time directly denies the Easterlin-like hypotheses.[2] Subsequent studies including these, found that the relationship between national income and happiness is quite close in analyses of various data on more countries (Diener et al., 2009: 85).

[2] In addition, there are criticisms regarding Easterlin's paradox for targeting only a small number of countries for comparison, adopting a one-time cross-sectional analysis rather than a time-series analysis, and only comparing between countries.

There are also approaches to resolve the conflict between the positions. In relation to the model for determining happiness, both positions can be viewed as corresponding to adaptation theory and reactivity theory, respectively (Graham et al., 2010). For example, Graham (2011: 17) found on average, wealthier countries are happier than poor ones (R-squared = 0.498). However, the level of happiness increases up to a certain level of national income, but does not increase beyond that, and it is difficult to find a clear correlation between income level and happiness even in low-income countries. Kroll (2008) argues that national income is important for happiness, especially in developing countries. However, it is reported that in the short term the relationship between GDP and happiness is positive, but in the long run, the relationship between the two is weaker, as the Easterlin Paradox found. Clark et al., (2008: 101) point out that the Easterlin paradox is about the relationship between national income and national happiness and that the results of conventional research on the relationship between personal income and personal happiness is based on the concept of relative income. As shown in Fig. 3, the increase in personal happiness due to the increase in income within a country is more significant than the increase in income and happiness at the national level. This can be seen from the fact that the slope (dotted lines) of the relationship between income and happiness is steeper than the slope (thick lines) of the relationship between income and happiness at the national level. However, the slope of the relationship between individual income and happiness within a country becomes flatter as the average income of the country increases (t0 → t1 → t2). This is because when the state and individual get rich (t2) the collective utility due to the high-income level of the country is minimized, but the status return due to the individual's higher income promotes the individual's well-being. Basically, Easterlin's paradox does not deny the general relationship between income and happiness at the individual level, but it shows that there is not an increase in the level of happiness corresponding to the increase in income at the national level.

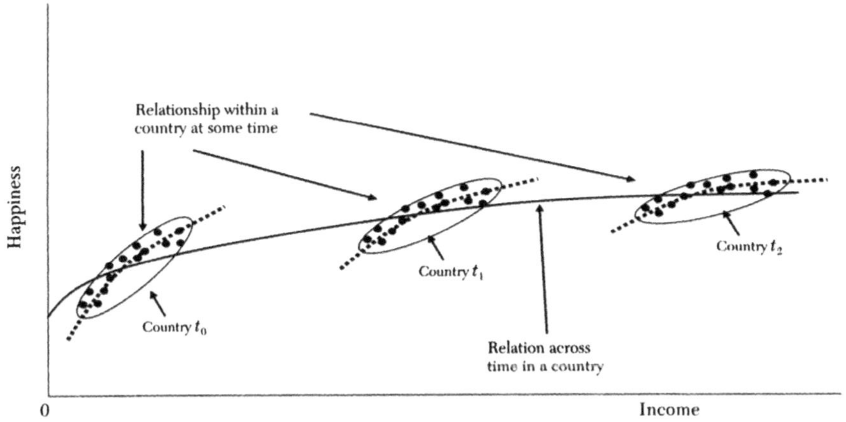

Fig. 3 Relationship between income and happiness: individual and national level (Clark et al., 2008)

In this regard, Clark et al.'s explanatory model is evaluated as a useful contribution to resolving the discrepancy between the Easterlin paradox and the existing theoretical view on the relationship between income and happiness.

The distribution of income (or inequality), as well as the income level of the country, is another important factor influencing people's wellbeing. However, positions differ regarding how income inequality affects national happiness. Several studies suggest that income inequality and happiness have a negative relationship. Graham and Felton (2006) found that income inequality negatively affects happiness in an analysis of the Latino-barometer survey. O'Connell (2004) assessed the interrelationship between wealth (GDP per capita), equality of income, and mean satisfaction for 15 EU countries between 1995 and 1998, and found that income distribution equality has a greater impact on satisfaction than absolute income. In addition, several studies reported that happiness decreases as income inequality increases (Delhey & Dragolov 2014; Gandelman & Porzecanski, 2013; Hagerty & Veenhoven, 2003; Jang, 2011; Kalmijn et al., 2005; O'Connell, 2004; Oshio & Kobayashi, 2011; Oshio & Urakawa, 2014; Ott, 2005).

On the contrary, some studies maintain that income inequality is not an impediment to happiness, but rather increases happiness. Clark (2003) used data from the British Household Panel Survey (from 1991 to 2002) and found that regional inequality and life satisfaction are positively correlated. He posited that for these respondents, inequality is a sign of opportunity. Eggers et al. (2006), in their study on the effect of regional unemployment rates on subjective wellbeing in post-Soviet Russia, found that respondents, both employed and unemployed, are happier in regions with higher unemployment rates. Their interpretation was that respondents in a troubled region lower their aspiration level ceteris paribus and perceive themselves to be better off in worse times.

Some studies have shown that income inequality is not a significant influencer, whether positive or negative, of happiness. Becchetti et al. (2014) analyzed the increase in happiness inequality between 1992 and 2007, by using the German Socio-Economic Panel (GSOEP) data base, and found that income inequality cannot be considered as a driver of happiness inequality. Haller and Hadler (2006) analyzed the data of the World Value Survey (1995–1997) and concluded that the economic wealth of nation and the distribution of income are more related to welfare state or political freedom than to happiness. Stevenson and Wolfers (2008) found that absolute levels of income are far more important in shaping happiness than relative income comparisons.

The relationship between income inequality and happiness can appear differently depending on group characteristics. Alesina et al. (2004) found that individuals are less happy when inequality is high, even after controlling for individual income, personal characteristics, and year and residence. But they also found that there are differences across groups. In Europe, the poor and the political left are unhappy about income inequality, whereas in the USA the happiness of the poor and politically left-leaning is uncorrelated with inequality. They explain this difference is due to the fact that Americans' expectations for social class mobility are greater than Europeans' expectations for social class mobility. Similarly, Kim (2016) found that in a study of Koreans, overall income inequality is negatively associated with happiness, but when the expectation for social class mobility is included as a moderator variable, the moderating effect was not evident in the group that perceived the possibility of social upward mobility to be high, but the negative relationship was aggravated in the group that perceived the possibility of social upward mobility to be low.

Borrowing from welfare theories, Verme (2011) proposes that the impact of income inequality on happiness can be positive (Hirschman & Rothschild, 1973) or negative (Runciman, 1966). The former, called the "tunnel effect theory," posits that income inequality has a positive impact on happiness by raising individual expectations for future social mobility, while the latter posits that income inequality has a negative impact due to relative deprivation. Verme used data from the European and the World Values Surveys between 1981 and 2004 to test the conflicting hypotheses and found that income inequality has a consistent, negative and significant effect on life satisfaction when a standard happiness model is used.

Nonetheless, he indicated that such results may vary due to multicollinearity depending on data sets, number of countries, and years of observations. In addition, he maintained that it may be due to this problem that the results of existing empirical studies on the relationship between income and inequality produce different results. In the end, Verme was not able to resolve clearly the conflict in existing research, but he properly suggested the direction for resolving the theoretical conflict.

Besides income and income inequality, scholars are analyzing the effects of several economic variables on happiness such as economic freedom, unemployment, inflation, labor market conditions, and taxes (Alesina et al., 2004; Bennett & Nikolaev, 2016; Di Tella et al., 2003; Frey & Stutzer, 2001, etc.).

Social and Cultural Factors

Socio-cultural factors are also studied as important influencing factors of happiness. The interest in social capital triggered by Putnam's (1995, 2000) seminal work has also been extended to happiness studies, and social capital occupies an important position in happiness studies. Helliwell (2003), using three successive waves of the World Values Survey between 1990 and 1997, revealed that social capital is directly and indirectly linked to wellbeing at the individual level and the social level. Kroll (2008) analyzed the impact of social capital on life satisfaction using World Value Survey data. The analytical result revealed that cognitive social capital (social trust) and structural social capital (membership and participation in associations) have a positive, significant but moderate effect on the life satisfaction, but linking social capital (trust in state institutions) did not have a significant effect. Overall, economic variables (e.g., GDP) was found to be a stronger influencing factor than social capital. Eren and Aşıcı (2018) found that in a survey analysis on the level of happiness in Turkey, even though Turkey's GDP increased for 10 years from 2004 to 2014, the level of happiness remained almost unchanged. It was argued that the cause was not an economic factor, but rather an informal social network.

In addition, various studies have examined the relationship between happiness and social–cultural factors such as social relationship, civic participation, social capital, and inequality in society (Bennett & Nikolaev, 2016; Eren & Aşıcı, 2018; Kalmijn et al., 2005; Ott, 2005; Paralkar et al. 2017; Rode, 2013; Welzel & Inglehart, 2008, etc.).

2.3 Summing up

Research on various influencing factors were presented above by dividing them into individual and collective dimensions. However, it is still not easy to comprehensively understand the research progress and results because various research results have been presented for a wide variety of correlates. In this regard, Veenhoven (1991a, 1991b)'s summary of the existing research results provides useful help in grasping the contour of the related research progress.

> "At the risk of simplifying too much, one could characterize the results as follows: Happy persons are more likely to be found in the economically prosperous countries, where freedom and democracy are held in respect and the political scene is stable. The happy are more likely to be found in majority groups than among minorities and more often at the top of the social ladder than at the bottom. They are typically married and get on well with families and friends. In respect of their personal characteristics, the happy appear relatively healthy, both physically and mentally. They are active and open minded. They feel they are in control of their lives. Their aspirations concern social and moral matters rather than money making. In matter of politics, the happy tend to be at the conservative side of the middle."

Apart from the basic understanding of the contents, some notes about the discussion on influencing factors of happiness are necessary. First, external factors may be influencing happiness, but they may also be the result of happiness. Therefore, it is necessary to examine the causal relationship between various external conditions and happiness. It is also important because identifying the cause of happiness is an essential prerequisite for the effectiveness of happiness policy. Second, although income is still an important influencing factor, various political, economic, and sociocultural factors other than income are also related to happiness. Therefore, broad interest in the cause of happiness is required. Third, factors at the individual level and at the collective level are related to happiness at the same time. However, whether it is a variable at the individual level or a variable at the collective level, external factors are not reflected in happiness without additional influence. This is because, as suggested by the adaptive theory, external conditions, whether large or small, will undergo an individual-level interpretation process. Therefore, in the discussion of influencing factors, the interaction between individuals and conditions should be considered (Diener et al., 1999). Fourth, even with the same influencing factors, the influence may vary depending on the target group, region, culture, etc. Therefore, a more detailed analysis is needed on what conditions the relationship between external factors and happiness changes. Fifth, since happiness is multidimensional, it is necessary to recognize that even the same influencing factors can be differentiated depending on the components of happiness.

The fifth item requires further discussion. Diener et al. (2010) presented evidence that material variables were more closely related to life satisfaction than affect. They stated that in analyzing the relation between income and subjective wellbeing, it is important to distinguish between the affective and judgmental components of subjective wellbeing rather than to rely on measures of happiness as a whole. Similarly, Costa and McCrae (1980) found that the effect of personal disposition on happiness depends on the components of happiness. That is, extraversion affects positive affect and neuroticism affects negative affect, respectively. These studies together have shown that even the same factors have different influences depending on the components of happiness, or that factors that influence happiness may differ depending on the components of happiness. Unlike these, most studies of happiness have approached the topic as if the same influencing factors function in the same way regardless of the components of happiness. This approach has a problem of overlooking detailed information for each component of happiness, notwithstanding the advantage of comprehensively understanding the effects of influencing factors. Also, such a problem can be an obstacle to the effective pursuance of the happiness policy. Suppose that a policy aiming at satisfaction, a component of happiness, is being implemented. In this case, the analysis of the influencing factor of happiness as a whole, instead of satisfaction, can hinder effective policy implementation by distorting the estimates of the causal relationship between the influencing factor and happiness. Therefore, in discussing the influencing factors of happiness, it is necessary to pay proper attention not only to happiness as a whole, but also to partial happiness as suggested by Diener et al. (2010).

In this regard, Lee and Lee (2017), using the survey data from the 2014 National Awareness Research on the Government Role and Quality of Life by the Center for Survey Research in GSPA, Seoul National University, performed an empirical analysis on the influencing factors of local residents' happiness. Political, economic, and social variables were adopted as independent variables, and overall happiness and three components of happiness (feeling, satisfaction, and life meaning) were included as an indicator of happiness, the dependent variable. In employing the dependent measures, this research is differentiated from most existing studies in that it encompasses not only affect or satisfaction but also meaning of life along with overall happiness. The analysis results presented in Table 2 show that the influence of the independent variable on happiness is different for each of the three components of happiness. Income has a significant relationship with satisfaction, but not with affect. Income inequality did not have a significant relationship with affect and satisfaction, but only with meaning. Other independent variables turn out to have differential associations depending on the overall happiness or the components of happiness. Such results reaffirm the necessity of paying attention not only to happiness as a whole, but also to partial happiness in research on the factors influencing happiness.

3 Analysis of Factors Influencing Public Happiness

In the study of factors influencing public happiness, the definition of the dependent variable is as important as the identification of independent variables. Unlike

Table 2 Differential effects of influencing factors of happiness on happiness components (Lee & Lee, 2017)

		Overall happiness	Satisfaction	Feeling	Life meaning
Income inequality		−0.112	−0.09	0.057	−0.247**
Average income		0.204**	0.27***	0.030	−0.016
Local economy		0.055	0.02	0.137	−0.003
Density		−0.422**	−0.44**	−0.176	−0.334
Traffic safety level		0.030	0.04	0.028	−0.041
Local safety level		−0.045	−0.04	−0.022	−0.075
Water supply		0.326**	0.34**	0.083	0.290*
Education		−0.178*	−0.17*	−0.100	−0.156
Culture		−0.079	−0.05	−0.118	−0.055
Medical		0.036	0.05	0.087	−0.040
Welfare		−0.191**	−0.17**	−0.170**	−0.134*
Transparency		0.176**	0.18**	0.152**	0.064
Civil servant		−0.102	−0.07	−0.311**	0.089
Financial independence		−0.002	0.03	−0.177	0.088
Region type	metropolitan	0.169	0.16	0.224*	0.030
	Rural	0.206	0.23*	−0.057	0.202
Obs.		223			

*$P < 0.1$, **$P < 0.05$, ***$P < 0.001$

research on personal happiness, in research on public happiness, distribution should be a research interest in addition to the level of happiness. This is because public happiness is not happiness enjoyed by isolated individuals, but happiness enjoyed in connection with members of the community. Also, considering the meaning of relative deprivation in human happiness (Runciman, 1966; Stouffer et al., 1949), distribution can be a more important factor than the level of happiness. Bennett (2016) provides the following reasons for interest in research on the distribution of happiness. First, looking only at the levels of happiness could be misleading. In situations where the level of happiness increases, the distribution of happiness may deteriorate. Second, the goal of public policy can include not only improving the level of happiness, but also improving the distribution of happiness. Third, happiness distribution, as well as income distribution, may be an important factor affecting society. Notwithstanding such a necessity, most existing studies focus on the level of happiness, and only some studies are studying the distribution of happiness.

Veenhoven (1990) was the first study to focus on the distribution of happiness in a cross-country comparison. He measured the inequality of happiness for 28 countries. It was found that the distribution of happiness among countries was not bi-modal but uni-modal, and the degree of happiness distribution among countries was significantly different. More specifically, inequality in happiness appeared to be greater in the socioeconomically equal countries, and smaller in politically democratic and economically developed nations. And inequality in happiness appeared to be more closely related to social equality among richer nations than among less rich ones. Bennett and Nikolaev (2017) analyzed the relationship between economic freedom and happiness inequality in the surveyed countries using World Value Survey data and found economic freedom was negatively associated with happiness inequality. That is economic freedom reduces happiness inequality. For measures of happiness distribution, mean absolute difference, interquartile range, Gini coefficient, coefficient of variation, and standard deviation, were used. It was found that the relationship between economic freedom and happiness inequality did not change significantly depending on the indicator type, unlike in Kalmijn and Veenhoven (2005) that suggested standard deviation as the optimal indicator.

Ott (2005) examined both the level and distribution of happiness. Using the data of World Value Surveys (1999–2001), he examined the relationship between happiness levels and distribution in 78 target countries. For measures, the average of life satisfaction was used for the happiness level, and the standard deviation of life satisfaction was used for the happiness distribution. The analytical result showed that there was a negative correlation between happiness level and happiness inequality ($r = -0.65$ for all nations). More specifically, the correlation between the two in rich countries was stronger than that in poor countries (−0.74 for rich nations, −0.29 for poor nations). The gap between the level of happiness and equality was greater in poor countries than in rich countries. In addition, Ott analyzed the effects of 14 public conditions related to the level of happiness and inequality. As a result, except for income inequality, it was found that factors related to happiness level or distribution of happiness were the same independent variables. Based on these results, Ott argued that harmony determines the level and distribution of happiness rather than tension, and therefore, the position of utilitarians emphasizing happiness level and the position of egalitarians interested in happiness distribution are reconcilable. Ott's research is one of few exceptional studies that deal with level and distribution simultaneously; although methodologically, it has a limit of relying on a simple correlation analysis. A few other studies (e.g., Bennett, 2016; Kalmijn & Veenhoven, 2005) also contributed to the progress of happiness research by expanding research interests to the distribution of happiness beyond the level of happiness. However, there is still a lack of full-scale analysis of issues such as how the influencing factors will change depending on the level and distribution of happiness, or how the influencing factors will change when the level and distribution of happiness are integrated.

In this regard, Lee et al. (2020), employing data from the World Value Survey (2008–2018), examined the relationship between the influencing factors of happiness and happiness in 130 countries. This study is a multivariate analysis that includes important variables in the fields of politics, economy, and socio-culture over a period of more than 10 years, for a majority of countries. In addition, from a more comprehensive standpoint, the study employed as dependent variables the level and distribution of happiness, and gross public happiness which combines the two, and attempted to show that influencing factors differ depending on the components of dependent variables. One of the dependent variables, gross public happiness, was compose by combining the level and distribution (inequality) of happiness, and thus, there may be disagreements about combining the level and distribution of happiness, which can be a separate dimension. However, by calculating the gross index by combining the level and distribution, it provides a more concise and integrated information on the national happiness status, beyond considering the level or distribution. Independent variables included variables in the fields of politics, economy, and social culture. Political factors include confidence in national government, corruption, political stability, and voice and accountability. Economic factors include GDP per capita, economic inequality, and unemployment. Social and cultural factors include social support, life expectancy, freedom to make choice, generosity, and aging. As an analysis method, panel regression analysis based on a probability effect model was applied.

The analysis results are shown in Table 3 and show that the influencing factors are different depending on the dependent variables. Three variables (confidence in government, unemployment, social support) were found to be significant influencing factors for all happiness variables (level, distribution, gross happiness), but other variables were not. Specifically, perceptions of corruption and income inequality had a significant relationship with the distribution of happiness and gross happiness, but not with the level. Political stability had a significant relationship with the level of happiness and gross happiness, but not with the distribution. GDP and civic participation had a significant relationship with the level of happiness and gross happiness, but not with the distribution. Life expectancy and aging had a significant relationship with the level and distribution of happiness, but not with gross happiness. Freedom was found to be related only to the level of happiness. This result is different from that of Ott (2005), aforementioned study, which reported that the influencing factors related to the level and distribution of happiness were identical, except for income inequality. It seems that this difference is not due to the difference in the validity of the hypotheses, but rather due to the difference of research designs between this study and Ott's including the differences in the period analyzed (single year vs. multiple years), the analysis methods (correlation analysis vs. multivariate analysis), and the list of independent variables, etc. At any rate, the results of this study suggest that it is necessary to consider not only the influencing factors but also the attributes of the dependent variable in the discussion of the relationship between the influencing factor of happiness and happiness. In addition, it suggests that not only the level and distribution of happiness, but also an approach to assessing happiness from a more comprehensive perspective by combining both may be useful.

Table 3 Analysis of factors influencing happiness (level, distribution, total happiness

		Model 1	Model 2	Model 3
Dependent variables Independent variables		Happiness level	Happiness distribution	Gross happiness
Political variable	Confidence in national government	0.6042***	−0.1965**	1.0540***
		(0.1642)	(0.9079)	(0.2829)
	Perceptions of corruption	−0.1119	0.3706**	−0.9818**
		(0.2393)	(0.1350)	(0.4181)
	Political stability and absence of violence/terrorism	0.1420**	−0.0107	0.1611**
		(0.0512)	(0.0287)	(0.0891)
	Voice and accountability	0.2076***	−0.0185	0.2258**
		(0.0752)	(0.0432)	(0.1328)
Economic variable	GINI index	0.2970	0.7696**	−1.7558**
		(0.5906)	(0.3399)	(1.04489)
	Log GDP per capita	0.3914***	−0.0091	0.3461**
		(0.0839)	(0.0490)	(0.0845)
	Unemployment	−0.0409***	0.0116***	−0.0445***
		(0.0063)	(0.0035)	(0.0063)
Socio-cultural variables	Social support	1.9294***	-0.7056***	3.4255***
		(0.3548)	(1.997)	(0.6188)
	Life expectancy	0.0336***	0.0183***	-0.1524
		(0.0106)	(0.0062)	(0.0191)
	Freedom to make choice	0.1174	0.4544***	−1.0178
		(0.2361)	(0.1307)	(0.4076)
	Generosity	0.3578**	0.1259	0.0388
		(0.1788)	(0.0997)	(0.3101)
	Aging	−0.0297**	−0.0135*	0.0071
		(0.0142)	(0.0082)	(0.02522)
Environmental variable	Population density	−0.0003	−0.0001	−0.0001
		(0.0002)	(0.0002)	(0.0005)
Constant		−1.8178	0.5589	97.2284
		(0.7136)	(0.4166)	(1.2728)
Number of countries		133	133	133
R-sq.	Within	0.2733	0.1022	0.1928
	Between	0.7912	0.2700	0.6224
	Overall	0.7478	0.3332	0.6021
		584.03***	80.65***	255.28***

Standard errors in parentheses *$p < 0.1$, **$p < 0.05$, ***$p < 0.01$

References

Alderfer, C. P. (1969). An empirical test of a new theory of human needs. *Organizational Behavior and Human Performance, 4*(2), 142–175.

Alderfer, C. P. (1972). *Existence, relatedness, and growth: Human needs in organizational settings*. Free Press.

Alesina, A., Di Tella, R., & MacCulloch, R. (2004). Inequality and happiness: Are Europeans and Americans different? *Journal of Public Economics, 88*(9–10), 2009–2042.

Anglim, J., Weinberg, M. K., & Cummins, R. A. (2015). Bayesian hierarchical modeling of the temporal dynamics of subjective well-being: A 10 year longitudinal analysis. *Journal of Research in Personality, 59*, 1–14.

Becchetti, L., Massari, R., & Naticchioni, P. (2014). The drivers of happiness inequality: Suggestions for promoting social cohesion. *Oxford Economic Papers, 66*(2), 419–442.

Bennett, D. L. (2016). Subnational economic freedom and performance in the United States and Canada. *Cato Journal, 36*(1), 165–185.

Bennett, D. L., & Nikolaev, B. (2016). Factor endowments, the rule of law and structural inequality. *Journal of Institutional Economics, 12*(4), 773–795.

Bennett, D. L., & Nikolaev, B. (2017). Economic freedom and happiness inequality: Friends or foes? *Contemporary Economic Policy, 35*(2), 373–391.

Binswanger, M. (2006). Why does income growth fail to make us happier?: Searching for the treadmills behind the paradox of happiness. *The Journal of Socio-Economics, 35*(2), 366–381.

Bjørnskov, C. (2005). Life satisfaction: Is there a role for policy? *EEI Policy Paper No. 6*. Brussels: European Enterprise Institute.

Bjørnskov, C., Dreher, A., & Fischer, J. A. (2007). The bigger the better? Evidence of the effect of government size on life satisfaction around the world. *Public Choice, 130*(3), 267–292.

Blanchflower, D. G., & Oswald, A. (2005). Happiness and the human development index: The Paradox of Australia. *Australian Economic Review, 38*(3), 307–318.

Bok, D. (2010). *The politics of happiness: What government can learn from the new research on well-being*. Princeton University Press.

Boyce, C. J., & Wood, A. M. (2011). Personality prior to disability determines adaptation: Agreeable individuals recover lost life satisfaction faster and more completely. *Psychological Science, 22*(11), 1397–1402.

Brickman, P., & Campbell, D. T. (1971). Hedonic relativism and planning the good society. In M. H. Appley (Ed.), *Adaptation-level theory* (pp. 287–305). Academic Press.

Brief, A. P., Butcher, A. H., George, J. M., & Link, K. E. (1993). Integrating bottom-up and top-down theories of subjective well-being: The case of health. *Journal of Personality and Social Psychology, 64*(4), 646–653.

Bruni, L., & Porta, P. L. (Eds.). (2005). *Economics and happiness: Framing the analysis*. Oxford University Press.

Bruni, L., & Zamagni, S. (2007). *Civil economy: Efficiency, equity, public happiness*. Peter Lang.

Choudhary, M. A., Levine, P., McAdam, P., & Welz, P. (2012). The happiness puzzle: Analytical aspects of the Easterlin paradox. *Oxford Economic Papers, 64*(1), 27–42.

Clark, A. E. (2003). Inequality-aversion and income mobility: A direct test. *DELTA Working Paper 2003–11*. https://worlddatabaseofhappiness-archive.eur.nl/hap_bib/freetexts/clark_ae_2003.pdf. Accessed May 2, 2020.

Clark, A. E. (2016). Adaptation and the Easterlin paradox. In T. Tachibanaki (Ed.), *Advances in happiness research* (pp. 75–94). Springer.

Clark, A. E., & Oswald, A. J. (1994). Unhappiness and unemployment. *The Economic Journal, 104*(424), 648–659.

Clark, A. E., Frijters, P., & Shields, M. A. (2008). Relative income, happiness, and utility: An explanation for the Easterlin paradox and other puzzles. *Journal of Economic Literature, 46*(1), 95–144.

Costa, P. T., & McCrae, R. R. (1980). Influence of extraversion and neuroticism on subjective well-being: Happy and unhappy people. *Journal of Personality and Social Psychology, 38*(4), 668.

Cummins, R. A. (2005). The domains of life satisfaction: An attempt to order chaos. In A. C. Michalos (Ed.), *Citation classics from social indicators research* (pp. 559–584). Springer.

Cummins, R. A. (2010). Subjective wellbeing, homeostatically protected mood and depression: A synthesis. *Journal of Happiness Studies, 11*, 1–17.

Cummins, R. A. (2013). Measuring happiness and subjective well-being. In S. A. David, I. Boniwell, & A. Conley Ayers (Eds.), *Oxford handbook of happiness* (pp. 185–200). Oxford University Press.

Cummins, R. A. (2018). *Measuring and interpreting subjective wellbeing in different cultural contexts: A review and way forward*. Cambridge University Press.

Cummins, R. A., Li, N., Wooden, M., & Stokes, M. (2014). A demonstration of set-points for subjective wellbeing. *Journal of Happiness Studies, 15*(1), 183–206.

Delhey, J., & Dragolov, G. (2014). Why inequality makes Europeans less happy: The role of distrust, status anxiety, and perceived conflict. *European Sociological Review, 30*(2), 151–165.

Diener, E. (1984). Subjective well-being. *Psychological Bulletin, 95*(3), 542–575.

Diener, E., & Biswas-Diener, R. (2008). *Happiness: Unlocking the mysteries of psychological wealth*. Wiley-Blackwell.

Diener, E., & Oishi, S. (2000). Money and happiness: Income and subjective well-being across nations. In E. Diener & E. M. Suh (Eds.), *Culture and subjective well-being* (pp. 185–218). The MIT Press.

Diener, E., Sandvik, E., Seidlitz, L., & Diener, M. (1993). The relationship between income and subjective well-being: Relative or absolute? *Social Indicators Research, 28*(3), 195–223.

Diener, E., Suh, E. M., Lucas, R. E., & Smith, H. L. (1999). Subjective well-being: Three decades of progress. *Psychological Bulletin, 125*(2), 276–302.

Diener, E., Lucas, R., Schimmack, U., & Helliwell, J. (2009). *Well-Being for public policy*. Oxford University Press.

Diener, E., Ng, W., Harter, J., & Arora, R. (2010). Wealth and happiness across the world: Material prosperity predicts life evaluation, whereas psychosocial prosperity predicts positive feeling. *Journal of Personality and Social Psychology, 99*(1), 52–61.

Di Tella, R., MacCulloch, R. J., & Oswald, A. J. (1999). How do macroeconomic fluctuations affect happiness. Harvard Business School, Mimeo.

Di Tella, R., MacCulloch, R. J., & Oswald, A. J. (2003). The macroeconomics of happiness. *Review of Economics and Statistics, 85*(4), 809–827.

Dorn, D., Fischer, J. A., Kirchgässner, G., & Sousa-Poza, A. (2007). Is it culture or democracy? The impact of democracy and culture on happiness. *Social Indicators Research, 82*(3), 505–526.

Duesenberry, J. S. (1949). *Income, saving, and the theory of consumer behavior*. Harvard University Press.

Easterlin, R. A. (1973). Does money buy happiness? *The Public Interest, 30*(3), 3–10.

Easterlin, R. A. (1974). Does economic growth improve the human lot? Some empirical evidence. In P. A. David & M. W. Reder (Eds.), *Nations and households in economic growth* (pp. 89–125). Academic Press.

Easterlin, R. A. (2001). Income and happiness: Towards a unified theory. *The Economic Journal, 111*(473), 465–484.

Easterlin, R. A. (2003). Explaining happiness. *Proceedings of the National Academy of Sciences, 100*(19), 11176–11183.

Eggers, A., Gaddy, C., & Graham, C. (2006). Well-being and unemployment in Russia in the 1990s: Can society's suffering be individuals' solace? *The Journal of Socio-Economics, 35*(2), 209–242.

Eren, K. A., & Aşıcı, A. A. (2016). The determinants of happiness in Turkey: Evidence from city-level data. *Journal of Happiness Studies, 17*, 1–23.

Eren, K. A., & Aşıcı, A. A. (2018). Subjective well-being in an era of relentless growth: The case of Turkey between 2004 and 2014. *Journal of Happiness Studies, 19*(5), 1347–1371.

Estaji, H. (2014). Flexible spatial configuration in traditional houses, the case of Sabzevar. *International Journal of Contemporary Architectur. "The New ARCH", 1*(1), 26–35.
Frey, B. S., & Stutzer, A. (2000). Happiness, economy and institutions. *The Economic Journal, 110*(466), 918–938.
Frey, B. S., & Stutzer, A. (2001). Beyond Bentham-measuring procedural utility. *CESifo Working Paper Series 492*. https://www.cesifo.org/DocDL/cesifo_wp492.pdf. Accessed May 2, 2020.
Frey, B., & Stutzer, A. (2002a). *Happiness and economics: How the economy and institutions affect human well-being*. Princeton University Press.
Frey, B. S., & Stutzer, A. (2002b). What can economists learn from happiness research? *Journal of Economic Literature, 40*(2), 402–435.
Frey, B. S., & Stutzer, A. (2010). *Happiness and economics: How the economy and institutions affect human well-being*. Princeton University Press.
Gandelman, N., & Porzecanski, R. (2013). Happiness inequality: How much is reasonable? *Social Indicators Research, 110*(1), 257–269.
Gao, S., & Meng, X. (2015). The Impact of Government Size on Chinese Elders' Life Satisfaction: 1998–2008. In F. Maggion (Ed.), *A new research agenda for improvements in quality of life* (pp. 135–161). Springer.
Graham, C. (2009). *Happiness around the world: The paradox of happy peasants and miserable millionaires*. Oxford University Press.
Graham, C. (2011). *The pursuit of happiness: An economy of well-being*. Brookings Institution Press.
Graham, C., & Felton, A. (2006). Inequality and happiness: Insights from Latin America. *The Journal of Economic Inequality, 4*(1), 107–122.
Graham, C., Chattopadhyay, S., & Picon, M. (2010). The Easterlin and other paradoxes: Why both sides of the debate may be correct. In E. Diener, J. F. Helliwell, & D. Kahneman (Eds.), *International differences in well-being* (pp. 247–288). Oxford University Press.
Hagerty, M. R., & Veenhoven, R. (2003). Wealth and happiness revisited–growing national income does go with greater happiness. *Social Indicators Research, 64*(1), 1–27.
Haller, M., & Hadler, M. (2006). How social relations and structures can produce happiness and unhappiness: An international comparative analysis. *Social Indicators Research, 75*(2), 169–216.
Halpern, D. (2010). *The hidden wealth of nations*. Polity.
Hartog, J., & Oosterbeek, H. (1998). Health, wealth and happiness: Why pursue a higher education? *Economics of Education Review, 17*(3), 245–256.
Headey, B. (2008). The set-point theory of well-being: Negative results and consequent revisions. *Social Indicators Research, 85*(3), 389–403.
Headey, B., & Wearing, A. J. (1989). Personality, life events, and subjective well-being: Toward a dynamic equilibrium model. *Journal of Personality and Social Psychology, 57*(4), 731.
Headey, B., & Wearing, A. J. (1992). *Understanding happiness: A theory of subjective well-being*. Longman Cheshire.
Helliwell, J. F. (2003). How's life? Combining individual and national variables to explain subjective well-being. *Economic Modelling, 20*(2), 331–360.
Helliwell, J. F., & Huang, H. (2008). How's your government? International evidence linking good government and well-being. *British Journal of Political Science, 38*(4), 595–619.
Herzberg, F., Mauser, B., & Snyderman, B. (1959). *The motivation to work*. Wiley.
Hirschman, A. O., & Rothschild, M. (1973). The changing tolerance for income inequality in the course of economic development: With a mathematical appendix. *The Quarterly Journal of Economics, 87*(4), 544–566.
Howell, R. T., & Howell, C. J. (2008). The relation of economic status to subjective well-being in developing countries: A meta-analysis. *Psychological Bulletin, 134*(4), 536.
Inglehart, R., & Klingemann, H. D. (2000). Genes, culture, democracy, and happiness. In E. Diener & E. M. Suh (Eds.), *Culture and subjective well-being* (pp. 165–183). The MIT Press.
Inglehart, R., & Welzel, C. (2005). *Modernization, cultural change, and democracy: The human development sequence*. Cambridge University Press.

Inglehart, R., Foa, R., Peterson, C., & Welzel, C. (2008). Development, freedom, and rising happiness: A global perspective (1981–2007). *Perspectives on Psychological Science, 3*(4), 264–285.

Jang, S. (2011). Political economy of happiness: Effects of perceptions of income inequality on the life-satisfaction among Koreans. *Korean Party Studies Review, 10*(2), 43–66 (Korean).

Kacapyr, E. (2008). Cross-country determinants of satisfaction with life. *International Journal of Social Economics, 35*(6), 400–416.

Kahneman, D. (1999). Objective happiness. In D. Kahneman, E. Diener, & N. Schwarz (Eds.), *Well-being: The foundations of hedonic psychology* (pp. 3–25). Russell Sage Foundation.

Kahneman, D., & Krueger, A. B. (2006). Developments in the measurement of subjective well-being. *Journal of Economic Perspectives, 20*(1), 3–24.

Kahneman, D., & Tversky, A. (1979). Prospect theory: An analysis of decision under risk. *Econometrica, 47*(2), 263–291.

Kahneman, D., Krueger, A. B., Schkade, D., Schwarz, N., & Stone, A. A. (2006). Would you be happier if you were richer? A focusing Illusion. *Science, 312*(5782), 1908–1910.

Kalmijn, W., & Veenhoven, R. (2005). Measuring inequality of happiness in nations: In search for proper statistics. *Journal of Happiness Studies, 6*(4), 357–396.

Kalmijn, M., De Graaf, P. M., & Janssen, J. P. (2005). Intermarriage and the risk of divorce in the Netherlands: The effects of differences in religion and in nationality, 1974–94. *Population Studies, 59*(1), 71–85.

Kaufmann, D., Kraay, A., & Mastruzzi, M. (2007). Governance matters VI: Aggregate and individual governance indicators, 1996–2006. *Policy Research Working Paper No. 4280*. http://info.worldbank.org/governance/wgi/pdf/govmatters6.pdf. Accessed May 2, 2020.

Kim, B., Kang, H., & Kim, H. (2015). A study on the moderating effect of quality of life on the relationship between public service satisfaction and citizens happiness. *Korean Journal of Public Administration, 53*(3), 29–56 (Korean).

Kim, H. (2016). Exploring the influence of perceived income inequality on happiness: Focusing on the moderating effect of perceived upward social mobility. *Korean Policy Studies Review, 25*(2), 559–587 (Korean).

Ko, M. (2013). Citizen satisfaction, government performance, and quality of life: focused on bottom-up Spillover approach. *Korean Public Administration Review, 47*(2), 1–30 (Korean).

Koo, K., Lim, J., & Choi, S. (2014). Determinants of happiness: Reevaluating the role of income and capability. *Korean Public Administration Review, 48*(2), 317–339 (Korean).

Kozma, A., Stone, S., Stones, M. J., Hannah, T. E., & McNeil, K. (1990). Long- and short-term affective states in happiness: Model, paradigm and experimental evidence. *Social Indicators Research, 22*(2), 119–138.

Kroll, C. (2008). *Social capital and the happiness of nations: The importance of trust and networks for life satisfaction in a cross-national perspective*. Peter Lang.

Lance, C. E., Mallard, A. G., & Michalos, A. C. (1995). Tests of the causal directions of global—Life facet satisfaction relationships. *Social Indicators Research, 34*(1), 69–92.

Larsen, R. J. (2000). Toward a science of mood regulation. *Psychological Inquiry, 11*(3), 129–141.

Layard, R. (2005). *Happiness: Lessons from a new science*. Penguin Books/Penguin Group.

Lee, S. J., & Lee, J. E. (2017). Differential effects of community income inequality on components of happiness. *A Paper Presented at the ISQOLS 15th Annual Conference*. Innsbruck, Austria.

Lee, S. J., Lee, S., & Jo, C. (2020). A study on the differential factors that affect public happiness level and distribution. *Korean Public Administration Review, 54*(1), 171–197 (Korean).

Lim, J., Koo, K., & Choi, S. (2016). Inequality and Happiness: The Mechanism of Inequality from Sen's Capability Perspective. *Korean Journal of Public Administration, 54*(3), 175–198 (Korean).

Lucas, R. E. (2007). Adaptation and the set-point model of subjective well-being: Does happiness change after major life events? *Current Directions in Psychological Science, 16*(2), 75–79.

Lucas, R. E., & Diener, E. (2009). Personality and subjective well-being. In E. Diener (Ed.), *The science of well-being: The collected works of Ed Diener* (pp. 75–102). Springer.

Lucas, R. E., Clark, A. E., Georgellis, Y., & Diener, E. (2003). Reexamining adaptation and the set point model of happiness: Reactions to changes in marital status. *Journal of Personality and Social Psychology, 84*(3), 527–539.

Lucas, R. E., Clark, A. E., Georgellis, Y., & Diener, E. (2004). Unemployment alters the set point for life satisfaction. *Psychological Science, 15*(1), 8–13.

Luttmer, E. F. (2004). Neighbors as negatives: Relative earnings and well-being. *National Bureau of Economic Research*. https://doi.org/10.3386/w10667

Lykken, D., & Tellegen, A. (1996). Happiness is a stochastic phenomenon. *Psychological Science, 7*(3), 186–189.

Maggino, F. (Ed.). (2015). *A new research agenda for improvements in quality of life*. Springer.

Maslow, A. H. (1943). A theory of human motivation. *Psychological Review, 50*(4), 370–396.

Max-Neef, M. A. (1991). *Human scale development: Conception, application and further reflections*. The Apex Press.

McClelland, D. C. (1961). *The achieving society*. Van Nostrand.

Michalos, A. C. (1985). Multiple discrepancies theory (MDT). *Social Indicators Research, 16*(4), 347–413.

Michalos, A. C. (2008). Education, happiness and wellbeing. *Social Indicators Research, 87*(3), 347–366.

Mizobuchi, H. (2017). Measuring socio-economic factors and sensitivity of happiness. *Journal of Happiness Studies, 18*(2), 463–504.

O'Connell, M. (2004). Fairly satisfied: Economic equality, wealth and satisfaction. *Journal of Economic Psychology, 25*(3), 297–305.

Oshio, T. (2017). Which is more relevant for perceived happiness, individual-level or area-level social capital? A multilevel mediation analysis. *Journal of Happiness Studies, 18*(3), 765–783.

Oshio, T., & Kobayashi, M. (2011). Area-level income inequality and individual happiness: Evidence from Japan. *Journal of Happiness Studies, 12*(4), 633–649.

Oshio, T., & Urakawa, K. (2014). The association between perceived income inequality and subjective well-being: Evidence from a social survey in Japan. *Social Indicators Research, 116*(3), 755–770.

Ott, J. (2001). Did the market depress happiness in the US? *Journal of Happiness Studies, 2*(4), 433–443.

Ott, J. (2005). Level and inequality of happiness in nations: Does greater happiness of a greater number imply greater inequality in happiness? *Journal of Happiness Studies, 6*(4), 397–420.

Ott, J. (2011). Government and happiness in 130 nations: Good governance fosters higher level and more equality of happiness. *Social Indicators Research, 102*(1), 3–22.

Pacek, A. C., & Radcliff, B. (2008). Welfare policy and subjective well-being across nations: An individual-level assessment. *Social Indicators Research, 89*(1), 179–191.

Pagán-Rodríguez, R. (2010). Onset of disability and life satisfaction: Evidence from the German socio-economic panel. *The European Journal of Health Economics, 11*(5), 471–485.

Pagán-Rodríguez, R. (2012). Longitudinal analysis of the domains of satisfaction before and after disability: Evidence from the German Socio-Economic Panel. *Social Indicators Research, 108*(3), 365–385.

Paralkar, S., Cloutier, S., Nautiyal, S., & Mitra, R. (2017). The sustainable neighborhoods for happiness (SNfH) decision tool: Assessing neighborhood level sustainability and happiness. *Ecological Indicators, 74*, 10–18.

Pavot, W., & Diener, E. (1993). Review of the satisfaction with life scale. *Psychological Assessment, 5*(2), 164–172.

Pugno, M. (2009). The Easterlin paradox and the decline of social capital: An integrated explanation. *The Journal of Socio-Economics, 38*(4), 590–600.

Putnam, R. (1995). Bowling alone: America's declining social capital. *Journal of Democracy, 6*, 65–78.

Putnam, R. (2000). *Bowling Alone: The Collapse and Revival of American Community*. Simon and Schuster.

Radcliff, B. (2001). Politics, markets, and life satisfaction: The political economy of human happiness. *American Political Science Review, 95*(4), 939–952.
Ram, R. (2009). Government spending and happiness of the population: Additional evidence from large cross-country samples. *Public Choice, 138*(3), 483–490.
Rode, M. (2013). Do good institutions make citizens happy, or do happy citizens build better institutions? *Journal of Happiness Studies, 14*(5), 1479–1505.
Rothstein, B. (2010). Happiness and the welfare state. *Social Research, 77*(2), 1–28.
Runciman, W. G. (1966). *Relative deprivation and social justice: A study of attitudes to social inequality in twentieth-century England*. Routledge.
Ryan, R. M., & Deci, E. L. (2000). Self-determination theory and the facilitation of intrinsic motivation, social development, and well-being. *American Psychologist, 55*(1), 68–78.
Sacks, D. W., Stevenson, B., & Wolfers, J. (2012). The new stylized facts about income and subjective well-being. *Emotion, 12*(6), 1181.
Schwarz, N., & Strack, F. (1999). Reports of subjective wellbeing: Judgmental processes and their methodological implications. In D. Kahneman, E. Diener, & N. Schwarz (Eds.), *Well-being: The foundations of hedonic psychology* (pp. 61–84). Russell Sage Foundation.
Scitovsky, T. (1976). *The joyless economy: An inquiry into human satisfaction and consumer dissatisfaction*. Oxford University Press.
Shin, S. (2015). The analysis on the determinants of happiness in Korea. *Kookmin Social Science Review 41*(2), 183–208 (Korean).
Sirgy, M. J. (2001). *Handbook of quality-of-life research: An ethical marketing perspective*. Springer.
Sirgy, M. J., Efraty, D., Siegel, P., & Lee, D. J. (2001). A new measure of quality of work life (QWL) based on need satisfaction and spillover theories. *Social Indicators Research, 55*(3), 241–302.
Solnick, S. J., & Hemenway, D. (1998). Is more always better?: A survey on positional concerns. *Journal of Economic Behavior & Organization, 37*(3), 373–383.
Stevenson, B., & Wolfers, J. (2008). Economic growth and subjective well-being: Reassessing the Easterlin paradox. *National Bureau of Economic Research*. https://doi.org/10.3386/w14282
Stevenson, B., & Wolfers, J. (2013). Subjective well-being and income: Is there any evidence of satiation? *American Economic Review, 103*(3), 598–604.
Stouffer, S. A., Suchman, E. A., Devinney, L. C., Star, S. A., & Williams, R. M., Jr. (1949). *The American soldier: Adjustment during army life. (Studies in social psychology in World War II)* (Vol. 1). Princeton University Press.
Subramanian, S. V., Kim, D., & Kawachi, I. (2005). Covariation in the socioeconomic determinants of self rated health and happiness: A multivariate multilevel analysis of individuals and communities in the USA. *Journal of Epidemiology & Community Health, 59*(8), 664–669.
Sugden, R., & Teng, J. C. Y. (2016). Is happiness a matter for governments? In S. Bartolini, E. Bilancini, L. Bruni, & P. L. Porta (Eds.), *Policies for happiness* (pp. 36–57). Oxford University Press.
Thin, N. (2012). *Social happiness: Theory into policy and practice*. Policy Press.
United Nations Development Programme. (2010). http://hdr.undp.org/en/. Accessed February 26, 2019.
Veblen, T. (1899). *The theory of the leisure class: An economic study of institutions*. Random House.
Veenhoven, R. (1990). Inequality in happiness: inequality in countries compared across countries. Resource document. Munich Personal RePEc Archive MPRA Paper No. 11275. https://mpra.ub.uni-muenchen.de/11275/. Accessed May 2, 2020.
Veenhoven, R. (1991a). Is happiness relative? *Social Indicators Research, 24*, 1–34.
Veenhoven, R. (1991b). Questions on happiness: Classical topics, modern answers, blind spots. In F. Strack, M. Argyle, & N. Schwarz (Eds.), *Subjective well-being: An interdisciplinary perspective* (pp. 7–26). Pergamon Press.
Veenhoven, R. (2000). The four qualities of life. *Journal of Happiness Studies, 1*(1), 1–39.
Veenhoven, R. (2004a). *The greatest happiness principle. Happiness as an aim in public policy. Positive Psychology in Practice*. Wiley.

Veenhoven, R. (2004b). Happiness as an aim in public policy: The greatest happiness principle. In P. A. Linley & S. Joseph (Eds.), *Positive psychology in practice* (pp. 658–678). Wiley.

Veenhoven, R., & Vergunst, F. (2014). The Easterlin illusion: Economic growth does go with greater happiness. *International Journal of Happiness and Development, 1*(4), 311–343.

Verme, P. (2011). Life satisfaction and income inequality. *World Bank Policy Research Working Paper No. 5574*. https://papers.ssrn.com/sol3/papers.cfm?abstract_id=1774421. Accessed May 2, 2020.

Vittersø, J. (2013). Introduction to psychological definitions of happiness. In S. A. David, I. Boniwell, & A. Conley Ayers (Eds.), *Oxford handbook of happiness* (pp. 155–160). Oxford University Press.

Weick, S. (2015). Subjective well-being after the onset of the need for personal assistance and care. In F. Maggion (Ed.), *A new research agenda for improvements in quality of life* (pp. 191–204). Springer.

Welsch, H. P. (2003). *Entrepreneurship: The way ahead*. Routledge.

Welzel, C., & Inglehart, R. (2008). The role of ordinary people in democratization. *Journal of Democracy, 19*(1), 126–140.

Winkelmann, L., & Winkelmann, R. (1998). Why are the unemployed so unhappy? Evidence from Panel Data. *Economica, 65*(257), 1–15.

Witter, R. A., Okun, M. A., Stock, W. A., & Haring, M. J. (1984). Education and subjective well-being: A meta-analysis. *Educational Evaluation and Policy Analysis, 6*(2), 165–173.

Yamamura, E. (2011). The Influence of government size on economic growth and life satisfaction: A case study from Japan. *Japanese Economy, 38*(4), 28–64.

Yeh, H. J., Hsieh, Y. S., & Tsay, R. M. (2015). Self-evaluation affects subjective well-being: The effects of socioeconomic status and personality in Taiwan. In F. Maggion (Ed.), *A new research agenda for improvements in quality of life* (pp. 109–134). Cham.

Chapter 6
Public Happiness Policy

1 The Need for a Happiness Policy

With the "beyond GDP" movements, countries have begun to newly understand the living conditions and wellbeing of their people, and in this regard, have begun to develop a framework to measure wellbeing. As a representative example, the OECD developed a framework for measuring wellbeing in 2011 based on the recommendations of the Commission on the Measurement of Economic Performance and Social Progress (Stiglitz et al., 2009) and consultations with member countries. Individual countries are also working to develop a framework for measuring happiness in this international trend. This effort to measure happiness is important for assessing the current quality of life and understanding what information needs to be shared for a better life, but providing information alone will not improve people's happiness. This is why active policy efforts beyond measuring happiness are required to promote happiness.

What is a happiness policy? If the series of government activities to achieve a public purpose or simply the government's purposeful activities are referred to as policies, the happiness policy is government activities to promote the happiness of people. Public happiness demands public responsibility for the promotion of happiness, and happiness policy is a major instrument responding to such demands for public responsibility of happiness. In this regard, Bruni's (2016) statement, "Public happiness is directly connected to governmental intervention for increasing common good," concisely indicates the demand for happiness policy. The direction of happiness policy is basically allowing public happiness to drive government policies. In a sense, this can be compared to Lowi (1964)'s attempt to shift the policy paradigm from the conventional paradigm that regards public policy as the output of politics to a new paradigm that regards policy as an independent variable of politics. In other words, in the past, it was assumed that policy determines happiness as a result, but in happiness policy, happiness drives policy decisions.

There can be two questions regarding the discussion of the need for a happiness policy. First, it may be questioned whether happiness can be adopted for the purpose

S. J. Lee, *Public Happiness*, Community Quality-of-Life and Well-Being,
https://doi.org/10.1007/978-3-030-89643-0_6

of government policy. Second, even if happiness is adopted as the purpose of government policy, it is questionable whether there can be a substantial change in the level of happiness through policy efforts. The former relates to the normative necessity of happiness, and the latter relates to the practical necessity of happiness. In view of this, the necessity of happiness will be discussed below in terms of normative and practical aspects. The necessity of happiness policy includes: (1) For the normative aspect, the government, which is a servant of the public as it is, has obligations to try to secure the right to pursue happiness as a basic right of the people. (2) For the practical aspect, it is also necessary to process happiness policies. The practical need encompasses the primary effect of promoting happiness (direct effect), the secondary effect of policy innovation (indirect effect), and the positive effect due to increased happiness (inductive effect). A more detailed discussion follows.

1.1 Desirability of Happiness Policies

Happiness policy is necessary because of the importance of happiness as a purpose value. First, happiness is a universal human need that does not require explanation and deserves the attention of the state (Layard, 2005: 145–157). The right to pursue happiness is recognized as a fundamental human right. As is widely known, the right to pursue happiness is included in the US Declaration of Independence and the French Declaration of Revolution, and is explicitly guaranteed in the constitutions of various countries such as Bhutan, Bolivia, Ecuador, Japan, and South Korea (Pellerin, 2016). Therefore, it is necessary to make policy efforts to assure such rights.

There is disagreement over the normativeness of the happiness value. For the Epicurians of ancient Greece or the Utilitarians of the nineteenth century, whether we should pursue happiness for a purpose was not a question. Their belief was that happiness is the supreme good, and it is therefore natural to pursue happiness. However, for example, those who were in the extension of the Stoic school in Greece, while placing value on pain and perseverance, regarded the pursuit of joy in life as not only a path to destroying themselves by desire but also undermining the social community due to individualism. The mainstream Asian philosophical ideology, which values satisfaction with a modest life (安分之足), seems to have some similarities with this position. However, if happiness is expanded to include the meaning of life, not just enjoyment, the reserved position for happiness is in fact not very different from the position pursuing happiness. Indeed, happiness is currently understood as including meaning as well as enjoyment.

Second, since individual happiness is affected by social conditions as well as by individual propensity, it should be considered as an object of public responsibility at least to that extent. This is not only because the influence of social conditions cannot be transferred to the individual's responsibility, but also because social conditions cannot be improved by the individual's ability alone. Of course, there are opinions that public intervention to promote happiness violates individual autonomy. However, the government's intervention for the promotion of happiness is focused on improving social conditions to support the pursuit of individual happiness, and it is neither aimed at nor is it capable of ensuring the final state of individual happiness. Rather, it should be recognized that the government's public intervention may help increase an individual's active freedom by expanding the individual's available resources with which individuals pursue their own life goals more easily. Of course, since individual freedom is an individual's basic right as important as individual happiness, it is necessary to secure a balance between happiness promotion and individual autonomy in public intervention. Although recognition of public responsibility for happiness and possible infringement of individual autonomy are closely related issues, it does not mean they have to be mutually exclusive.

Third, as Maslow (1943)'s multilayered needs theory or Alderfer (1972)'s multi-focal needs theory for example suggests, human needs are diverse, so humans can live a happy and meaningful life when their various needs are satisfied. Satisfaction of various needs means not only the satisfaction of economic needs, but also the satisfaction of non-economic needs. Although the same is true of economic needs, the satisfaction of non-economic needs is largely related to social conditions. Therefore, improvement of social conditions must also be made in an effort to balance between economic and non-economic aspects. In the industrial state in the past, the expansion of the total economy was important. Even in the age of the welfare state, economic growth was important to expand welfare. However, in a post-industrial society in which basic economic demand has been secured to some extent, the importance of total economy in relation to people's lives is not the same as in the past, and the importance of non-economic factors has increased that much. Pursuing the improvement of social conditions in response to these demands is an object of public responsibility as above mentioned. In addition, public efforts to improve social conditions from a more balanced standpoint are policies aimed at happiness.

1.2 Happiness Promotion Effect (Direct Effect)

Government policy is necessary because it has a direct effect on the promotion of happiness. However, some are skeptical about whether the level of happiness can be significantly changed by the government's intervention to promote happiness. This is the position of those who emphasize the effects of adaptation or social comparison to changes in external conditions, where mainly psychologists occupy the center (e.g., Akerlof, 1997; Clark et al., 2008; Dusenberry, 1949; Frank, 1985; Lykken & Tellegen, 1996; Oswald, 1997).

This skepticism can be summarized as follows. First, it is difficult to manipulate policy intervention effectively because there are so many factors that influence happiness, and accordingly, the policy process becomes irrational, more like a political rhetoric, or a repackaging of the existing policy (Bache et al., 2016). In this regard, Duncan (2010) argues that since the values and priorities of happiness differ from individual to individual, happiness is not generally appropriate as an object for policy decisions that are basically processed by groups rather than individual units.

Second, it is difficult for improvement of external conditions to be channeled into the improvement of happiness. This is because, as argued in the adaptation theory or top-down theory, happiness is dominated by human personality traits, and changes in external social conditions do not have significant effects on happiness. In addition, the effect of improving external conditions is considered to be counterbalanced by the operation of adaptation mechanisms such as aspiration control or social comparison. Besides, happiness and unhappiness show a pattern of happiness–unhappiness–happiness cycles, and therefore, the claim that happiness and unhappiness in the long term are zero sums is a claim in the same context. This is because the cycle of happiness and unhappiness continues regardless of changes in external conditions.

On the other hand, some argue that happiness is enhanced through policy intervention to improve external conditions. This is the position of many social scientists and focuses on the influence of external conditions on happiness rather than individual adaptation or social comparison (e.g., Bok, 2011; Layard, 2005; Radcliff, 2001; Veenhoven, 1991, etc.). According to them, human happiness can be influenced by personal disposition as suggested by the adaptation theory, but this does not completely block the influence of external conditions. In other words, the influence of external conditions on happiness still remains, and therefore, a happiness policy to improve social conditions is effective. For example, Bok (2011) argues that government policy is an important means to affect happiness to the extent that one of the six factors that determine happiness (marriage, human relations, work, health status, religion, quality of government), in addition to innate personality and material success, is government policy.

In the same context, the following explanation by Veenhoven (1991) seems appropriate. Basically, happiness is influenced more by socioeconomic conditions than by psychological factors. The low correlation between socioeconomic conditions and happiness does not mean that socioeconomic conditions have nothing to do with happiness, because there are limits to individual adaptation. This can be verified from the fact that the happiness level of developing countries with poor social conditions is lower than that of developed countries. In addition, external conditions include not only economic conditions or social position, but also political systems, cultural characteristics, and civic networks, which are closely related to happiness. Since inner sources, such as individual wisdom and vigor, also affect happiness through interaction with external conditions. The argument that internal factors dominate happiness does not sufficiently reflect the interaction between internal factors and external conditions. Along with this, he indicates the limitations of the argument for social comparison. That is, regardless of the objective conditions, social comparison is related to the evaluation of life, but its effect is not so meaningful. He also indicates that comparisons are not only made in the social aspect but are made in various domains as suggested by the multiple discrepancy theory demonstrated by Michalos (1985), and social comparison is not the most important domain. He adds that serious deprivations due to war, hunger, social disorganization and so on decrease the enjoyment of life drastically.

Overall, the position that emphasizes adaptation is unreceptive to the happiness policy, and the position that emphasizes reactivity is more supportive of the happiness policy. However, it is difficult to find any evidence that happiness policy decreases happiness. In this situation, it is not desirable to reject any and all happiness policy by dismissing happiness as the problem of an individual's propensity or adaptation. This would be neglecting the possibility of promoting the happiness level of people through happiness policies. Although there may be a problem with the magnitude of the effect, it is clear that happiness can be promoted at a meaningful level through appropriate policy efforts. Of course, the adaptation effect emanating from the individual's disposition to external conditions is widely recognized. However, adaptation does not necessarily overwhelm the influence of external conditions, and thus, there is no need to exaggerate the effect of adaptation because the degree or mode of adaptation also differs between individuals. This judgment also corresponds to the revision direction of the adaptive theory that Diener et al. (2009: 103) properly suggested.

It should also be noted that the evidence against adaptation theory has accumulated substantially. Exemplary findings include: it is difficult to adapt to serious events (e.g., Lucas, 2007), happiness levels in early childhood, unlike in adulthood, are sensitive to the influence of external conditions (e.g., Veenhoven, 1991), happiness and unhappiness are not in a circular relationship (e.g., Fordyce, 1972: 151 from Veenhoven, 1991), etc. In addition, as Duncan (2010) argues, it is not necessary to exclude happiness from policy objectives because of differences in individual values of happiness. Although government policies are carried out based on the unit of groups or regions due to considerations of efficient use of resources and convenience of policy implementation, it does not mean that consideration of individual deviation is impossible in the policy process. For example, it is possible to alleviate the problem due to differences in values and priorities among individuals by expanding the range of individual choices in policy design. That is, the value of happiness is an issue to be considered in relation to the design and application of policies but not to be presented as a basis for opposing happiness policies.

In fact, the statement that changes in external conditions will have a significant impact on individual happiness can be understood with common sense without having to prove it. Otherwise, there is no way to explain why people seek better external conditions, such as income, status, reputation, and health. A more fundamental problem is that individuals do not have enough and equal resources to improve external conditions, rather than whether or not they are significantly influenced by external conditions. In such a situation, the government's policy intervention should be recognized as necessary as an effort to respond to or supplement the needs of individuals who want to improve their external conditions for a better life. In this regard, a short argument by Veenhoven (1991) deserves attention: "In summary, there is sense in trying to improve human happiness. Better living conditions and wiser, more sensible living can contribute to more enjoyment in life. Though not all recipes work, many improvements are possible. The challenge for future research is not to question the obvious any longer, but to find out which improvements promise the greatest yields."

As Veenhoven suggests, it is desirable to promote an effective happiness policy beyond unnecessary controversy over the necessity of policy by clearly clarifying the causal relationship between improvement of social conditions and happiness.

However, unfortunately, research on which social conditions have a meaningful and sustainable effect on happiness is still in its infancy, and therefore, the relevant knowledge and understanding are in dearth. The appropriate response for this situation is clear. First of all, it is necessary to build the knowledge foundation for policy enactment to improve social conditions by proliferating more in-depth research on the relationship between social conditions and happiness. And on this basis, it is necessary to flexibly pursue happiness policies to improve external conditions. In pursuing happiness policies, excessive confidence in its effectiveness is not desirable. As already mentioned, not only is there a limit to the efficiency of investment for happiness policy due to individual adaptation, but there is also a concern for infringement of individual autonomy by excessive policy intervention. In this regard, it is necessary to pay attention to the discussion by Bache et al. (2016) on the dilemma of the happiness policy. They indicate four dilemmas regarding happiness policy: First, the reliability problem that wellbeing cannot be adequately measured and so should not be relied upon for public policy purposes. Second, the responsibility problem that government is not the most appropriate or effective vehicle for promoting wellbeing. Third, the trust problem that politicians will be inclined to manipulate data and thus cannot be trusted with wellbeing data. Lastly, the distraction problem that the pursuit of wellbeing by government will lead to government failing to address other concerns.[1] They argue that the happiness policy is likely to take a partial, provisional approach and pursue coherent action instead of a final solution because of such a dilemma, and suggest that accordingly more deliberative, more knowledgeable, and more incremental approaches are needed to promote the happiness policy. Although the dilemmas they raised were from the standpoint of skepticism, and mixed with exaggerations that are difficult to accept as it is, it should be noted that their comments and suggestions are not to fundamentally deny the necessity of the happiness policy but rather suggest an appropriate prescription for the direction of the happiness policy.

Moreover, it should be indicated that happiness must be measured for effective enactment of the happiness policy. As discussed in Chap. 4, happiness can be scientifically studied and measured despite some limitations. In fact, many countries and academics are making efforts to measure happiness today, and it is expected that more reliable and valid measurements can be established in the future (Sachs, 2019). The increasing possibility of scientific measurement of happiness is another factor supporting the necessity of a happiness policy.

[1] A good example for this is Dalingwater et al. (2019) implying that the Bhutan government neglected other important policy tasks such as economy, unemployment, and education as an excuse for the happiness policy.

1.3 Policy Development Effect (Indirect Effect)

Happiness policy is necessary because we can expect not only the direct effect of happiness promotion but also the effect of policy development in the policy process. Until now, discussions on happiness policies have focused mainly on the effects of happiness policies on the promotion of happiness, but there has been little interest in the effect of policy development emanating from happiness policies. Of course, the effect of happiness promotion is important as a basic argument for supporting the necessity of the happiness policy. However, an equally important effect of the happiness policy is that, we can expect development of the policy itself from pursuing the happiness policy. This effect may be as important as the direct effect on happiness. It is because an effective happiness policy as a tool for promoting happiness can only be secured when policy development takes place as a prerequisite, and even if it does not, policy development itself has an important meaning.

Accordingly, even those who do not support the happiness policy have a reason to pay attention to this additional effect of the happiness policy. Aside from the happiness policy, inefficiency, unresponsiveness, and injustice in the policy process have been criticized as a public problem that cannot be easily corrected across times and countries, and thus, research interests have increased in academic fields such as political science, public administration, and public policy in which governments are the major research objects, on how to secure efficiency, democratization, and equity in the government policy process. If there is a possibility to alleviate such core problems of a policy process by pursuing a happiness policy, it is of course worthy of attention. Nevertheless, happiness studies so far have prioritized promoting happiness and thus have not exhibited adequate research interest in the effect of such policy development emanating from the happiness policy process. However, if there is a virtuous cycle that the enactment of happiness policy induces policy development, and the policy development contributes to the effectiveness of happiness policy, it is necessary to pay serious attention to such additional effects of the happiness policy on policy development beyond on the increase of happiness.

In this regard, Helliwell et al. (2019) have presented four items as an advantage of pursuing the happiness policy, such as improving the policy evaluation method, increasing cooperation among government agencies, expanding interest in the scope of policy benefit, and the provision of effective policy performance evaluation criteria. Although simple, it is noteworthy that they explicitly mentioned the effect of the happiness policy on policy development. However, assuming that the core value of the policy includes not only efficiency or effectiveness but also democracy and equity (Lee, 2014: 483), the list is limited in that it does not cover all the core policy values. A more comprehensive and detailed explanation was necessary. In this regard, the following section discusses the effects of policy development expected with the pursuit of happiness policies, by categorizing them into efficiency, responsiveness, and equity.

Contribution to policy efficiency

The happiness policy is expected to enhance policy efficiency through reinforcement of policy cooperation between institutions, change in policy evaluation method, and change in policy paradigm. First, by setting happiness as a high-level policy goal that penetrates the various institutions, it provides an opportunity for lateral communication among various government agencies and contribute to the facilitation of cooperation among government agencies. Organizational sectionalism based on institutional selfishness is one of the most chronic problems in the government process. As the goals of individual institutions are prioritized over goals of the entire government, and competition is prioritized over cooperation between institutions, synergies of various institutional activities are not secured, resource allocation is distorted and overall policy efficiency is deteriorated. Such a phenomenon can be regarded as a substitution of objectives for means, and in this situation, as Helliwell (2019) suggests, by setting happiness as a common goal that applies across the institutions, cooperation between agencies to achieve the common goal can be encouraged. Of course, it is also possible to argue that the same effect can be secured if other common goals such as national development, freedom, equality, or human rights are adopted as goals instead of happiness. However, other values are too abstract compared to happiness (e.g., national development), or are limited in universal applicability to institutions with different functions (e.g., human rights), or are means for happiness (e.g., freedom or equality). There seems to be a limit to discussing these in the same line as happiness. Of course, even if we set happiness as a common policy goal, we will not be able to eliminate the chronic institutional sectionalism at once. Nevertheless, it is expected that at least serious sectionalism between governmental agencies will be alleviated by stimulating communication for achieving the common goals. This expectation is by no means insignificant considering the seriousness of the problem of sectionalism among governmental agencies.

Second, by creating policies with the goal of happiness, the input or process-based policy paradigm is converted to a goal-oriented paradigm, and accordingly, policy effectiveness is enhanced by having a consistent interest in the relevance of the policy goals. That is, instead of policies driven by vague common sense or ideology, goal-driven policies can be promoted based on scientific evidence of the relationship to happiness. In contrast, public policies in the past have basically shown a tendency toward input-centered process management. The implicit assumption that increased input of resources such as finance, personnel, facilities, and information, rather than relevance to goals, will lead to better policy outcomes has been dominant. However, increasing input does not guarantee policy performance. In order to improve policy performance, interest in the causality between policies and objectives should be strengthened, and resource input or policy evaluation should be made on the basis of evidence for the causal relations with policy goals. Pursuing a happiness policy aimed at happiness is to respond to such a demand. Of course, policy goals have also been presented in the past. However, the goal was generally an input or process goal and not the ultimate goal of policy, such as happiness or a good life. If the relationship between policy input and the final goal of the process is increased, the systematic relationship between the policy process and the goal becomes strengthened, the management of policy results becomes easier, and accordingly, the overall policy performance is expected to be improved.

Third, the policy evaluation method can be improved through the enactment of the happiness policy. In the past, policy evaluation focused on the evaluation of economic performance based on cost–benefit analysis, so there was a limit in the evaluation of non-economic performance. In addition, comparative evaluation between economic and non-economic performance was difficult. However, policy evaluation based on happiness includes not only economic performance but also non-economic performance such as health and social trust as evaluation targets, as long as it functions as a positive factor for happiness (Helliwell, 2019). It becomes more possible to evaluate non-economic performance for which the performance evaluation criteria were ambiguous.[2] Cost–benefit analysis can also be applied as an instrument to analyze not only economic performance but also non-economic performance based on the effect on happiness. Such a change in the evaluation method increases the validity of evaluation by allowing the policy performance according to the same criteria across various institutions with different functions. This is a factor contributing to the improvement of policy performance in the non-economic sector, which was particularly difficult to evaluate due to the difficulty in securing relevant measures, and accordingly, the overall performance of the policy can be improved. On the other hand, even if happiness is adopted as the policy evaluation criterion, a question remains: Is it possible to operate happiness as a criterion for performance evaluation? This question is important because one of the difficulties in performance evaluation is the difficulty in setting performance standards. However, as Helliwell (2019) points out, happiness standards such as life satisfaction are an easily understood measure of the quality of life, which is much simpler, more intuitive, and more comprehensive than fragmented measures of social conditions. Of course, the development of happiness indicators is not yet sufficient (especially measuring factors such as life meaning), but it is expected that the utilization of happiness as an evaluation criterion will increase as happiness measures are continuously improved. Overall, there needs to be a policy evaluation system that places happiness as the upper level variable and other meaningful social conditions as factors influencing happiness.

Contribution to policy democratization

The happiness policy will contribute to the improvement of democracy in the policy. Happiness is, after all, a subjective emotion that each citizen feels subjectively, so policymakers must increase contact with citizens and listen to public opinion in the process of making happiness policy. In the past, policymakers tended to carry out policies that they thought were good for citizens by making their own judgments without contacting citizens or collecting opinions from citizens. In pursuing policies for citizens, policymakers have continued their undemocratic policy behavior without seriously asking or listening to what citizens really want.

However, when happiness is the policy goal, the attitude of such policymakers should change. Because the goal of the policy is the happiness of the citizens, which is a matter for the citizens to evaluate, policymakers have new reason to value public

[2] For example, Porta & Scazzieri (2007: 99) propose to apply enabling conditions, measured levels of happiness, opportunities and competencies, as policy evaluation criteria.

opinion gathering and consultations with citizens in the policy process. As for citizens, although they do not have specialized knowledge about the policy process, they can form a relevant opinion on satisfaction with the policy and thus take a more effective and meaningful response to the gathering of public opinion and policy discussions. Furthermore, if public opinion gathering and cooperation with citizens are emphasized in the policy process, cooperation between policymakers and citizens becomes more active. Also, in such a process, the sovereignty of citizens can be improved. In all, public policy should be for the citizens. However, in the conventional policy process, citizens were only the targets of policy or cumbersome requesters. In fact, policies were often more for policymakers than for citizens. Under an authoritative regime, such a tendency is stronger. This is one of the chronic problems that are difficult to find a solution in government research. However, the pursuit of the happiness policy will provide an opportunity to alleviate such problems. It is expected that the undemocratic policy process can be transformed into a more democratic policy process with the change in motives of policymakers, the change of citizens' motives and increased bilateral contacts between them.

The democratization effect of happiness policy does not stop with itself. Democratization of policy enhances citizens' political efficacy in the more interactive policy process and also citizenship by augmenting citizens' understanding of policy issues. Citizens will shift from a passive citizen who unilaterally makes a demand to the government to a citizen as a coproducer or prosumer who engages in policy cooperation with active participation. A public citizen or a cultured citizen will refrain from imprudent demands for happiness and contribute to the public interest. Such changes have the effect of improving policy performance along with changes in the behavior of policymakers. In the end, policy democratization due to the happiness policy is expected to bring not only the democratization effect but also the effect of improving policy performance.

A question can be raised about this effect. For example, Ormerod (2012) is concerned that local decisions or individual freedoms will be overridden by central experts in the happiness policy process. That is, he is arguing that the happiness policy may bring the harmful effects of anti-democracy or centralization. However, as will be described later, in order to successfully implement the happiness policy, it is necessary to carry out consumer-oriented tailored policy in a small unit close to the citizen. That is, the happiness policy in nature is closer to democratic and decentralized policy practice than authoritative and centralized policy practice. This was proved in Frey and Stutzer (2002), which reported that in an empirical analysis of 26 Cantons in Switzerland, democracy increased happiness by 11% and local autonomy by 3.2%. For the happiness policy, customized or tailored policies through small-scale and decentralized policies must be strengthened rather than a national initiative alone. The case of Korea provides a good example. The happiness policy was adopted under the name of Government 3.0 during the Park Geun Hye Administration (2013–2017). In doing so, Local Government 3.0 was also implemented in parallel with the national initiative, to promote the policy at the local level. Nevertheless, if the happiness policy is carried out in the manner of authoritative or centralized leadership, it may either be an early phenomenon that inevitably occurs in the launching process of the happiness policy or the case of expanding a centralization rhetoric while pursuing a pseudo happiness policy rather than a genuine happiness policy.

Contribution to policy equity

First, the pursuit of the happiness policy alleviates policy inequality through the integration of policy evaluation criteria and balance of influences between institutions. Earlier, it was mentioned that the introduction of the happiness policy has the effect of increasing the validity of the evaluation by applying the same evaluation criteria including economic and non-economic performance. This change in evaluation method will have a greater impact on non-economic institutions than on economic institutions. This is expected to contribute to equalization of influence among government agencies. When the evaluation is performed mainly based on economic performance as in the present, economic institutions naturally have a relatively superior position and non-economic institutions have a relatively inferior position. As a result, there is a risk of creating a power gap between institutions and inequality in resource allocation, which differentially affects the morale and work commitment of public officials, and also creates an imbalance in policy performance across sectors. However, when happiness is set as a common high-level goal that applies across institutions, it is expected that cross comparison between various institutions will be feasible, the gap in influence among government agencies will be mitigated, and the balance between various policies will be improved. This is because policies not only in the economic sector but also in the non-economic sectors are expanded as a subject of policy evaluation, and the comparative standards are integrated based on the level of achievement of the happiness goal.

Second, by pursuing the happiness policy, the policy effect not only brings benefits to the direct beneficiaries of the policy but also to secondary beneficiaries. The social diffusion of such policy benefits refers to a phenomenon that happiness is acquired and spread in social context rather than exclusively possessed in isolation (Helliwell, 2019). Of course, in the case of other policies also, policy benefits are not limited to direct beneficiaries, and external effects occur. Welfare benefits, for example, not only improve the lives of beneficiaries but also alleviate the burden on those in relationships with welfare beneficiaries. However, such effects are limited in proportion to the size of the benefits and are limited compared to the external effects of happiness embedded in social networks. On the other hand, since the effect of the happiness policy is amplified through the social network as a medium, a high degree of external effects can occur beyond the input of resources. In this regard, Helliwell et al. (2019) indicated that if the happiness policy is not implemented, such secondary effects will not be captured in the policy process. In this way, the diffusion of policy benefits according to the happiness policy contributes to policy equality by incorporating neglected targets of policy interest into policy-oriented internal customers.

1.4 Positive Social Function (Inductive Effect)

As discussed in Chap. 2, happiness is not only desirable in itself, but at the individual level, it exhibits positive functions for longevity, health, work, human relations, cooperation, and citizenship, and at the social level, it functions positively for the health, reciprocity, democracy, and prosperity of society. In positive psychology, the pursuit of happiness is understood as having a positive function in society by mitigating the impact of negative life events. Although there is some controversy about the positive function of happiness policy, Bartolini et al. (2016)'s response is a good reference:

> Interestingly, both the advocates of policies for happiness and their opponents seem to share the view that happiness is a desirable goal.... the reason probably is that, plausibly. happiness is a leading aspiration of human beings. The only objection to the desirability of happiness as a policy goal that has been raised in the debate concerns a possible conflict between happiness and moral norms. According to this view, happiness should not prevail over moral goals such as justice, fairness, or freedom. .... However, one of the most remarkable results of happiness research is that no trade-off exists between happiness and ethics. The way to happiness includes prosocial behaviors such as civic-mindedness, tolerance, generosity, civic engagements, kindness, solidarity, helpfulness. (Another) ethical aspect... lies in posing a problem of intergenerational equity, that is, a problem of intertemporal ethics.... However, the empirical evidence shows no conflict between intertemporal ethics and happiness, Bartolini and Sarracino (2013) ...find that individuals' current wellbeing is sharply and negatively (positively) influenced by a negative (positive) expectation of the future. This suggests that problems of sustainability must be due to some other factor than the human intertemporal greed.

In this way, if happiness plays a positive role both personally and socially, it is expected that happiness will eventually be promoted through the happiness policy, and a virtuous cycle that positively affects happiness will begin by positively affecting social conditions and personal attitudes. This inducing effect is another reason to pursue the happiness policy.

To sum up the discussion so far, the happiness policy is not only a desirable and legitimate demand but is necessary primarily for the promotion of happiness, secondarily for policy development, and in addition, for positive social functions. Skepticism has been raised about the effectiveness of the happiness policy and ethical issues, but it is difficult to find the results of research that completely deny the normative demand or effect of the happiness policy. Instead, there are a substantial number of studies supporting the effectiveness of the happiness policy, which suggest that the happiness policy should not be neglected. In particular, when considering the potential effect of happiness policy on policy development or the positive function of happiness in society, support for happiness policy should be further increased. This is because focusing only on the direct effect of the policy is to undervalue the overall effect of the happiness policy. Therefore, a future task is to pay more attention to what direction, what level of goal, and how to promote the happiness policy beyond the discussion of the need for a happiness policy. Of course, in doing so, we must pay attention to the ethical issues and issues of practical effect that reservationists raise with regard to the happiness policy. Especially, consideration of the government intervention for the happiness policy and the conflict with individual autonomy are issues to be noted not only for individual autonomy but also for enhancing the effectiveness of the happiness policy.

2 Purpose of the Happiness Policy

If a happiness policy is needed, what is the primary goal of the happiness policy? Is it the ultimate happiness state of the people? Or is it creating social conditions in which the people will be happy? The answer is the latter. The basic purpose of the happiness policy is not to secure the final happiness but to create social conditions (living conditions) that support the individual activities of pursuing happiness (cf., Graham, 2011: 25). Frey (2008: Chap. 13) provides a more detailed discussion of this, taking the national happiness index as an example. First, for the reason the promotion of happiness itself can be promoted as a policy goal, he indicated the following: the national happiness index includes the subjective wellbeing factor (which is an immaterial factor of happiness), reflects the result of input factors included in the concept of GDP, presents a new vision for the government, allows the evaluation of government performance based on the satisfaction of the people, and places equal weight on everyone's preferences. On the other hand, for the reason it is difficult to adopt the promotion of happiness itself as a policy goal, he suggests the following: there is a controversy over the comparison of the utility between individuals, the social welfare function is related to dictatorship, happiness may not be the ultimate goal, the effect of external factors on happiness can be short-term, and falsehood can be involved in measuring happiness.

Basically, a policy aimed at happiness and a policy that guarantees final happiness do not mean the same thing. The former means that the government supports personal happiness activities through improvement of social conditions and as a result seek to promote happiness, but the latter means that the government directly pursue the increase of personal happiness. The former is based on the fact that not only the government's contribution but the individual contribution is important, but the latter assumes that the final happiness can also be secured by the government's contribution only. The problem is that the guarantee of final happiness through policy may be an ideal goal, but it is not achievable. Therefore, in reality, the goal of happiness policy is to improve social conditions that lead to happiness. Nevertheless, when the final state of personal happiness, which is an unrealizable goal, is set up as the policy objective, there is not only concern about indoctrination or manipulation based on patriarchal authority over the public as feared by Frey (2008) but also even a possibility that the happiness issue itself will lead to default due to concerns of excessive input of resources and infringement of individual autonomy. Therefore, it is not only practical but desirable to aim for improvement of social conditions as the goal of happiness policy rather than pursuing an unrealizable goal. By nature, such a happiness policy is not a direct method that aims to promote happiness itself, but an indirect method through improvement of social conditions, and is a method that focuses on providing opportunities rather than results. The effect will be greater as the proportion of social conditions in the factors influencing happiness increases, and the more certain the causal relationship between social conditions and happiness is.

The argument that the happiness policy purports to improve social conditions first does not deny that the ultimate goal of the happiness policy is the promotion of happiness itself. Happiness policy naturally seeks to promote public happiness as its final state. That is, it exerts to raise the level of happiness of members and equalize the distribution of happiness in the community. However, it does not assume that final happiness will be guaranteed by the policy effort alone. It recognizes that securing ultimate happiness by policies may be an ideal goal, but it is not a feasible goal. It is because the level of happiness enjoyed by individuals varies depending on the individual's disposition and efforts, and public policies are basically implemented in groups or regions rather than individuals. In the end, the final happiness of an individual can only be determined by the sum of the government's contribution and the individual's contribution. Therefore, the happiness policy has little choice but to pursue the improvement of social conditions as the primary policy goal, rather than the final happiness of individuals. Fortunately, the provision of an opportunity to pursue happiness by improvement of social conditions is likely to have a positive influence on the final happiness compared to doing otherwise. In particular, it is possible to contribute positively to the distribution of happiness as well as the level of happiness by reinforcing consideration for the underprivileged in improving social conditions. However, since individual variables (personality, effort) are still inherent in such a process, the provision of opportunities is not transmitted to the final result as it is. For this reason, we say that the goal of promoting happiness is not the same as the goal of guaranteeing final happiness. In other words, the happiness policy moves toward the promotion of happiness, but that alone does not secure the ideal state of happiness.

The premise of pursuing the happiness policy is that although improvement of social conditions does not entirely determine happiness, it will contribute to the promotion of happiness by satisfying a substantial part of individual demand. As Veenhoven (1991) properly pointed out, if happiness is determined by factors other than need, such as comparison, fixed disposition or traits, or personal cognitive construct, as suggested by the adaptation theory, such improvement of objective social conditions is meaningless. However, happiness is not entirely determined by comparison or fixed personal personality. Basically, happiness is not a psychological goal secured by aspiration or self-control. Therefore, there is inevitably a limit to how happy one can be based on the suggestions of many liberal arts books about happiness (e.g., "Reduce desires!"). Of course, there may be individual differences in happiness depending on psychological tendencies, but basically, it is far more influenced by objective conditions. Therefore, even if happiness is affected by factors other than need to some extent, it is necessary and desirable to improve social conditions as a basis for happiness because happiness is considerably affected by needs gratification. At the same time, such a policy goal is also an inevitable choice given the limited government resources and the expandability of human desires.

It should be emphasized that in order to promote an effective happiness policy, more active research on the causal relationship between social conditions and happiness must be carried out in parallel. In the absence of knowledge on this relationship, policies for improving social conditions are no different from general welfare policies. It is because general welfare policies also purport to improve social conditions. The problem is that the causal relationship between social conditions and happiness is not always certain because of the failure to identify such causality, the vulnerability of the causal relationship due to adaptation or other intervening factors, or the individual difference in disposition and effort. Until now, of course, substantial studies have verified that personal factors such as income, employment, marriage, and health, as well as various collective factors such as economic conditions, democracy, social values, and government quality, have a significant influence on happiness. However, research on the causal relationship between social conditions and happiness is still incomplete, and it is hoped that the basis for the effectiveness of the happiness policy be strengthened as more related research is conducted in the future. This discussion on the relationship between the conditions of happiness and the promotion of happiness also means that evidence should be an important consideration in pursuing the happiness policy. It is because a policy promoted without evidence on how the resource input for the establishment of certain conditions is indeed related to happiness is likely to be inefficient and wasteful.

There may be a question as to whether the purpose of the happiness policy targets only objective social conditions or individual values as well. This question can arise from the fact that despite the same social conditions, the level of happiness can be different because of individual characteristics. In fact, if personal characteristics are a significant factor that influences the effect of a policy to some extent apart from the magnitude of the effect, it may be considered that it contributes to the promotion of happiness through adjustment of such individual factors. Also, normatively, public happiness is not of an isolated individual, but of a group member, so there is room for the legitimacy of policy efforts to increase the congruence between public and individual values. In this regard, Layard (2005) proposed specific policy alternatives such as limiting harmful advertisements and implementing moral education. This is a policy proposal related to individual values. If so, in the same context, similar policies such as economic education, support for civic movements, social capital formation activities, and support for cultural activities could be included in the alternative. However, there is also a strong argument to oppose such a proposal on the basis of personal autonomy. For example, Sugden and Teng (2016) indicate the policy proposed by Layard as patriarchal and a direct intervention in individual values. According to them, such a policy regulates people's choices from a patriarchal standpoint, assuming that the government knows happiness better than people. They argue that even if individual motivations are wrong, direct regulation of them should be avoided. Instead, the government should communicate with the public based on scientific evidence. For example, in order to restrain the preference for unhealthy smoking, rather than imposing a tobacco tax, the harmful effects of smoking should be shared as a social message based on scientific information.

Furthermore, as seen earlier, scholars such as Duncan (2010) even question the suitability of happiness policies per se based on individual differences in happiness values. Such a reserved position can be understood in that it is desirable that the correspondence between individual and public values is naturally achieved by social norms or communications of members of society prior to interventive policies. However, even if the value of individual autonomy is revered, it seems difficult to completely deny public efforts to close the gap between individual and public values. The excessive gap between individual value and public value will limit the public effect of achieving happiness by improving social conditions, because it has the nature of a public problem in itself. Even Sugden and Teng (2016), mentioned above, are not denying the necessity of policy effort itself to reduce the gap between public and personal values. In addition, even when a direct interventive policy is not enacted related to individual values, social conditions affect individual values to some extent, resulting in a change in the congruence between individual values and public values. It is because the objective external conditions and the individual's subjective perception are bound to interact each other. In other words, whether direct or indirect, personal values are inevitably affected by external conditions, and if so, it is more desirable to attempt to manage them properly rather than disregard them. In this regard, Thin (2012: 60)'s statement on the public relevance of personal values is worth referring to as a logical support for the necessity of public policy regarding personal values.

"(P)eople have always pondered and debated the trade-offs and relative prioritization between efforts to manipulate our innerselves and efforts to change our external circumstances. … (W)e need to combine assimilation (adapting our surroundings to suit us) with accommodation (adapting ourselves to fit our surroundings). As humans, we must accept that our main environmental consideration is other people. So ongoing happiness projects must operate at both individual and social levels. As individuals, we constantly trying to adjust others' behavior and attitudes toward us, but also adjusting ours to them. Collectively, we adjust our non-social environments to fit our social preferences, and adjust our societies in the hope that we will interact better with our non-human environments. But, unlike other species, we have the unique ability to modify the way in which both our social and non-human environments affect our happiness."

As such, if individual values affect the performance of happiness policy, and social conditions are also consistently related to individual values, it may be desirable to pursue the happiness policy in an appropriate tension between individual autonomy and public values, while checking the social conditions related to individual values and vice versa. In other words, policies within a limited range to increase congruence between individual values and public values without excessively infringing on individual autonomy are worth pursuing. In the end, public policy related to individual values needs to be recognized as a question of how and to what extent to promote it rather than whether or not. However, it would not be desirable to prioritize the pursuit of policies related to values over policies for the improvement of other social conditions. It is because excessive intervention in individual values can not only infringe on basic rights and freedom, but also cause other controversy, leading to derailing the entire happiness policy.

It should be indicated that whether to accept happiness as a policy goal and whether to adopt it as the only policy goal may be a separate issue. The objection to adopting happiness as a policy goal is often against adopting it as the only overarching policy goal. In other words, they worry that if happiness is pursued as the highest exclusive policy goal, it can undermine legitimate interest in other important values such as freedom, equality, and human rights (e.g., Duncan, 2010; Sugden & Teng, 2016). However, there are few cases in which the proponents of the happiness policy argue that happiness should be the only exclusive policy goal. In general, proponents of the happiness policy argue that it is necessary to pursue happiness for specific policy objectives, which has been insufficient in practical efforts compared to normative support for happiness. Therefore, they do not oppose the parallel promotion of other appropriate values besides happiness, such as freedom, equality, human rights, and safety. Moreover, the happiness policy purports to improve social conditions for happiness rather than maximization of happiness as the final result. Therefore, there is a limit to the critical opinion on the happiness policy that presupposes happiness as an exclusive higher policy goal. Furthermore, the criticism that presupposes happiness not as an exclusive higher goal but as a policy goal parallel to other values also has limitations for the following reasons.

First, if happiness is adopted as a parallel goal with other values, there arises a problem of diluting the policy interest that fits the importance of happiness. Opponents of the happiness policy criticize that excessive interest in happiness undermines appropriate interest in other values. However, unless other values are removed from the policy goal and happiness is the sole policy goal, such criticism is weakened. In other words, if happiness is recognized as an important policy value similar to other values and accepted as a parallel policy goal, the counter-argument that the value of happiness is undermined due to the adoption of other values is also valid, just as the criticism that happiness should be excluded from the goal because it undermines other values is valid. Of course, if happiness has a lower value than other values, or when negative opinions about happiness are ubiquitous, such objections are difficult to maintain. However, it is difficult to find that even critics of the happiness policy argue that happiness is a sub-value of other values or deny the value of happiness at all (Bartolini et al., 2016: 13). Exceptionally, some studies suggest a reserved position on the policy value of happiness. For example, Duncan (2010) argues, "The fact that we want to be happy does not ineluctably lead to the conclusion that happiness-maximization should be our ethical guide. Indeed, there are respectable branches of moral philosophy that argue that it should not be, and instead principles such as freedom, human rights, duties, virtue, capabilities or fairness may be more relevant." However, such a reserved position on happiness is interpreted as having in mind the hedonic approach which sees happiness as pleasure. However, if happiness is approached as including Eudamonic elements such as the meaning of life, beyond the evaluation of pleasure and life, such criticism is difficult to establish. Moreover, as discussed above, the happiness policy does not seek to maximize happiness.

Second, by adopting happiness as the highest policy goal that transcends other values, it is possible to prevent the problem of conflict with other values. If happiness is the highest policy goal, values such as freedom, equality, human rights, and safety have the characteristics of intermediate goals in the journey to happiness, and in this case, pursuing happiness does not undermine interest in other values. Rather, interest in other values can be strengthened to promote happiness. Therefore, in this case, it is difficult to maintain a criticism that targeting happiness undermines interest in other values. The question is, does the value of happiness take precedence over other values? It may not be without controversy, but the value of happiness basically has the character of the ultimate goal of the highest priority over other values. This is a self-evident basic human need that does not need to be explained.

For example, "To be happy" can be the answer to the questions, "Why freedom?" or "Why safety?" In other words, other ideological values such as freedom and equality can become instrumental goals for a happy life. In this regard, leading happiness theorists such as Layard (2005) advocate that happiness will be self-evident as the only policy goal, while Sen (2009), who advocated the capability theory, acknowledged the importance of happiness, but opposed that happiness become the only policy goal. It makes sense for Sen to stand in such a position because his primary interest lies in the ability to enable individuals to make autonomous choices prior to their final welfare. In the comparison of the two scholars, Thin (2012: 12) emphasizes the value of happiness as the policy goal by pointing out that the problem is not excessive interest in happiness, but insufficient interest. Thin's judgment seems to be valid considering that serious interest in happiness is a recent phenomenon.

In sum, it is desirable to adopt happiness as the highest value that takes priority over other values and to reflect on the connection with other values. However, it is not easy to convert the happiness goal into the highest national policy goal in a short period of time. More progress will be made with more policy implementation and research. The case of the Park Geun-hye administration in Korea in the past is a good reference. In the case of the Park Geun-hye government, "national happiness" was presented as the highest goal overarching the entire government policy in the preparation stage of the government's inauguration, but in the process of adjusting the goal afterward, it became a policy goal in line with other policy values. It is a good example of the happiness goal having been adjusted downward. However, the value of happiness was not downgraded to a value that is inferior to other values. This is because the happiness policy was declared and applied as a policy stance that applies both to the central government and localities (Lee & Oh, 2013). Through such an example, we can simultaneously see the possibilities and limits of the happiness goal at the present stage.

References

Akerlof, G. A. (1997). Social distance and social decisions. *Econometrica, 65*(5), 1005–1027.

Alderfer, C. P. (1972). *Existence, relatedness, and growth: Human needs in organizational settings*. Free Press.

Bache, I., Reardon, L., & Anand, P. (2016). Wellbeing as a wicked problem: Navigating the arguments for the role of government. *Journal of Happiness Studies, 17*(3), 893–912.

Bartolini, S., & Sarracino, F. (2013). *Twenty-five years of materialism: do the US and Europe diverge?* (No. 689). Department of Economics, University of Siena.

Bartolini, S., Bilancini, E., Bruni, L., & Porta, P. L. (Eds.). (2016). *Policies for happiness*. Oxford University Press.

Bok, S. (2011). *Exploring happiness: From Aristotle to brain sciences*. Yale University Press.

Bruni, L. (2016). Public happiness and relational goods. In S. Bartolini, E. Bilancini, L. Bruni, & P. L. Porta (Eds.), *Policies for happiness* (pp. 263–282). Oxford University Press.

Clark, A. E., Frijters, P., & Shields, M. A. (2008). Relative income, happiness, and utility: An explanation for the Easterlin paradox and other puzzles. *Journal of Economic Literature, 46*(1), 95–144.

Dalingwater, L., Costantini, I., & Champroux, N. (2019). Wellbeing: Political discourse and policy in the anglosphere. Introduction. Revue interventions économiques. *Papers in Political Economy, 62*, 1–15.

Diener, E., Lucas, R., Schimmack, U., & Helliwell, J. (2009). *Well-being for public policy*. Oxford University Press.

Duncan, G. (2010). Should happiness-maximization be the goal of government? *Journal of Happiness Studies, 11*(2), 163–178.

Dusenberry, J. S. (1949). *Income, saving, and the theory of consumer behavior*. Harvard University Press.

Fordyce, M. W. (1972). *Happiness, its daily variation and its relation to values*. ProQuest Dissertations Publishing, United States International University. https://www.proquest.com/docview/302583798?pq-origsite=gscholar&fromopenview=true. Accessed June 5, 2010.

Frank, R. H. (1985). *Choosing the right pond: Human behavior and the quest for status*. Oxford University Press.

Frey, B. S. (2008). *Happiness: A revolution in economics (Munich Lectures in Economics)*. The MIT Press.

Frey, B. S., & Stutzer, A. (2002). What can economists learn from happiness research? *Journal of Economic Literature, 40*(2), 402–435.

Graham, C. (2011). *The pursuit of happiness: An economy of well-being*. Brookings Institution Press.

Helliwell, J. F. (2019). Measuring and using happiness to support public policies. *National Bureau of Economic Research*. https://doi.org/10.3386/w26529

Helliwell, J. F., Sachs, J. D., Adler, A., Bin Bishr, A., de Neve, J. E., Durand, M., Layard, R., & Seligman, M. P. E. (2019). How to Open Doors to Happiness. In J. D. Sachs, A. Adler, A. B. Bishr, dN. Jan-Emmanuel, M. Durand, E. Diener, J. F. Helliwell, R. Layard, & M. P. E. Seligman. *Global happiness and wellbeing policy report 2019* (pp. 9–26). Sustainable Development Solutions Network.

Layard, R. (2005). *Happiness: Lessons from a new science*. Penguin Books/Penguin Group.

Lee, S. J. (2014). *Local autonomy*. Parkyoungsa (Korean).

Lee, S. J., & Oh, Y. (2013). *National happiness and Government 3.0: understanding and application*. Hakjisa (Korean).

Lowi, T. J. (1964). American business, public policy, case-studies, and political theory. *World Politics, 16*(4), 677–715.

Lucas, R. E. (2007). Adaptation and the set-point model of subjective well-being: Does happiness change after major life events? *Current Directions in Psychological Science, 16*(2), 75–79.

Lykken, D., & Tellegen, A. (1996). Happiness is a stochastic phenomenon. *Psychological Science, 7*(3), 186–189.
Maslow, A. H. (1943). A theory of human motivation. *Psychological Review, 50*(4), 370–396.
Michalos, A. C. (1985). Multiple discrepancies theory (MDT). *Social Indicators Research, 16*(4), 347–413.
Ormerod, P. (2012). The folly of wellbeing in public policy. In P. Booth (Ed.), (2012). *And the pursuit of happiness-wellbeing and the role of government* (pp. 39–58.) Institute of Economic Affairs.
Oswald, A. J. (1997). Happiness and economic performance. *The Economic Journal, 107*(445), 1815–1831.
Pellerin, C. (2016, February 16). Constitutional considerations of happiness. *Columbia Undergraduate Law Review.*
Porta, P. L., & Scazzieri, R. (2007). Public happiness and civil society. In L. Bruni & P. L. Porta (Eds.), *Handbook on the economics of happiness* (pp. 95–109). Edward Elgar Publishing.
Radcliff, B. (2001). Politics, markets, and life satisfaction: The political economy of human happiness. *American Political Science Review, 95*(4), 939–952.
Sachs, J. (2019). Introduction. In J. Sachs, R. Layard, & J. F. Helliwell (Eds.), *Global happiness and wellbeing policy report 2019* (pp. 4–7). Sustainable Development Solutions Network.
Sen, A. (2009). *The idea of justice.* Harvard University Press.
Stiglitz, J., Sen, A., & Fitoussi, J. P. (2009). *The measurement of economic performance and social progress revisited. Reflections and overview.* Resource document. Commission on the Measurement of Economic Performance and Social Progress. https://hal-sciencespo.archives-ouvertes.fr/hal-01069384/document. Accessed June 15, 2020.
Sugden, R., & Teng, J. C. Y. (2016). Is happiness a matter for governments? In S. Bartolini, E. Bilancini, L. Bruni, & P. L. Porta (Eds.), *Policies for happiness* (pp. 36–57). Oxford University Press.
Thin, N. (2012). *Social happiness: Theory into policy and practice.* Policy Press.
Veenhoven, R. (1991). Questions on happiness: Classical topics, modern answers, blind spots. In F. Strack, M. Argyle, & N. Schwarz (Eds.), *Subjective well-being: An interdisciplinary perspective* (pp. 7–26). Pergamon Press.

Chapter 7
The Factors of a Successful Happiness Policy

1 Demands of the Happiness Policy

If happiness is accepted as the goal of national development, of course, public policy must be transformed into a happiness-driven policy. In the past, we have focused on happiness as the output of policy, but now, on the contrary, the development goal of happiness should determine policy. Then, what conditions are required for the successful pursuit of such a happiness policy? To answer this, an understanding of the characteristics of happiness as a policy goal must be preceded. As shown in Table 1, the characteristics of happiness as a policy goal can be summarized as follows: (1) the establishment of a policy paradigm that enables the pursuit of happiness as the goal (because it is difficult to pursue happiness as a policy goal in the existing policy paradigm); (2) an individual's subjective emotion is important (because happiness is a subjective attribute); (3) individuals are important policy units (because happiness is basically what an individual feels); (4) the government's active efforts to construct the conditions for happiness are essential (because the government has an obligation to secure the right to pursue happiness, but there is a limit to promoting happiness only with the efforts of individuals with insufficient resources); (5) for the promotion of happiness, the government's efforts alone are insufficient, and individual efforts are also needed (because happiness cannot be secured only by external conditions); and (6) cooperation between policy participants is necessary (due to the limitation of input resources and the connectedness of individual happiness).

From these characteristics of the happiness goal, some conditions for the successful implementation of happiness policy can be derived. As shown in Table 1, such conditions include: (1) transition of policy paradigm (from process-based to goal-based), (2) establishment of consumer-centered policy orientation (balanced, microscopic, and preemptive), (3) micronization of policy of units, (4) restructuration of governance, (5) enhancing government capabilities, and (6) strengthening citizens' capabilities (Lee & Oh, 2013: 47). Though these conditions are interrelated, (1) policy paradigm and (2) consumer-centered policy orientation are conditions related to "policy," and (3) the policy execution unit, (4) government capability,

S. J. Lee, *Public Happiness*, Community Quality-of-Life and Well-Being,
https://doi.org/10.1007/978-3-030-89643-0_7

Table 1 Happiness goal attributes and requirements for policy orientations

Characteristics of happiness as a policy goal	Conditions for the successful implementation of the happiness policy
Importance of happiness goals	Transition of the policy paradigm from process-based toward goal-based
Importance of subjective satisfaction	Consumer-oriented policy orientation – Balance between economic and non-economic policy – Microscopic policy (tailored services) – Preemptive services (outreach service)
Importance of individual dimension	Micronization of policy enactment unit or governance unit
Importance of governance	Establishing good governance
Importance of government intervention	Strengthening governmental competence
Importance of individual responsibility	Strengthening civic competence

(5) citizen capability, and (6) governance are conditions related to "governance" for policy enactment. Reflecting this, the discussion below divides these conditions into policy-related conditions and governance-related conditions.

2 Directions of Happiness Policy

2.1 The Basic Directions of Happiness Policy

Transition of Policy Paradigm: From Process-Based to Goal-Based

The most basic condition for the successful implementation of the happiness policy is that not only is happiness set as an explicit policy goal, but the policy paradigm must be shifted in a direction that responds to it. Even if happiness is adopted as a policy goal, if the past policy paradigm continues, there should be a high concern that happiness will end up as a nominal policy goal or political rhetoric rather than being pursued as a substantial policy goal. This concern is particularly important because the happiness goal has more subjective, personal, and abstract properties, but existing policies have been pursued for goals with more objective, collective, and specific properties.

Furthermore, the general policy paradigm has evolved to a process-oriented paradigm rather than a goal until now. In other words, the dominant policy paradigm so far has focused on the issue of how to manage human, material, and information resources more efficiently than policy goals. Even when interested in the goal, priority was given to process values such as democracy, efficiency, and equity as an intermediate goal rather than an interest in a good life, which is the ultimate goal of policy. As such, policies so far have tended to act as barriers to the policy goals by prioritizing the policy process rather than focusing on the policy goals. This process-based paradigm has always been an approach that was limited in that policy itself is not an end but a means to achieve a goal. This applies to all policies in general, but is particularly important for the pursuit of happiness policy. This is because, as indicated earlier, the causal relationship between the policy and the goal in happiness policy is more uncertain than the relationship between the process and goal in general policy due to the lack of accumulated related knowledge and the involvement of the individual's interpretation process. Because the causal relationship between policies and the happiness goal is uncertain, a transition from the conventional process-based paradigm to the goal-based paradigm is required in pursuing the happiness policy.

Establishing a Consumer-Centered Policy Approach

Happiness is related to subjective satisfaction or evaluation at the individual level, and in order to respond to this, it is necessary to convert the conventional supplier-centered policy approach toward a consumer-centered policy approach. As a consumer-centered policy approach, the following three suggestions can be made. First, it is necessary to balance economic and non-economic policies. Happiness is related to the satisfaction of human needs and is composed of various needs, in both the economic and non-economic aspects. Therefore, not only economic policy but also balanced attention to non-economic aspects is necessary. The pursuit of happiness does not mean that economic interest should be neglected. The economy is still an important influencer of happiness. Therefore, promoting the happiness policy does not mean avoiding economic policy, but demanding a policy balance between the economic and non-economic aspects.

Second, in order to adequately respond to demands of consumers at the individual level, a micro-policy approach should be emphasized rather than a macro-policy approach. In other words, rather than establishing and pursuing policies at the national or large group level, relative attention should be paid to the responding individual level. This is because standardization and generalization are prioritized in macro-policy, so consideration of locality and individuality will inevitably be neglected compared to the case of micro-policy. The micronization of policy has the same meaning as tailored service in the sense that it responds to individual demands at the individual level. Through tailored services, individuals will be able to satisfy their needs at a higher level, and the level of happiness will be improved accordingly. Of course, due to the innate characteristics of public policies for a large number of individuals or groups, there may be limitations in that individuality or specificity can be considered sufficiently, but at least in a relative sense, it is possible to change the conventional policy approach, which is characterized by uniform treatment, to a more microscopic approach. Such transition efforts can be made easier by progress in information technologies, coordination of policy units, and strengthening the capacity of public officials and citizens.

Third, a preemptive policy approach is necessary. In order to effectively respond to individual demand, the government should proactively identify individual service demands prior to individuals approaching the government and adopt preemptive service efforts in providing public services (cf., Denhardt & Denhardt, 2003). Such preemptive service (or active service) is also an essential element for the effective implementation of micro- or customized policies. This is because it is difficult to realize a micro-policy or a customized policy without a preemptive approach. The core of the preemptive service is the government's own active contact efforts prior to the voluntary contact action of the consumer. The reason for demanding the government's proactive contact with citizens is that citizen participation has inherent constraints due to costs, such as time, money, knowledge, and information, and the unequal distribution of these resources acts as a deteriorating factor for social equity. In other words, the government's active outreach is encouraged prior to civic participation because it has advantages in reducing potential costs for participation, reducing concerns about social inequality, and accumulating trust and cooperation between the government and citizens. Preemptive services in which the government approaches the people first will become a practical preemptive policy when the following four elements (C.A.R.E) are included: (1) Make sure that trustworthy, not formal, contact is made (credible). (2) Provide access to services so that they are easily accessible to all citizens (access). (3) Ensure sustainability in the policy process (responsible). (4) Maintain fairness in policies so that they do not alienate anyone due to physical reasons or lack of information (equitable).

2.2 Contents of the Happiness Policy

List of Happiness Policies

For the direction of the happiness policy, the establishment of a goal-centered policy paradigm and the consumer-centered policy stance (policy balance, micronization, and preemption) were discussed above. Here, the contents of the happiness policy will be discussed in more detail.

In order to establish a comprehensive and systematic list of happiness policies, it is desirable to develop policy alternatives based on appropriate types of happiness policies rather than sporadically presenting fragmented policy suggestions. This is because the appropriate policy typology can be used as an instrument to prepare a more comprehensive and systematic policy list according to the scope or perspective of the typology, or to establish and promote differentiated policies for each policy target or unit. An example of presenting a policy list based on the typology of happiness policy is Diener and Biswas-Diener (2019), which presented a happiness policy based on the size of a policy unit as a category. After classifying the policy units into societal level, local level, and individual level, they presented specific policy items for each category: health, income, corruption, and pollution as societal-level policies; domestic violence, governmental corruption, and tight-knit neighborhoods as local-level policies; and skills and habits of individuals as individual-level policies. This categorization will help policymakers to prioritize policies relevant to the respective units.

Table 2 Types of happiness policy

		Policy target (demand side)	
		Macro-approach	Micro-approach
Policy unit (supply side)	Wide area (national and regional)	A. Wide macro-policy	B. Wide micro-policy
	Narrow area (local and community)	C. Narrow micro-policy	D. Narrow micro-policy

Here, we present a policy typology based on the supply and demand aspects of the happiness policy from a more comprehensive perspective (Table 2). First, the demand side of the policy is divided into a macro-approach and a micro-approach based on the scope of the policy target. The former is a policy targeting the entire population or residents of a wide area, and the emphasis is on universality. The latter targets the residents of local governments or community residents, and specificity is emphasized. The supply side of the policy is divided into a wide area unit and a narrow area unit based on the policy execution unit. The former may refer to a country, state, or province, and the latter may refer to a province or community. Four policy types can be derived by overlaying these two criteria. Type A is a wide macro-policy. That is, this type of policy is a policy pursued by the state or regional government with the entire population or residents of a large region as a policy unit and may include macroeconomic policies, SOC policies, etc. Type B is a wide micro-policy. That is, this type of policy is a policy pursued by the state or regional government with the entire state or individual residents of a large region as a policy unit and may include health insurance, public assistance, etc. Type C is a narrow macro-policy. That is, this type of policy is a policy pursued by the local or community government with the entire local or community residents as a policy unit and may include local health, support for community activities, etc. Type D is a narrow micro-policy. That is, this type of policy is a policy pursued by the local or community government with each local or community resident as a policy unit and may include support for individual psychological treatment and emergency life support.

This typology is an example, but it can be used as a framework that can promote a differentiated happiness policy according to the policy organization and policy target.

Which type of policy should be prioritized? Basically, happiness is multidimensional, and therefore, various social conditions can have a significant effect on happiness. This means it would be undesirable to focus only on certain types of policies. Nevertheless, the emphasis of a policy that values happiness can be shifted from type A policies toward type D policies considering that policies in the past have focused exclusively on the economy, giving priority to type A policies.

Also, more detailed policies can be derived for each type. For example, Diener and Biswas-Diener (2019) categorized happiness policies into individual, local, and social levels as seen above and presented detailed individual-level wellbeing intervention programs for each policy category, based on suggestions from positive

Table 3 Examples of wellbeing interventions

Thinking	Social	Biological	Listing, Labelling, and Describing
Cognitive Behavioral Psychotherapy	Altruism	Learning Deep Relaxation Techniques	Strengths Identification
Mindfulness Training	Forgiveness & Gratitude	Exercise	Narrative Writing
Loving Kindness Meditation	Social Recreation	Sleep	Counting Kindnesses & Blessings

Source Diener and Biswas-Diener (2019), p. 100

psychology. Specifically, as shown in Table 3, they divide policy interventions for individual happiness into four areas, such as thinking happier, social happiness, physical happiness, and listing and labeling, and list detailed policy items for each policy area. First, in the field of happy thinking, it is suggested that policy efforts to expand psychotherapy opportunities to more people beyond the mentally ill are necessary, because psychological intervention is effective not only for the mentally ill but also for general people. Second, in the area of social happiness, it is suggested that policy efforts to create a social atmosphere are necessary to ensure the happiness effect of altruism since giving helps happiness. Third, in the area of physical happiness, it is suggested that policy efforts to create conditions for physical fitness training and health maintenance are necessary, because bodily wellbeing affects psychological wellbeing. Fourth, in the area of listing, labelling, and describing, it is suggested that policy efforts to ensure that such actions occur in a stable way because recording or acknowledging positive things such as good luck, empathy, and good deeds helps to promote happiness.

Overall, such individual-level policies focus on psychotherapy as interventions to directly increase the level of happiness, and accordingly, a more direct and prompt policy effect is expected than efforts to promote happiness through improvement of social conditions. On the other hand, in the process of direct intervention with individuals, there are concerns of excessive public intervention harming privacy and individual autonomy, so efforts to find a balance point between the two will be necessary. In addition, as they also mentioned, the happiness policy is not limited to policies at the individual level but encompasses policies at the collective level. There is a need for additional efforts to suggest systematic policy proposals for the improvement of social conditions.

Survey items of existing happiness-related surveys can help establish an overall list of happiness policies. This is because the survey items cover a variety of social conditions. In this regard, the survey items of existing surveys, such as the Better Life Index, World Value Survey, and Gross National Happiness, have already been introduced in Chap. 4. In this section, I introduce the measurement items of the Community Wellbeing Index since this indicator system covers various fields of social conditions on the basis of six capitals and can be used to derive a policy list from a more comprehensive perspective. The six capitals, which are applied as the criteria to derive survey items, include human development (education, health, welfare), economy (employment and regional economy), society (community relations, citizenship, trust, culture), environment (physical and ecological environments), infrastructure (housing, ICT, transportation, safety), and governance. As shown in Table 4, the specific survey items consist of 17 domains and a total of 47 indicators.

Stages of Happiness Policy

It was previously suggested that, for the successful implementation of happiness policies, a happiness-driven and consumer-oriented policy approach should be maintained. At a more specific level, Helliwell et al. (2019) provide a good reference by presenting eight stages of successful happiness policies as follows.

(1) Securing support and establishing an objective: It is necessary to secure broad support from stakeholders for the happiness-based policy orientations. In particular, it is important to obtain support from policymakers. It is also necessary to present accepted objectives supported by data and analysis.
(2) Turning talk into action: When support and data and analysis supporting the happiness policy are secured, the transition to action becomes easier. Good examples (leading examples) should be available to encourage innovation or include practice at the operation level.
(3) Enabling collaboration within portfolios: The policy process should be one that can build trust or liking capital among members of different levels of organizations. A horizontal cooperative process is preferable to a vertical command system.
(4) Enabling collaboration across ministries and disciplines: A silo-linking process spanning related organizations, departments, and expertise should be promoted, overcoming the sectionalism of government departments or experts.
(5) Pursuing innovation: Innovation should be induced based on experimentation and evaluation of policy effects. It is recommended to take a step-by-step approach to spreading success cases after implementing it in a small range at the beginning.
(6) Facilitating consistent policy choices: It is important to maintain consistency in policy choices, and for this, wellbeing evaluation criteria for various outcomes in various areas must be secured. In doing so, care should be taken to reduce the inequality of the wellbeing distribution. In addition, rather than focusing on resolving some misery, it is better to pursue policies with the entire population in mind and focusing on creating positive circumstances. Policies for improving social conditions can benefit those in misery even more.
(7) Assuring continuity: If positive leadership is not secured in the happiness policy, it is difficult to maintain it. For this, it is necessary to clarify the long-term vision for happiness policy, disseminate information about the benefits of happiness policy, and conduct education and training to maintain and foster leadership.
(8) Reporting of results: The diffusion of policy innovation does not occur naturally, so active efforts must be made for transmission of policy results. By doing

Table 4 Indicators of the community wellbeing index

Capital	Domain	Indicator
Human development capital	Education	Public libraries
		Lifelong education services (local community education programs, etc.)
		Schools (elementary, junior high, senior high)
	Health	Medical service
	Welfare	Service for the elderly care
		Service for the handicapped
		Childcare service
		Overall education, health, and welfare levels
Economy capital	Employment	Availability of jobs of the local community
		Unemployment assistance of the local community
	Local economy	Revitalization of the local economy
		Living costs
		Overall employment and local economy levels
Social capital	Community activity	Participation in community associations
	Community tie	Community ties
		Communication and interaction with neighbors
	Civic awareness	Citizen participation in community affairs
		Civic awareness
		Respecting community interests
	Trust	Trust in local residents
		Trust in local government
		Trust in local politics
		Trust in national government
		Trust in national politics
	Cultural activity	Leisure and recreations
	Community cultural heritage	Cultural facilities and programs
		Inheritance of traditional cultural values

(continued)

Table 4 (continued)

Capital	Domain	Indicator
		Overall community bond, civic awareness, trust, and culture level
Environment capital	Environment	Recycling facilities and refuse collection
		Air pollution
		Parks and open space
		Quality of lakes, rivers, and sea
		Overall environment levels
Infrastructure capital	Dwelling	Living conditions
		Water supply and sewerage
	ICT	Information and communication service
	Transportation system	Public transport
		Road conditions
	Safety	Disaster/safety management
		Prevention of infectious diseases
		Response to infectious diseases
		Public order and police services
		Overall dwelling, transportation, information and communication, and disaster response level
Governance capital	Governance	Quality of local government administration
		Public officials' attitude toward service
		Public officials' administrative capacity
		Overall public service level

Source 2020 Community Wellbeing Survey, Global Community Institute

so, it is possible to facilitate the diffusion of happiness policy across regions and narrow the inspiration and knowledge gap for happiness policy.[1]

[1] For the diffusion of policy innovation, in addition to active efforts, it is necessary to strengthen the automatic mechanism for the diffusion of policy innovation through reform of the government structure. For the automatic diffusion of innovation, the decentralized governing structure is more advantageous than the centralized governing structure. In the centralized structure, the diffusion of policy innovation may occur in a short period of time, but uniform application of innovation may cause inefficiencies, and policy continuity problems may arise depending on the effectiveness of monitoring and acceptance of the governing unit. On the other hand, in a horizontal decentralized structure, the speed of diffusion of innovation may be comparatively slow, but there is an advantage of diffusing innovative policies suitable for local conditions by an automatic control mechanism

The steps of the happiness policy Helliwell et al. (2019) suggest do not necessarily have to be executed in this order, but they present important factors to keep in mind during the execution of the happiness policy. Two things are added to this. First, it is important to reflect citizens' demand in the happiness policy. For this, it is necessary to perform a national priority survey on social conditions related to happiness. Such information is necessary for prioritization among various policies, resource input, and distribution, which are crucial elements for enhancing the effectiveness of happiness policy. Of course, such a priority survey can be understood as being included in the data or analysis mentioned in the first policy step. However, since securing information on people's priorities is one of the core elements in executing happiness policy, it is necessary to be included in the policy stage more explicitly.

Second, the evaluation of the policy should be included as an additional step. In order to improve happiness policy and secure its sustainability, improvement efforts through evaluation of policy performance must be made cyclically. This process should be repeated in the policy process rather than one time at the end of the policy process. In such policy evaluations, communication with citizens should be emphasized. This is because policy improvement should basically reflect the will of citizens who are the subject of happiness policy. The consumer-centered policy presented earlier implicates this.

Third, the government does not have to monopolize intervention efforts to promote happiness, and cooperation between stakeholders is necessary in the process of happiness policies. The process of the happiness policy requires, beyond the government's solo efforts, governance based on cooperation between stakeholders. In this regard, Helliwell et al. also show the same recognition by emphasizing partnerships. Specifically, they argue that the successful implementation of the happiness policy depends on the ability to secure collaboration and cooperation while allowing deniability for the happiness policy on the one hand and maintaining desirability for it on the other hand. At the same time, they argue that excessive commitments to happiness are not desirable because they induce opposition and hinder happiness policies. They emphasize partnership in the happiness policy arguing that the success cases of various interventions for happiness are bottom-up or cooperation cases based on private intervention rather than the government's monopoly policy. They argue that (national) governments should play a role in maintaining and creating partnerships for the promotion of happiness through function and financial support. A question is how actively the government should be in forming partnerships. Those concerned about excessive government intervention and emphasizing civil autonomy will argue that the role of the government should be limited to subsidiary roles that support citizens' bottom-up efforts. In contrast, those emphasizing the active role of the government will argue that government should take the initiative in making policies and maintain a cooperative relationship with citizens. Both have a same

---

for policy diffusion among decentralized governing units. That is, in a situation where the innovation policy is not forced downward, good policy innovation initiated by one policy unit is widely diffused due to the voluntary acceptance of neighboring or other units, but bad policy changes are automatically blocked due to the rejection or indifference of neighboring units, thereby enabling sustainable policy diffusion that fits the local situation (Gray, 1973; Lee, 2004; Walker, 1969).

form of partnership or governance, but their emphasis is different. Which position to take? Happiness policy is basically an effort of the government to improve social conditions that are difficult to solve with only individual resources and capabilities, so the commitment of policymakers and active involvement of government organizations and finances are necessary. At the same time, communication and cooperation with citizens must be maintained in such government intervention. That is, it is necessary to accept the opposing positions in a balanced way. However, it should be indicated that it is not desirable to go beyond this balanced position and excessively limit the role of the government in partnership. Such restrictions may be misused as rationales for exempting the government from responsibilities regarding the promotion of people's happiness. To a great extent, discussions of the happiness policy are inevitably premised on the active role of the government. This discussion is basically related to the question of how to understand governance, which will be discussed in more detail later.

2.3 Caveats to the Happiness Policy

Before concluding the discussion on the contents of the happiness policy, I add a few things to keep in mind in the happiness policy process. First, economic policy as well as non-economic policy is still important in happiness policy. As the driving force behind the happiness policy comes from the awareness that human happiness is not guaranteed by the economy alone, it is natural that more attention is paid to the non-economic aspects of the promotion of the happiness policy. However, happiness policy should not be misunderstood as synonymous with non-economic policy. The reason for promoting the happiness policy is not because the economy is not related to happiness, but because the economy is not the sole determinant of happiness. The economy is still an important factor in happiness. Moreover, when economic stability is threatened by an economic crisis or by the spread of a pandemic as in recent years, the economy is bound to emerge as an important factor. Therefore, the economy should not be undervalued on the list of happiness policies. However, in terms of the importance of economic factors, it is necessary to pay increased attention to life stability and alleviating economic inequality rather than economic growth. This is because, when approached from the perspective of happiness, stability or inequality becomes more important than growth among economic factors. Therefore, there is a need to increase attention to policies that strengthen social safety nets or alleviate economic inequality, such as the minimum wage system, basic pension system, basic income system, negative income tax, emergency assistance, and reorganization of the tax structure, beyond the policy to increase income. The problem is that such policies affecting the structure of distribution in society are difficult to promote because of conflict along the lines of political ideology. However, such policies with embedded conflicts may also provide an opportunity to reach a new agreement beyond political ideological lines by approaching public happiness as a new standard, which can be another motivating factor for pursuing the happiness policy.

Second, the happiness policy should focus primarily on improving social conditions rather than individual psychological changes. A policy that focuses on the individual's psychological or disposition can be a valid approach in that individual happiness is subject to the individual's psychological disposition. The effect of psychological policies is direct and immediate if policy effects can be secured. Meanwhile, the change of happiness through improvement of social conditions takes time, and even the causal relationship is uncertain. Therefore, in extreme cases, it is conceivable to pursue a policy that focuses on the individual's psychology only, without an effort to improve social conditions. However, such an approach has limitations. Happiness policy should basically support the improvement of social conditions so that individuals can carry out their desired activities to pursue happiness on that basis. Such policy efforts, in the expression of Sen (1999), are to provide the capability or opportunity for individuals to pursue happiness. Efforts to promote happiness only by changing individual attitudes without such improvement in capabilities are not sustainable. In this regard, it should be noted that an individual's attitude is significantly influenced by external conditions. Therefore, it is important to improve external conditions as much as external conditions affect individual attitudes or as external conditions affect happiness. If the importance of social conditions as an object of happiness policy is neglected, there is a concern that the happiness policy may be frustrated by weakening the government's will to improve social conditions or the social impetus to reflect on social conditions in relation to happiness. In particular, the government, which has limited resources to put into happiness policy, may be tempted to dismiss happiness as a psychological problem for individuals to solve. Of course, this does not mean that policies related to individual psychology should be excluded from the list of happiness policies. Instead, it emphasizes that the happiness policy should focus primarily on improving social conditions even when accepting policies related to individual psychological changes.

Third, the happiness policy does not have to be a policy that is completely distinguished from general policy. Of course, there may be cases where new policy development is necessary with regard to happiness, but if the primary purpose of the happiness policy is to improve social conditions, there is no fundamental difference between the happiness policy and general policies in that the existing policies also purport to improve social conditions. In other words, the happiness policy is not a policy that is completely different from existing ones, but a policy that renews the goal and process of the existing policies in consideration of the causal relationship with happiness, adjusts the priority of resource input, and reinforces policy management based on evidence. However, promoting such a happiness policy is not an easy task. This is because it has the same form as existing policies, but is substantially different in content. In the past, the policy of the growth state was sufficient to pursue growth maximization, and the policy of the welfare state to pursue welfare maximization. However, the policy of a happiness state is not enough to pursue the maximization of growth or welfare. It is because a discussion on how growth or wellbeing is related to happiness must be accompanied in the policy process. In other words, when it comes to the relationship with happiness, it may be more important not to maximize growth or welfare but to optimize the balance between growth and welfare, or to satisfy other social conditions. Accordingly, the policy problem in the process of pursuing a happiness state has the attribute of a more difficult task compared to those of the growth state or welfare state. The acquisition of policy support for new policy goals, restrictions on resource input, and uncertainty in policy effects are additional constraints. In this respect, the happiness policy has the character of a new challenging task that requires higher policy capabilities compared to those of the past. In the future, the rich country or the welfare state may not be the most advanced country, but a country that has the capacity to effectively respond to such difficult demands of happiness policies will remain the advanced countries or become new advanced countries.

3 Realizing Good Governance

3.1 Governance and Good Governance

What is Governance?

For the successful implementation of the happiness policy, an appropriate governance system for policy implementation must be established. Even if the policy direction is correct, it will be difficult to expect policy results unless a governance system to support policy implementation is properly established. However, compared to the abundant discussion on measurement of happiness and fragmentary discussions on happiness policy, it is difficult to find a full-fledged discussion on governance related to the implementation of the happiness policy, and interest in it is needed in the future. For the successful execution of the happiness policy, cooperation between the participants is necessary beyond the government's unilateral effort in the policy process. (In other policies, cooperation between the government and private actors including individuals and markets is necessary. However, in relation to the happiness policy, cooperation between the government and citizens should be especially emphasized, because the subject of happiness is the individual. Therefore, in discussing governance, the focus is on citizens without excluding market factors.) The reason cooperation between participants is important is that there is a conflict between the limit of governmental resources as a supply factor and unlimited individual desires as a demand factor, and thus, adjustments for the balance between the two are necessary. In addition, the fact that the government's efforts to improve social conditions are not entirely linked to the increase of happiness, and that it is influenced by the interpretation of individuals is a cause that demands cooperative efforts between the government and citizens. Such an expansion of cooperation between the government and citizens means the expansion of governance.[2]

[2] The concept of technodemocracy is useful to understand the justification of governance based on cooperation between the government and civil society. The ideal society can be said to be a technodemocracy, a political system in which technocracy based on expert judgment of technocrats

What is governance? In the 1990s, the reflection of the government's failure on the one hand and the growth of the market and civil society on the other increased the criticism of the government's monopoly on decision-making. Demands and discussions for governance as a bottom-up or horizontal decision-making method were widespread. The resumption of interest in the state that emerged in the 1980s is also one of the reasons for this change (Skocpol, 1985). Governance basically means that the role of the private sector other than the government increases in solving public problems. That is, in governance, as the participation of non-governmental actors (businesses, civil society) increases in the decision-making process which has been monopolized by the government, the participation and consensus of related groups becomes more valued. Supposing that society is composed of government, market, and civil society, governance emphasizes the interaction and partnership between them and is an expanded concept than the traditional concept of government. Governance is a term used collectively for not only public governance related to the government but also private governance related to the private sector. However, here, the discussion focuses on public governance in relation to the promotion of the happiness policy. Another reason for doing so is that the interest in governance was originally raised as a new way of managing public affairs in parallel with the critique of the limitations of nationalism or the rise of marketism represented by neoliberalism. However, the discussion of public governance is significantly related to private governance. This is because public governance is closely related to private governance by sustaining and regulating private activities (cf. Bevir, 2012: 1).

The concept of governance is not clearly established, and it is used in various ways depending on the author. In this regard, Rhodes (1996: 653) distinguishes six uses of the term: the minimalist state, corporate governance, New Public Management, good governance, a sociocybernetic system, and self-organizing networks. As Doeveren (2011) aptly points out, it seems that in the absence of a dominant definition of governance, scholars adopted any definition they pleased as long as it pertained to a decision-making process or the outcome of a decision-making process. Take some conceptualization examples. First, there is a position that understands governance as comprehensively related to governmental institutions and governmental processes. For example, the World Bank defines governance as the traditions and institutions by which authority in a country is exercised, which includes the process by which governments are selected, monitored, and replaced; the capacity of the government to effectively formulate and implement sound policies; and the respect of citizens and the state for the institutions that govern economic and social interactions among them (Kaufmann & Kraay, 2008: 7). On the other hand, there are positions that emphasize that governance is a different form of governance than government. For

---

and democracy based on public opinion are harmonized (De Sario & Langton, 1987). Such a society is neither a limited democratic society as supported by elitists, nor is it a populistic society in which participation is maximized as supported by democrats. In a technodemocratic society, it is expected that public happiness can be pursued more effectively by appropriately harmonizing the stability and demands of society, avoiding the arbitrary domination of professional bureaucrats or the seditious driving of public opinions. Such a technodemocratic society can be called cooperative democracy in that it is based on cooperation between the state and citizens (Lee & Kim, 2018: 582).

example, Peters and Pierre (1998) define governance as a method of governing with elements such as networks rather than government, exercise of influence rather than direct control, blending of public and private resources, and utilization of multiple instruments; Rhodes (1997) understands governance as a voluntary interorganizational network characterized by reciprocity, resource exchange, rules of the game, and autonomy from the state. Similarly, Lee (2002a, b) defines governance as a new way of governance that encompasses the characteristics of actors' autonomy, network management, and goal orientation of the system.

Other scholars focus on the process of coordination or collaboration among various actors. For example, Campbell et al. (1991) define governance as the political and economic processes that coordinate activity among economic actors, and provide six ideal-type mechanisms of governance, such as markets, obligational networks, hierarchy, monitoring, promotional networks, and association. Likewise, the Commission on Global Governance (1995: 2) understands governance as the continuing process through which conflicting or diverse interests of individuals and institutions, public and private, may be accommodated and cooperative action may be taken. More similar definitions include: "a political process in which various actors, including the state, coordinate and solve common problems through discussion and negotiation in an autonomous and interdependent process" (Kim, 2005), "a large number of participants working together toward a common purpose," "The process of governing" (Choi, 2002), "mechanism of cooperation between the government, the market and civil society" (Kim et al., 2002), "mechanism of social coordination to solve common problems" (Lee, 2002a, b), etc.

Some conceptualizations focus on decision-making. For example, Kooiman (2003: 2) describes governing as "the activities of social, political and administrative actors that can be seen as purposeful efforts to guide, steer, control or manage (sectors or facets of) societies" and governance as the pattern that results from these governing activities. More examples of conceptualization of the same position include: "The action or manner of governing" (Lynn, 2010: 671), "A process whereby societies or organizations make their important decisions, determine whom they involve in the process and how they render account" (Graham et al., 2003), "A process of setting, applying, and enforcing rules" (March & Olsen, 1995: 6), "All stages of the dynamic processes of political decision-making" (Doeveren, 2011), etc.

Notwithstanding the various definitions, at least some commonalities can be found among them. In other words, most governance concepts do not limit governance to the monopolistic actions of the government, but expand it to cooperative decision-making between the government and the private sector (market and civil society) to solve common problems. Therefore, a concise conceptualization effort is needed to escape the labyrinth of unnecessary concepts while preserving these commonalities. In response to this request, this book briefly defines governance as an "extension of the boundary of decision processes." That is, the decision process, which has been monopolized by the government, is now spread to external participants, and therefore, decisions are made as a result of the interaction between the participants extended.[3]

Here, the extension of the decision process includes dual meanings. One is the extension of participants in the decision process, and the other is the extension of methods in the decision process. First, the expansion of participants in the decision process means that the scope of participants in the decision process is expanded to include the private sector (citizen and market) beyond the government. That is, it is a shift from government monopoly to cooperation with private participants. Therefore, if governance is classified based on decision-making actors, governance encompasses not only government-centered but also market-centered and civil society-centered governance. Since such governance includes participants other than the government, it can be used to include not only public governance related to the government but also private governance related to private policies within the private sector. In addition, governance can be used for public governance confining it to the relation between the central government, local governments, and public institutions, and can also be applied to global governance across national boundaries by expanding the scope. Second, the expansion of decision methods means that the decision methods change to include market and network as well as hierarchy, where hierarchies rely on authority and central control, markets rely on prices and dispersed competition, and networks rely on trust across associations (Bevir, 2012: 16–30).[4]

As such, conceptually, the meaning of governance can be divided into the aspect of decision-making actors (or participants) and the aspect of decision-making methods. This is because when the government is the main actor, the hierarchy centered on the bureaucracy will function; when the market is the main actor, the market mechanism will function; and when civil society is the main actor, the network will function. In other words, the dual meaning of governance is only a difference in approach and emphasis, so it would be reasonable, from an integrated perspective, to define

---

[3] The extension of the "decision process" can be expressed as an extension of the boundary of "policymaking process." This is because, like decision-making, "policy" is a term applied not only to decision-making in the public domain, but also to decision-making in the private sector. Therefore, in fact, in defining governance, whether it is expressed as "decision" or "policymaking" is basically a matter of terminology, and virtually there is no difference in content. Nevertheless, policy is often understood as an abbreviation of public policy, and in that case, the conceptualization of governance expressed as "policymaking" may be misunderstood as referring only to public governance, excluding private governance. To prevent this misunderstanding here, governance is defined using the term "decision." However, in defining the concept of governance, this paper intentionally avoids using the term "governing" as in many literatures. This is because such a definition seems to have some tautological connotations. Of course, considering that the core of governing lies in decision-making, and that governing has a wider semantic scope than decision-making, it is not wrong to define governance using governing. Also, there is little difference in meaning between the two. However, I prefer to define governance by using the term "decision" than "governing," focusing on the brevity and clarity of conceptualization.

[4] Pierre and Peter (2000) distinguish between "governance as structure" and "governance as process." "Governance as structure" refers to the different institutional arrangements and the inclusion of societal actors under new conditions, and "governance as process" refers to the interactions among structures. This distinction largely corresponds to the distinction between the actor aspect and the decision method aspect presented here.

governance as the expansion of the boundary of the decision process or the expanded decision process.

Governance is a concept similar to governing in that it refers to the process of decision-making, but at the same time it is distinguished from governing, which has a neutral meaning, in that it includes a shift as the extension of the decision-making process of the government monopoly. In other words, governance has the character of extended governing beyond simply governing. Governance is also different from traditional government. Unlike the conventional government, which focuses more on political institutions, governance is more concerned with the governing (decision-making) process (Bevir, 2012:1). However, the difference between the two is not clear. This is because government also contains the meaning of process. The bigger difference between government and governance is that government refers to a closed policy process centered on the government, whereas governance refers to a diffused decision-making process involving participants other than the government.

Apart from the conceptualization of governance, it needs to be indicated that there is confusion between governance and new governance in the use of the term governance. In some cases, governance and new governance are distinguished. For example, Pierre (2000) calls governance in which partnerships and networks between the government and civil society play a leading role, as new governance, and distinguishes it from old governance, in which the government plays a leading role. Similarly, Peters and Pierre (2012), Denhardt and Denhardt (2003), and Bevir (2012) characterize new governance as a social problem-solving method that relies less on hierarchies and more on markets and networks. Some view new governance more narrowly, while distinguishing between governance and new governance. For example, Lee (2002a, b) sees governance as a mechanism for coordinating social problems and understands new governance by limiting it to network-based governance. Basically, this position focuses on the decision process per se rather than the change in decision process in understanding governance. In this case, old governance refers to a government-centered decision process in the aspect of decision actors and a hierarchy-oriented decision process in the aspect of decision methods; new governance refers to a market- or civil society-centered decision process in the aspect of decision actors, and a market- or network-oriented decision process in the aspect of decision methods. In addition, new governance is often equated with democratic governance or participatory governance.

Unlike these, there are many scholars who do not distinguish between governance and new governance and use them interchangeably (e.g., Jessop, 1997; Rosenau, 1992; Stoker, 2000). In other words, this position understands governance in a narrow sense by focusing on "change" in which actors in decision processes are expanded and decision methods are diversified. For them, the conventional government-centered and hierarchy-based government is not governance. Only governing with a non-governmental market or network is recognized as governance.

The use of terminology is not a matter of right or wrong, but a matter of choice. This paper grasps governance in a broader sense that is not limited to new governance. In other words, governance is understood as a term that includes old governance (government) and newly raised new governance. The reason for doing so is that governance has been used as a term to refer not only to new governance but also to traditional government, that traditional government, to some extent, does not entirely exclude collaboration with mayors and citizens, and that regardless of the type of governance, the government functions as a central actor, otherwise known as private governance.

Types of Governance

Based on various understandings of the concept of governance, diverse types of governance are proposed according to authors. Examples include: minimalist state, corporate governance, good governance, New Public Management, sociocybernetic system, and network (Rhodes, 1996); corporate governance, New Public Management, good governance, interdependent international relations, a sociocybernetic system, new political economy, and self-organizing networks (Rhodes, 2000); market model, participation model, elastic model, and deregulation model (Peters, 1996); hierarchical system, rational system, open system, and autonomy model (Newman, 2001); market, network, hierarchy, monitoring, and association (Campbell et al., 1991); traditional government, market government, participative government, flexible government, and deregulated government (Peters, 1996); old public administration, New Public Management, and new public service (Denhardt & Denhardt, 2003); hierarchy, market and networks (Bevir, 2012); government-oriented governance, market-oriented governance, and civil society-oriented governance (Kim et al., 2002; Lee, 2016), etc.

Most typologies suggest the typology of governance by combining actors or coordination methods of governance alone or in combination. I prefer a typology that, focusing on actors, classifies governance into government-centered, market-oriented, and citizen-centered. This typology has the advantage of identifying decision actors and decision-making methods depending on the actors.

Government-centric governance is a type in which the government takes the lead in managing the market and civil society, and the principle of decision process is hierarchy based on authority and central control. Market-centric governance is a type that expands market participation in order to secure efficiency, and the principle of decision process is market mechanism based on competition and customerism. Civic-centric governance is a type emphasizing the active participation of citizens in order to supplement the limitations of the representative system, and the principle of decision process is participatory democracy.[5]

It should be indicated that, regardless of the type of governance, it is difficult to deny the centrality of government in practice. This is because the government plays the role of coordinator for resolving public problems as the largest reservoir of resources necessary for resolving public problems and as the possessor of the official authority to make decisions. Based on this fact, several commentators express skepticism about governance, for example, that governance exaggerates a

[5] Market-centric and citizen-centric governance can be integrated into society-centric governance. For example, Robichau (2011) classifies these two types as society-centric governance in contrast to state-centric governance.

new phenomenon, that there is little evidence that governance is actually taking place, that the ability of governance to eclipse government is not certain, that the governance discussion is nothing more than pure scholarly debate, etc. (Cho, 2005; Heinrich et al., 2010; Kjæer, 2004; Lynn, 2010). However, governance is not entirely deniable. Even without addressing the arguments of positive proponents about the reality of governance (e.g., Bevir, 2012; Kooiman, 2003; Rhodes, 1996), the assessment that governance is a purely academic debate seems overblown. It is because, as Robichau (2011) pointed out, there is substantial agreement that the current governance decision-making method includes networks, hierarchies, and markets, and such an agreement would not be possible in the absence of any substance of governance. But this does not mean that governance has replaced the government. As Kjær (2004) properly indicates, governance does not take place without government. Therefore, it is appropriate to approach the governance typology in a relative sense. For example, market-centered governance or citizen-centered governance should be understood as accepting market principles or civil society participation to a significant extent compared to traditional government rather than defining it as governance dominated by market principles or civil society participation in a situation in which the government is excluded. Likewise, government-centered governance should be understood as a governance form of enhanced centrality of the government compared to other forms of governance, rather than being understood as a form of decision-making that excludes market principles or citizen participation in the governance. That is, as far as the centrality of government is concerned, it is appropriate to understand the classification of governance as "more or less" rather than exclusive categories. This is especially true in developing countries where civil society and market growth are relatively weak.[6]

[6] This relative nature often induces confusion about the distinction between types of governance. For example, Denhardt and Denhardt describe governance as old public administration, New Public Management (NPM), and new public service (NPS). These correspond to government-centered, market-oriented, and citizen-centered governance, respectively, and each type has its own characteristics. In the old public administration, the decision mode is hierarchy, the role of the government is rowing, and civic status is clients or constituents. In NPM, the decision mode is market, the role of government is steering, and civic status is customers. In NPS, the decision mode is collaboration (or network), the role of government is serving, and civic status is citizens. This distinction has the advantage of making it easy and concise to understand the differences between types of governance. A problem is whether everyone agrees to equate NPM with market-type governance. Basically, the NPM is an administrative paradigm that is open to market principles while maintaining the centrality of government, and thus, it can be said that it has an intermediate character between old public administration and market-oriented governance (Yoo, 2012: 176). If we pay attention to the introduction of marketism in government, we will understand the characteristics of NPM as market-oriented governance, and if we pay attention to that, notwithstanding the ingraftment of marketism, traditional government is the main body, we will understand the characteristics of NPM as government-centered governance. Considering that market-oriented governance focuses on the relationship between government and the market, whereas NPM focuses on management issues within the government, NPM may be classified as a government-centered governance. However, regardless of the type of governance, the centrality of the government is maintained to a considerable extent. Then, although NPM focuses on internal management issues of the government, and the centrality of government maintains in the decision process, it can be understood to be closer to

Aside from the discussion of the centrality of government, an important issue is which type of governance is more effective as governance for the happiness policy. There does not seem to be a fixed answer to this. Of course, considering that there is a greater need to actively reflect the will of citizens, who are the main agents of happiness due to the nature of the happiness policy, it can be expected that open and participatory governance will be more effective than traditional government which is less open and less participatory. In other words, there is a possibility that a governance type in which the centrality of government is not excessive is a relatively effective governance type. Nevertheless, since the degree of suitability will vary depending on the situation, it is difficult to generalize which type of governance will be more effective. For example, the type of governance suitable for Western developing countries with advanced market and civil society and developing countries with relatively insufficient market and civil society may not be the same. While Asian countries are relatively positive about the centrality of government, Western developed countries are relatively skeptical.

What is Good Governance?

For the successful implementation of the happiness policy, good governance is required as substantial governance beyond external or formal governance. The core of governance is the extension of policymaking power from the government monopoly to external participants. Such governance is widely welcomed as a phenomenon that alleviates the harmful effects of alienation and distortion from decision-making by the government monopoly in the past. In addition, there is a possibility that it will contribute more to the promotion of citizen's happiness as it reflects the needs of citizens more in the policy process. However, the expansion of such decision process alone does not guarantee that the happiness policy will be automatically executed and the happiness of citizens will be promoted accordingly. It should be indicated that governance can be detrimental to happiness enhancement if the capacity of governance participants is poor. For example, an encounter between a corrupt government and a greedy business will lead to collusion between politics and business, and an encounter between an incompetent government and selfish citizens will result in a populistic policy, which will hinder the implementation of happiness policy. In addition, a decision-making method that does not fit the social conditions will hinder the effective implementation of the happiness policy. For example, in a society where the market function is not well functioning, the expansion of market-oriented decision modes will not work properly. That is, external or formal governance may be a necessary but not a sufficient condition for the successful implementation of the happiness policy, and accordingly, evolution to a substantial governance type that can contribute to happiness beyond external governance is required. There is a difference between external governance and substantial governance. While external governance focuses on the process of extension of decision participants and decision methods, substantive governance focuses on the outcome of governance that contributes to policy

---

the market-oriented type. This discussion is due to the fact that the centrality of the government is substantially maintained regardless of the type of governance, albeit different degrees.

objectives. Such substantive governance requires cooperation between competent government and citizens, and creative application of decision methods that fit real-world conditions. Only under such governance will the successful implementation of the happiness policy be feasible. In this case, such substantive governance is good governance in the sense that it contributes to the implementation of the happiness policy and further to the enhancement of happiness, which is the ultimate goal of the policy. However, good governance in this sense is somewhat different from the prevailing understanding of good governance, so further discussion on this is required.

The concept of good governance was first used by the World Bank in the Long-Term Perspective Study on Sub-Saharan Africa in 1989. In the 1980s, in relation to aid to developing countries, bad governance was criticized as a cause of national or economic development failure. As a symmetric concept, good governance received attention (Crawford, 2006; World Bank, 1989). Basically, good governance is a general concept that suggests an ideal direction for what governance should be, but with such a background, it is often used narrowly in relation to developmental strategies.

Good governance is defined in various ways. First, to take the example of international organizations, the World Bank operationalized bad governance as personalization of power, lack of human rights, endemic corruption, and unelected and unaccountable governments, and accordingly, good governance is the natural opposite (Weiss, 2000). Initially, the World Bank suggested public sector management, accountability, a legal framework for development, and transparency and information as the dimensions of good governance (World Bank, 1992: 3), but some years after, revised the six dimensions of good governance to voice and accountability, political stability and the absurdity of violence, government effectiveness, regulatory quality, rule of law, and control of corruption (Kaufmann et al., 2008). Despite these changes, the World Bank's approach to good governance has maintained a liberal and market-friendly position since the 1990s. Such marketism of the World Bank is confirmed by its consistent attitude that even the successful cases of state-based East Asian development are regarded as market-friendly development (Crawford, 2006).

The United Nations Development Program (UNDP, 1997) spells out five principles: legitimacy and voice (participation and consensus orientation), direction (strategic vision), performance (responsiveness, effectiveness, and efficiency), accountability (accountability and transparency), and fairness (equity and rule of law) (Graham et al., 2003). UNDP's approach to good governance differs from the World Bank's approach to good governance, which focuses on the efficient management of the public sector from a market-oriented perspective, in that UNDP provides relative support for democratic values such as civic empowerment and decentralization (Kim, 2011; Weiss, 2000).

The European Commission (EC 2001: 10) presented openness, participation, accountability, effectiveness, and coherence as elements of good governance. The International Monetary Fund (IMF) presents ensuring the rule of law, improving the efficiency and accountability of the public sector, and tackling corruption as essential elements of good governance, and the Organisation for Economic Co-operation and Development (OECD) accepts the IMF's approach as it is. The Organization for Security and Co-operation in Europe (OSCE) emphasizes multilateral cooperation among governments, the private sector, and civil society for good governance. Specifically, support for capacity building through education and awareness campaigns, facilitation of cooperation and coordination between institutions, prevention of corruption, education to prevent conflicts of interest, development of code of ethics and asset reporting system, increasing public service integrity, protection of whistle blowers, promotion of transparency and citizen participation, regulatory reform, etc., are presented as strategies for good governance. Besides, several international organizations employ good governance criteria in their considerations about the distribution of development aid.

The concept of good governance presented by academia tends to emphasize the democratic decision-making process from a more comprehensive point of view, compared to the market-friendly approach of many international aid organizations. For example, Minogue et al. (1998) argue that good governance is not only efficiency but also a strategy of government reform that increases the capacity of civil society and makes the government accountable and democratic. Rhodes (2000) understands good governance as formal processes of both private companies and governments for auditing, ensuring transparency, and information disclosure. Rothstein (2012) argues that good governance has meaning as regulation in the provision of public goods by the government and is closely related to state capacity, quality of government, and common-pool resources. Also, as good governance involves the government's interactions with the various private sectors, the government does not function alone, but needs cooperation with other organizations. Besides, Lander-Mills and Serageldin (1991) propose political and bureaucratic accountability, freedom of association, objective and efficient judiciary, freedom of information and expression, efficient public institutions; Manasan et al. (1999) present political transparency and voice for all citizens, efficient and effective public services, the health and wellbeing of its citizens, and a favorable climate for stable economic growth as elements of good governance.

In such a situation wherein various views on the components of good governance are presented, Doeveren (2011) helps to gauge the breadth of understanding good governance through comparison of the approaches to good governance of international organizations and researchers. Objects included in the analysis are: the European Commission (EU, 2001), the OECD (2007; IMF, 1996), the World Bank (Kaufmann et al., 2008), the UN (1997, 2009), Hyden and Court (2002), Smith (2007), and Weiss (2000). As a result of comparative analysis, he found that good governance concept has overtime suggested multiple and sometimes contradictory meanings, but nevertheless remarkably converge around five components of good governance: accountability, efficiency and effectiveness, openness and transparency, participation, and rule of law. He also reported that the details of the elements that share such commonalities exhibit significant discrepancies, and differences among other components were not small. As such, the fact that the understanding of good governance shows similarities in some areas but still shows many inconsistencies reflects that it is difficult to agree on goodness in governance, and that it has to be different depending on the social context.

As we have examined various understandings of good governance above, good governance has meaning as a prescription for the desirable direction that governance should aim for. From this point of view, it is evaluated that the current dominant approach to good governance has limitations, such as the content of prescriptions being scattered, inconsistent, and weak in relation to the results of governance.[7] More specifically, various items are suggested as governance components. This has the advantage of suggesting various possibilities for the direction of governance. However, presenting too many components causes confusion when applied as a guideline for good governance. The list of components needs to be more concise.

Second, contradiction between the proposed components appears. In general, Western developed countries understand liberal democratic governance as good governance. This approach is based on the phenomenon of taking Western developed countries as a model, and it is easy to understand considering that good governance is a concept that has emerged in relation to the development strategies for developing countries of international organizations led by Western developing countries. However, there is a difference in specific content. While some emphasize competitive elections, accountability, and the rule of law, others emphasize pluralism, human rights, and political participation (Bevir, 2012: 105). The former is the approach taken by the World Bank or OECD, and the latter by the UN and the EU. Although they are in the same position as liberal democracy, they differ in that some emphasize more market factor, while the other emphasize more civil society factor. The problem is that these differences confuse the direction of good governance. In this regard, Doeveren (2011) specifically indicates that it is a problem that market liberalization policies are encouraged by the World Bank, whereas the same policies might be classified as bad governance by the United Nations on the grounds that citizens have not been involved in the decision-making process.

Conflicts between items suggested as components of good governance occur not only between institutions but also among the components within the same institution. In this regard, Graham et al. (2003), citing UNDP's good governance principles (legitimacy and voice, strategic vision, performance, accountability, and fairness) as an example, criticize that these principles often overlap or are conflicting at some point, that they play out in practice according to the actual social context, and that applying such principles is complex. Inconsistencies between good governance components also appear on higher levels. As aforementioned, the currently dominant concept of good governance is liberal democratic governance, but the problem is that the universal applicability of this approach is limited. In particular, the World Bank's market-friendly approach is criticized in that it may not be appropriate as a development prescription for developing countries where the state is vulnerable. This is

---

[7] Similarly, Doeveren (2011) criticizes that existing scholars and aids donors paid less attention to defining their components, identifying the possible trade-offs between their components, specifying their optimal values, and result of governance.

because prescriptions such as weakening of state power, strengthening the market, and decentralization of power can lead to bad governance.

Third, current approaches to good governance generally focus attention on the rationality of the decision process, such as efficiency, transparency, and fairness. This tendency is the same regardless of whether the emphasis is on market factors, civil society factors, or state factors. The problem is that, notwithstanding the importance of such process elements as policy values, if you approach good governance by leaning toward such process elements and downplay the relevance to the results or goals of governance, there is a limit that hinders the achievement of the goals of governance to that extent. This is because the process itself is not the goal of public policy. Therefore, in order for good governance to be an effective instrument to support the achievement of policy goals, it is necessary to reapproach it based on interest in the results or goals of governance in presenting components of good governance. In other words, it should be approached with interest in how much of a prescription for the decision process such as strengthening market factors, strengthening civil society, and weakening the state can contribute to policy outcomes as a goal of governance. In doing so, good governance should be governance that contributes to good life, not governance supported by a specific political ideology or fixed view of development. Of course, for example, governance supported on the basis of liberal democracy has the potential to bring desirable results compared to governance that is not, but it should be recognized that liberal democracy itself is at best a process value, not the goal value of good governance.

These discussions require a shift from the narrow definition of good governance which has focused so far on process values such as rule of law, decision-making capacity, legitimacy, transparency, accountability, participation, anti-corruption, and decentralization, to a wider definition of good governance which pays attention to good life or wellbeing as a result of governance. Although there have been many discussions about the process aspect of decision-making in the discussion of good governance so far, it is difficult to find a discussion about the outcome or purpose of such a process. This can be explained as the existing understanding of good governance is basically approached focusing on the rationality of the process rather than the goal of governance.

The problem is that rationalization of processes is not the goal of governance, and does not automatically guarantee substantial contributions to the goals of governance. In this regard, the point of Doeveren (2011) is noteworthy: "Argentina could have ended up with a healthy economy as the result of following IMF guidelines, but instead of economic recovery awaited a severe economic crisis. Meanwhile, the newly industrialized countries of Asia created vast economic growth with policies that violated all the common principles of good governance. As these examples show, one cannot assume that a decision-making process that lives up to good governance principles also produces results for the common good."

As such, even if the decision-making process in governance is rationalized, if it is difficult to achieve the goal value through the process, it is difficult to call such governance good governance. Therefore, good governance needs to be understood based on the close relationship with the results of governance.

Relatedly, it should be indicated that the prevailing understanding of good governance at present seems confused with governance in terms of content. In other words, there are cases where good governance is discussed while calling it governance, and governance is discussed while calling it good governance. Specifically, similar to how governance refers to the extension of participants and methods in the decision process, good governance also focuses on cataloging the extensible elements (participants and methods) of the governance process. However, such cataloging does not differ significantly between the discussion of governance and good governance. In general, they both refer to the extension of decision process to the market and citizens beyond the monopoly of decision process by the government. If there is a difference, the discussion of governance focuses on the description of the phenomenon of expansive change in the decision process, while the discussion of good governance presents such a change as a prescription for solving the public problem. Confusion of good governance with governance seems unavoidable, as both basically focus on changes in the decision-making process. Preferably, good governance needs to focus on the outcome of the process or its relevance to governance goals rather than focusing on the process and vice versa. This is because good governance has a primary meaning as a prescriptive tool that provides a direction for governance beyond specifying the process of governance.

To summarize the discussion above, good governance is a concept that has the characteristics of a practical prescription for governance. Considering the function of good governance, the prevailing prescriptions for good governance have the following limitations. First, by suggesting too many principles for good governance, the prescription entails a problem of diffuse prescriptions for good governance. Second, contradictions between the suggested components of good governance create inconsistent prescriptions for good governance. Third, by focusing on process values rather than on the relevance to governance results, the prescription exhibits a problem of uncertain prescriptions for good governance. These limitations are basically due to the fact that the existing approaches to good governance enumerate a number of process values that are difficult to agree on regardless of the results.

3.2 *Conditions for Good Governance*

In order to prescribe the desirable direction of governance, a new approach to good governance is required. What governance is good governance? What are the conditions for good governance? Its requirements should be primarily explored in relation to the results of governance. In the governance of the happiness policy, happiness enhancement through the successful implementation of the happiness policy is the result and goal of governance. Furthermore, it is necessary to pay attention to the core elements of governance. As mentioned earlier, governance is an extensive change in the decision process and includes two key elements: the expansion of the scope of decision participants and the expansion of the decision methods. Good governance should be an appropriate prescription for such shifts to work in the desired direction. That is, the expansion of the participants and the expansion of decision-making methods should be changed in a desirable direction. To this end, in terms of participants, it should not be simply a rendezvous between the government and the private sector, but cooperative decision-making between the competent government and capable private actors, and in terms of the decision method, flexible application of the decision-making methods depending on the social context is necessary, not the uniform transition from the hierarchy to the market or network method. If such a request is not secured, it will be difficult to implement a successful happiness policy and thus to achieve happiness as a goal of the happiness policy. Such concerns are easily understood if we foresee the results in governance of the collusion between an irresponsible government and greedy citizens or the application of a uniform decision-making method that unfits the social context. This is the reason the discussion on the governance of the happiness policy should pay attention to the participants and methods in the decision process. In particular, it would be useful to approach good governance from this point of view for the successful implementation of the happiness policy in which subjective evaluation occupies a greater proportion compared to other policies. Based on this discussion, paradigm shift in governance, innovation of participants (government and citizen), and methods of governance are presented as conditions for good governance below.

Governance Paradigm Shift: From Process Toward Purpose

As mentioned earlier, for successful implementation, the happiness policy needs to be converted from a process-based to a purpose-based policy. In line with this, the governance paradigm as a policy implementation system for good governance should also be changed from a process-based to a purpose-based paradigm. However, the current discussion of good governance has not paid much attention to the purpose (or the result) of governance. They have shown much interest in presenting the rational value that governance should aim for as a process, but neglected how the process value is related to the goal of the policy. Such a governance has limitation to be called as good governance in terms of contribution to the purpose, because the relationship between process values and policy goals is unclear. It should be emphasized that in the case of happiness policy, good governance means that the result of governance should contribute to happiness (through the promotion of happiness policy). In other words, in order to be good governance, the results of governance must be connected with the goals. And in order to respond to such a request, the governance paradigm must be changed from a process-oriented paradigm to a goal-oriented paradigm.

Current dominant governance paradigms include government-centered traditional governance, market-centered governance, and civic-centered governance, as shown in Table 5.

These paradigms basically give priority to the policy initiative or role between actors in the policy process. In short, the core of the discussion is who among the three actors (governments, market, and civil society) is leading the policy or plays a greater role in the policy process. Interest in whether or not government policy goals are achieved is rather secondary, and the focus of discussion is primarily on defining the scope of participants in the policy process. Discussion of the initiative of participants

Table 5 Governance paradigm comparison

Governance paradigm	Representative democratic government	Old governance	Market-centered governance (New Public Management)	New governance (network, new public service)
Period	19C	Early 20C	Late 20C	Late 20C
Government's role	Democratic representation	Rowing	Steering	Partner and serving
Civic attitude toward governments	Neglect	Active loyalty	Exit and passive loyalty	Voice
Core values	Electoral accountability	Responsibility, expertise, political neutrality	Efficiency and openness	Democracy (participation, cooperation, decentralization)
Limits	Factionalism and favoritism	Unresponsiveness	Private interest prevailing	Responsibility blurred
Citizenship	Voter and constituent	Beneficiary and client	Customer	Citizen and partner
Core actors	Politicians and voters	Bureaucracy	Business and government	Citizen and government
Decision method	Electoral control and delegation	Hierarchy and authority	Markets and competition	Networks and reciprocity

Source Compiled based on Denhardt and Denhardt (2003: 28) and Bevir (2012: 17). Denhardt and Denhardt divided the old public administration, NPM, and NPS, and Bevir divided the two into hierarchy, markets, and networks

in the policy process also tends to be defined uniformly regardless of the achievement of policy goals.[8] Thus, it is assumed that the policy is promoted by the bureaucratic hierarchy if the government is the leader, by the market mechanism if the market is the leader, by the civic participation and network if the citizen is the leader. In doing so, the focus of the discussion is on how much government initiative or monopoly is mitigated, since the government has generally taken the lead in the policy process. Also, as an extension of this, discussions related to methodological ideologies such as whether the policy process is democratic or efficient, participatory or exclusionary become central topics. As such, the existing governance paradigm has relatively neglected its focus on the achievement of policy goals, rather focusing on the policy process. Thus, although a certain policy orientation may be happiness-friendly, it is only consequential or accidental.

[8] It is also argued that governance theory, unlike traditional theory on government, makes no prejudgment about which social actors are most central to the pursuit of collective goals (Peters and Pierre 2012). However, in most cases, governance theory focuses on expanding the role of private actors other than the government uniformly.

Overall, these paradigms show differences in the relative role of actors and decision methods, but have process-based paradigms in common that focus on the decision process regardless of the policy goal, and exhibit limitations as the governance paradigm for the goal of development. It is because the transition of the national goal to happiness requires that governance be reoriented toward the goal of public happiness as a system for delivering happiness policies. That is, if policies are reoriented to goal-driven, governance as a policy delivery system must be reoriented to a goal-based paradigm accordingly.

In the goal-based governance paradigm, unlike in the conventional process-based paradigm, the role of governance actors is not predetermined, but different roles are accepted among participants based on the possibility of contribution to the goal achievement. In the goal-based paradigm, since the priority is given to the achievement of policy goals rather than the role initiative among governance participants, who becomes the leader of the policy is rather a secondary subject of interest. It does not matter whether it is traditional governance, New Public Management, or new public service, as long as it helps to achieve the goal. Unlike the process-based governance paradigm, which tends to regard other paradigms as superior to the traditional paradigm, the purpose-based paradigm does not predetermine superiority and inferiority between governance paradigms. Therefore, the relative superiority of governance forms may vary depending on the circumstances. For example, when a crisis or conflict is newly encountered in the situation where the government's policy initiative is being reduced, the government's leading role can be accepted to achieve the policy goal. This discussion applies equally not only to the participants in governance, but also to the aspect of decision-making methods in governance. In other words, in the goal-based paradigm, the decision-making method in governance is not predetermined, but a different decision-making method is accepted based on the possibility of contributing to the goal achievement. This is because the scope of participants and decision-making methods are closely connected in governance.

Although a combination of various actors and decision methods is possible in the decision process, basically, the goal-driven paradigm is primarily concerned with letting the policy purpose determine the decision process rather than the decision process itself. Even in the case of interest in the relationships participants in the decision process, as for the relationship between the participants in the policy process, since the focus is on goal achievement rather than the initiative between actors, liaison and cooperation are prioritized over participation or exclusion between actors. The same is true for decision methods. This can be said to demand a shift from "governing with" toward "governing for" in the governance discussion, just as interest shifted from "power over" toward "power to" in the power research. In short, if the ultimate goal of public policy is to promote public happiness, there is a fundamental limit to the process-oriented governance paradigm that is developed while neglecting the goal. Although rationalization of the policy process itself is important, desirable governance should be established based on an explicit interest in which policy processes and methods are effective in promoting public happiness. In addition, the goal-based governance paradigm presented here is expected to be a basis to resolving the conflicts of existing paradigms through flexibility of the model,

Table 6 Comparison of process-based governance paradigm and goal-based governance paradigm

	Process-based paradigm	Goal-based paradigm
Core value	Process rationalization	Goal achievement
Actor relation	Roles between actors (power over)	Interrelation between actors (power to)
Focus	Participation or exclusion	Competition or cooperation
Policy ideologies	Efficiency and responsiveness	Effectiveness
Performance	Performance undetermined	Process undetermined
Evaluation	Procedural performance	Goal achievement

while providing a more macro-direction to policies and governance promoting public happiness as a new development objective. For reference, the process-based governance paradigm and goal-based paradigm discussed so far are summarized in Table 6 (Lee, 2016).

Strengthening the Competence of Governance Participants

Assuming that governance participants include the government, which is an official participant, and the market and civil society, which are informal participants, for the effective operation of governance, that is, the realization of good governance, the capabilities of these governance participants must be secured. Good governance will be achieved if cooperation between competent participants occurs, but otherwise it will result in poor or bad governance. If governance that prescribes cooperation between the government and the private sector in the policy process is a necessary condition for good governance, cooperation between the competent government and the private sector is a sufficient condition. This point indicates that governance, which includes the expansion of the participants in the decision process as a core principle, does not automatically lead to desirable results, which is why we need to discuss good governance beyond governance. This request also applies to governance for the happiness policy. In other words, good governance must be secured for the promotion of happiness, and for good governance to be achieved, the capabilities of governance participants must be secured. Nevertheless, in the existing discussion of good governance, instead of paying attention to the relationship between governance participants as a requirement for good governance, interest in the participants' competence is relatively insufficient. The World Bank (1994) exceptionally mentions the quality of bureaucrats and citizens along with other process values, but in most cases, they do not pay much attention to the competence of governance participants. However, as a core requirement for realizing good governance, more serious attention to innovation efforts to strengthen the capabilities of participants is necessary.

Strengthening Government Competence

For good governance, efforts to strengthen the competence of the government, which are the official policymakers, are important. This is because public happiness is affected not only as a result of public policy but also by public evaluation (image) of government competence (Bok, 2010: 179). In this regard, Bovaird and Löffler (2009: 229–230) suggest that for there to be good governance there must be good government.

What is competence? The concept of competence has been presented with various definitions since the introduction of McClelland (1973), but it is generally understood to include material competence, which means overall resources and capabilities of an organization, and personal competence, which means internal characteristics of individuals (Lee & Yoon, 2005). The concept of competence was initially limited to human competence, an internal characteristic of an individual (Boyatzis, 1982; McClelland, 1973; Mirabile, 1997), but was later expanded to include physical competence, which means overall resources and capabilities of an organization, as related research progresses (Sparrow, 1996). Accordingly, government competence can be defined as including the human capacity of public officials constituting the government and the material capacity as the organization and resources of the government.[9]

What are the tasks to strengthen government competence? First, efforts are required to strengthen the competence of public officials. Public officials' competence is human competency and includes the ability and will of public officials. In this competence, expertise in terms of ability is important, but in terms of perception, an active will to contribute to the improvement of individual happiness is also important. This demand is nothing but a request for a change of perception of public officials from a passive policy to an active policy. The proactive service discussed before or the service emphasized by Denhardt and Denhardt can be considered in the active policy category. Such activeness in public policy is particularly important in happiness policy which requires attention to how well the policy satisfies the subjective happiness of an individual beyond simply delivering the policy. However, an active policy that considers the causal relationship between the result of the policy and happiness beyond the delivery of the policy inevitably comes as an additional work burden on public officials. This is because individual needs and responses must be taken into consideration beyond a policy based on group-based consideration. In addition, in order to pursue such a policy, a more open attitude and willingness to serve are required than in other conventional policies. This is the reason for emphasizing not only professionalism but also positive attitude in the competence of public officials to deliver happiness policies. In fact, as the government's role is ubiquitous in the delivery of all public policies, such an active awareness of public officials is an important factor for effective governance. On the other hand, in order to deliver an active

[9] Competence is used interchangeably with capacity. In the dictionary sense, competence refers to the potential to perform work effectively, and capacity refers to the magnitude of the potential to perform work. But the distinction between the two is not always clear, and the practical benefit of the division is not great.

policy, resource consumption inevitably increases, and thus, resource constraints may act as an additional limiting factor for the policy process. In this regard, strengthening the competence of public officials should be given importance because it can function as a factor to overcome such resource constraints.

How can we secure such public capacity? It is not a simple matter, but efforts such as control over public officials, reinforcement of education and training, and rationalization of the evaluation system will be helpful. In this effort, flexible methods such as information disclosure and self-regulation should be actively developed in addition to control instruments such as incentives and disincentives. In education and training, prior to the enhancement of professionalism, it is necessary to prioritize the promotion of public service ethics such as democratic openness and positive attitude to serve. It needs to establish an evaluation system based on results rather than process evaluation.

Second, governmental organizations and policy systems should be reorganized in line with the happiness policy. It is necessary to take actions for the innovation of government organization, including the establishment of a control tower that manages happiness policies, and the introduction of a happiness policy management and evaluation system are necessary. It is necessary to utilize various alternative service delivery methods. The use of an alternative method is to expand the government-exclusive service delivery in the direction of enhancing the participation of the private sector, and it corresponds to the service delivery method that meets the needs of governance. From the viewpoint of happiness policy, it is necessary to pay attention to the development and utilization of service delivery methods based on citizen participation prior to market-based privatization methods in order to enhance the subjective satisfaction of citizens. It is also necessary to secure the material resources necessary for pursuing the happiness policy. To this end, the government needs to adjust the priorities of material resources.

Third, leadership that propels the happiness policy must be established based on the confidence in the happiness policy. Happiness policy requires innovative measures such as change of policy direction, reorganization of organizations, mobilization of resources, and acquisition of support, and such measures are difficult to sustain without strong support from leadership.[10]

[10] Overall, these efforts can be expressed as government innovation efforts. Government innovation is defined in various ways. For example, Berry (1994) defines government innovation as a series of processes for recognizing government policy and administrative issues, discovering and producing information or knowledge, and employing administrative programs or policies. Osborne et al. (1998) understand government innovation as a fundamental reform of a government organization or public service system to enhance the effectiveness and efficiency of public organizations. According to them, government innovation is not about changes in the political system (e.g., electoral campaigns, parliamentary reform, etc.), nor does it mean just the reorganization or reduction of government organizations. It does not mean the abolition of administrative waste or an efficient government, nor is it the same as privatization either. Government innovation should be understood as an effort to strengthen the competence of the government as a whole, including meaningful changes in the structure, personnel, functions, and policy processes of the government.

Strengthening Civic Competence

If governance is a cooperative mechanism between the government, the market, and civil society, the competencies of governance actors in each area must be guaranteed for the realization of good governance. When these prerequisites are not met, governance will not function properly or will be reduced to a lame form of governance by monopolizing control in some areas. Strengthening government capacity alone is insufficient. Efforts to strengthen civic competence are required to position citizens as partners in governance together with the government.

Civic competence refers to the quality of a citizen as a member of a political community, i.e., citizenship. More specifically, civic competence requires the ability and willingness to participate in and make suggestions in public affairs as a member of a political community, along with fulfilling the rights and obligations as a citizen in legal and ethical dimensions. What is required for strengthening civic competence is not much different from what is required for a so-called good citizen. For example, active political participation, ethical and moral responsibility, acceptance of state authority, political knowledge, social order, and social solidarity are suggested as the virtues of a good citizen (Dalton, 2008: 24–26), and these virtues are commonly raised items in discussions of citizenship. Citizens, as members of the political system, have certain rights and responsibilities for the political system to which they belong. Such civic competence, that is, citizenship, can be defined as a series of rights and obligations traditionally defined in the political, social, and economic fields in the formal relationship between the individual and the state (Ghose, 2005).

The focus of the discussion here is on what citizenship is required in relation to the governance of the happiness policy. First of all, it should be pointed out that there is no agreed list of desirable citizenship or required citizenship, and various virtues are suggested (Lee & Kim, 2018: 181–184). For example, Stivers suggested an active citizenship is desirable whose attributes include the four elements: authoritative participation in public decision-making based on simple judgment, consideration of the public interest, political learning, and maintenance of mutual relationships as members of a political community. Ghose (2005) also mentioned that it is necessary to move away from passive citizenship to active citizenship in the name of flexible citizenship. Schachter (1995) proposed a paradigm shift in citizenship from a client-centric perspective to an owner's perspective. She argued that the more effective citizenship among the two is the owner's perspective because citizens with this consciousness will exert efforts to achieve change for the development of the government of which they are owners. Gyford (1991) suggested that citizens should strive to have a sovereign status over the political process by exiting from the objective status of the political process. More specifically, he suggested that citizens are to transform from the conventional ratepayer to the shareholder, from a client to a consumer, and from a voter to a citizen. Disagreements exist over liberal virtues. For example, Galston (1988), under the premise that liberal virtues are important, presented civic consciousness, such as discernment and respect for the rights of others, judgment on the talents and character of political candidates, unwillingness to demand public services beyond national capabilities, willingness to pay for benefits, and participate in public discourse as desirable.[11] However, as Conover (1991) points out, free citizens are not necessarily democratic citizens. If the liberal element is overemphasized, citizens do not have to participate in politics, to sacrifice their private interests for the public good, and to accept the consensus of the majority, and so, there is a risk of harming the public interest.

As such, the values of desirable citizenship are diverse and difficult to define uniformly. Here, instead, awareness of participation, public interest consciousness, civic dignity, and civic temperance are presented as citizenship values required from the viewpoint of governance in pursuit of happiness. First, the awareness of participation as a civic duty for governance should be emphasized. Awareness of participation as a duty is the will to actively participate in community decision-making for the public good and is necessary for maintaining governance. Awareness of participation is not easily cultivated. It is because the will of citizens to participate can be dampened by the fact that humans tend to be selfish, passive, and indifferent to public affairs. Unlike the city-states of ancient Greece, the size of the modern nation-state makes it difficult for active participation, and the activities of generalized interest groups overwhelm the participation of ordinary citizens in modern society. In relation to social stability, the negative view of active participation is formidable. Nevertheless, it is important to secure the willingness of citizens to participate as an essential element of good governance. In ancient Greece, Athens, everyone went to an ecclesia to make a collective decision—politics was pursued by all citizens. In this process, citizenship was emphasized, which was recognized as an active meaning of participating in the public decision-making process as a duty and right, not as a passive meaning that one can enjoy the right and freedom not to be interfered with by others (Greenberg, 1983). Etymologically, a citizen means a legal member of a political community, and a citizen as a legal member is considered to be naturally accompanied by rights and obligations to the political community such as participation (Barbalet, 1988). This consciousness has significant meaning in relation to the happiness policy, because happiness is not regarded as a matter of individual domain, but rather serves as a basis for recognition as a community member to pursue happiness for the whole community.

Second, it is necessary that each citizen participating in governance has a sense of public interest. In general, the sense of public interest can be understood as a collective concern for the interests of the whole community (Ranson, 1988) or the treatment of all persons affected by a policy in an equal manner with an emphasis on equality as an important factor in the public interest (Barry, 1967). Having a sense of public interest does not mean that the pursuit of private interests should be restrained. In general, the public interest does not necessarily conflict with private or individual interests. Public interest ignoring private interest cannot fully represent the interest of citizens, and conversely, private interest ignoring public interest cannot fully represent the interest of citizens. This is easy to understand when considering that there can be no development of citizens as members without the development of

[11] In this regard, Barber (2003: 21) argues for the importance of political discourse in asserting participatory democracy.

the community, and that there can be no development of the community without the development of the members. The two are interrelated, and the public interest is not the same as a collection of private interests, but it will bear significant similarities. The consciousness of public interest in this sense is connected with the virtue of so-called golden mean (mesotés) which Confucius and Aristotle also suggested as a virtue to be pursued. The golden mean refers to taking the virtuous middle position without biasing either side of the polarities of excess and deficiency. But the golden mean is different from neutrality, which means the renunciation of opposing values. Rather, the golden mean refers to an attitude that pursues developmental unity of these values on the premise of understanding and accepting each of the opposing values. Thus, citizens with a sense of the golden mean will be able to contribute to the maintenance and development of the community by pursuing the public interest but not ignoring the private interest, and pursuing the private interest but not denouncing the public interest. This consciousness becomes an important cognitive asset in carrying out the happiness policy which is based on the recognition of individual-level happiness as a public issue.

Third, for good governance, civic dignity is necessary in addition to the awareness of participation and public interest. Civic dignity refers to a balanced consciousness of both the willingness to participate and the sense of public interest based on proper knowledge of public issues. The reason for the need of such a sense of balance is that if only the awareness of participation is emphasized, the content and results of participation may be disregarded as the focus is only on the quantitative expansion of participation, and if only the sense of the public interest is emphasized, participation may be restrained. From this point of view, civic dignity becomes a factor for forming a new citizenship in that it expands the quantity and quality of participation in governance, and shares responsibility for the results of participation. Dignity citizens contribute to good governance by aiming for a cooperative solution of social problems rather than prioritizing only individual needs in their participation. With regard to the happiness policy, they pursue the happiness of symbiosis based on their own active efforts to promote happiness and the understanding of public happiness and policies. However, the participation of citizens with a low sense of participation or public interest can hinder the formation of good governance and thus the promotion of happiness will be driven by demands based only on partial interests. In this regard, Barber (2006), a representative participatory theorist, warns the possibility that civil society's public discourse may become barbaric. That is, civil society can fail as much as the government and the market fail (Kim et al., 2002: 15), so it is necessary to emphasize the participation of competent citizens rather than regard civic participation as unconditionally correct. Civic dignity here does not mean high education level and possession of material assets. Therefore, the discussion of it has nothing to do with cases, for example, where the right to vote was restricted based on gender, property, or knowledge.

Fourth, in relation to the happiness policy, it is necessary to emphasize civic temperance as an independent item of civic competence. Although civic temperance is not frequently mentioned as a virtue of civic qualities as much as a sense of participation or public interest, civic temperance is recognized as an important civic virtue. Thomas More had earlier suggested the ideal of civil temperance in his Utopia. Although fictitious, the citizens of Utopia do not seek luxuries beyond the demands of everyday life, seeing gold or jewelry as a sign of shame or childishness. Galston (1988) suggested civic temperance as important virtues, along with discernment and respect for the rights of others, and the will to participate in public discourse as political virtues that a democratic citizen should possess. He specifically suggested that the will to not demand public services beyond national capabilities and payment for benefits are necessary. Regarding individual happiness, Seligman (2002a, b) suggested that temperance, which is found in self-control, prudence, and humility, is a virtue that can lead to the realization of happiness and flourishing. Civil temperance is a civic quality that is particularly required in pursuing happiness policies at the public level beyond the pursuit of individual happiness. This is because happiness policy is basically related to infinite human desires, and it is infeasible to satisfy the infinite needs of individual people with the limited capability of the government. Moreover, there are some needs that the government does not have to satisfy or should not. Examples are excessive desires (e.g., luxury goods) or illicit desires (e.g., drugs) that deviate far from the average level of individuals. If civic moderation is secured in such a situation, it will be possible to satisfy the needs of more citizens with limited public resources, and it will increase the possibility of enjoying a more equitable level of happiness for all members of the community. This is the reason why civic moderation is included as a civic virtue in addition to public mind and participatory consciousness.

So far, we have discussed the civic competence or civic virtues required for good governance, but if civic competence is emphasized too much, alienation or inequality problems may occur in governance participation. Even so, it is difficult to support irresponsible populist participation in governance regardless of civic competence, because it interferes with good governance. It should be understood that the demand for civic competence is not for discrimination, but for sufficing the minimum condition of good governance for the happiness policy. This necessity is in line with Schachter (1995)'s proposal of "reinventing ourselves" in response to Osborne and Gaebler (1992)'s proposal of "reinventing government" from a New Public Management perspective. She argued that citizens should be reformed from passive citizen-as-consumer model in the past to citizens conforming to the active citizen-owner model. Indeed, citizens who possess an owner-type citizenship are expected to play the role of a prosumer beyond the passive beneficiary of public services, with knowledge and understanding of public issues. And they are also expected to contribute to the good governance of the happiness policy by assuming the balancing role between the limitations of public resources and the attributes of human desire.

How to strengthen civic competence? In order to enhance the governance capacity of citizens, civic education should be taught. Citizen education is an educational activity aimed at cultivating civic qualities in a broad sense and stabilizing the political system in a narrow sense (Lee & Kim, 2018: 190). Citizen education can be achieved not only through school education, but also through various methods such as lifelong education in local communities and workplaces. However, based on the recognition that the best means of civic education is participation itself, increased interest in expanding participation opportunities is necessary. Civic participation is also an essential part of the governance per se. It is necessary to pay attention to deliberative democracy as a method of civic education through participation. In general, deliberative democracy is suggested as an effective democratic political institution that combines the advantages of direct democracy and indirect democracy (Mathews, 1999), and is expected to serve as a useful educational instrument for citizens who participated in the discussion to increase their willingness to participate and adopt a balanced recognition of public issues and for public officials to increase their receptivity of civic participation (Carson & Hartz-Karp, 2005). In particular, by bringing citizens and policymakers into contact during the deliberation process, it is expected that the effectiveness of civic education will increase as well as the effectiveness of governance.

Civic participation can be realized more easily at the local or community level than at the national or regional level. Also, as will be discussed later, in the governance of happiness, the importance of governance in a smaller unit like a locality or a community is greater than that of a country or a wide region. In this regard, service learning gathers attention as a new field-oriented educational method that connects service provision activities and educational activities at the community level. Service learning is based on the influence of John Dewey's pragmatic educational philosophy in the early twentieth century and the rise of universities and community-based organizations as a result of the civil rights movement in the 1960s. Service learning can be said to be an evolutionary innovation that seeks to link knowledge education of schools with community practice based on the grassroots organization of the local community (Stanton et al., 1999). Specifically, students, by participating in community service provision activities, learn how to apply and integrate knowledge in practice, have the opportunity to evaluate their own knowledge and methods (Duley, 1981), and develop skills and understandings for political and social activities that require active citizenship (Stanton, 1983). Service learning is generally a civic education method for students of regular educational institutions, but it is possible to expand the practical civic education method for adults. For example, volunteer activities and civic education can be linked as a service learning opportunity.

As discussed above, the instrument for effective civic education is the practice of participation, and in order for participation to take place, it is necessary to extend the opportunities for participation. However, although opportunities for participation are created by the efforts and demands of citizens themselves, they must be provided by the government before citizens ask. A problem is that the government is not active in the practical expansion of participation opportunities mainly due to distrust of citizens. At the same time, citizens' trust in the government is also weak, leading to cynicism or deviancy to participation (cf., Nye et al., 1997). In the end, due to mutual distrust, the expansion of participation opportunities or actual increase of participation does not take place. Such a vicious circle can be transformed if there is an improvement of government's trust in its citizens. This is because government's trust in citizens increases the government's receptivity to civic participation and thus has the potential to expand civic participation (Yang, 2005). Of course, not only the trust of government in citizens, but also citizens' trust in government can increase the government's receptivity to participation, thereby creating a virtuous cycle. However, in terms of possibilities, it will be easier to secure the trust of the government, which is an integrated group, than citizens that exist in a dispersed state. Such a request is included in the effort to strengthen the competence of public officials.

Finally, in relation to civic competence, morality should be emphasized as the competence of NGOs. NGOs are institutions representing civil society to such an extent that they are often equated with civil society in a situation where civic participation is practically dormant, and NGOs' contribution potential for good governance is high. NGOs' basic mission is to contribute to the development of society as a whole by assuming the role of an equalizer in the power relationship between the government, the market, and the citizens. In a situation where the government or the market operates as an exploiter based on superior resources in relations with citizens, and the citizens' defense power is suppressed due to the vulnerability of fragmented resources, such a role of NGOs is important as an intervening power to fill the gap (Mott, 1993). In many cases, NGOs actively assume such a role with the participation of sacrificial volunteers. However, some NGOs are criticized for not meeting these expectations properly. In this regard, the results of Knight et al. (2002)'s survey of 10,000 people in British Commonwealth countries are noteworthy. The result reports that respondents in this survey think NGOs advocate for the survival of their own organizations rather than advocate for civic interest and thus paradoxically that they expect an untrusted government to serve the civic interest rather than NGOs. As such, today, some NGOs are criticized for serving their own organizations rather than civic interests, being bureaucratized, or being captured by the government or corporations, failing to fulfil their innate roles, and losing morality as an equalizer. Of course, some criticism of NGOs stems from the high level of expectations for NGOs rather than the actual deviant behavior of NGOs. However, there is no need to disparage such positive prejudice. This is because it is natural for NGOs to be judged at a higher moral level in order to play the role of a balancer among the government, the market, and citizens. This is why the morality of NGOs, important actors in the domain of civil society, is emphasized in governance. For this, self-controlling efforts within the NGO, expansion of general support from citizens and public resources instead of government or corporate ad hoc subsidies, and activation of resident organizations by ordinary citizens are required.

Strengthening Market Competence

For good governance, it is necessary to strengthen the competence of governance participants, the government as the official policymaker and the private sector as the unofficial participants. Since the private sector includes citizens and market, the competence of not only citizens but also the market must be strengthened. A market is not a specific place, but an area in which goods and services are exchanged between suppliers and consumers, and price and competition are the basic operating principles (Bevir, 2012, 22; Kooiman, 2003: 160).

There are different views on the market in terms of good governance. Proponents of neoliberalism or neoclassical economics are market-friendly. The World Bank's position on good governance is representative of this stance. However, the market is not a perfectly competitive market as suggested by Adam Smith, and there is always a possibility of market failure. Thus, a reserved position is raised to a market-friendly position in relation to good governance. Kiely (1998) criticizes the World Bank's market-friendly interpretation and prescription for the development of East Asian countries such as Korea and Taiwan, and concludes as follows, "States can of course be inefficient and oppressive, in both socialist and capitalist contexts. However, states are not necessarily inefficient. Markets, on the other hand, are unequal, hierarchical and incapable of working without the existence of states." As such, market participation in governance does not automatically guarantee good governance and accordingly the capabilities of market actors should be strengthened for good governance.

What competencies are required? In this regard, Campbell et al., (1991, from Kooiman, 2003, 162) suggest efficiency, technology, control, culture, and even policies of the state as driving forces that affect market operation, and desirable changes in these factors could have a significant impact on good governance. However, I focus on the conditions required of market actors in relation to good governance of the happiness policy. First, entrepreneurial competencies are required for businesses or entrepreneurs participating in governance. Entrepreneurial competence includes not only technological competence as a supplier, but also creative and challenging attitudes to new demands. Market participation in governance refers to the increase of the market role in the policy process. For example, in service provision, in addition to the traditional government provision method, various alternative service delivery methods that utilize market capabilities such as contracting, voucher, franchise, subsidy, and so on are expanded (Stein, 1990, 49). In order for this service delivery method to be effectively employed, the creative entrepreneurial capabilities of newly participating market actors must be strengthened. In addition, the market's active response to the environmental challenge including the Fourth Industrial Revolution, global warming, and pandemics is necessary. Such requests naturally include not only market actors as existing suppliers, such as businesses, but also citizens as producers and consumers who play a new supplier role. Overall, such entrepreneurial competency is a basic requirement for market revitalization and is necessary for increasing available resources to promote happiness. This is because available resources affect the level of happiness.

Second, excessive self-interest pursuance by businesses needs to be restrained. Of course, a business's main reason for existence is to make a profit. However, from the viewpoint of governance of happiness, there is a problem that businesses participating in public decision-making will pursue profits excessively. It has the side effect of infringing on cooperative governance among market actors. Therefore, not only the capital accumulation function of the business but also the social legitimation function should be emphasized at the same time (O'Conner, 1973; Offe, 1984). In relation to the latter, an expanded role for corporate social responsibility is necessary. It will be particularly demanding in developing countries with poor markets and high-income inequality (Azmat & Coghill, 2005). Overall, not only competition in the market, but also cooperation should exist in tandem. To this end, while ensuring market autonomy and the principle of competition, regulations at the adequate level are needed to promote public happiness.

Third, openness that pays attention to horizontal collaboration and contributions from the government and civil society is required in the governance process. Such openness includes the expansion of horizontal communication between suppliers and consumers. The necessity to extend horizontal communication is in line with the fact that governance has the characteristics of an effort to compensate for the traditional government's closedness. In other words, just as the government extends its decision-making to the private sector, businesses are also required to avoid unilateral decision-making as a supplier in their relationship with consumers and move on to cooperative decision-making.

Fourth, the competencies of consumers should also be strengthened. In this regard, as suggested in the discussion on civic competence above, it is necessary to move from the one-sided position of the consumer to the position of co-producer or prosumer by enhancing the sovereignty of the consumer.

3.3 Flexibility of Governance Method

Governance was described as the extension of decision methods, wherein markets and networks are being proposed as additional decision-making methods beyond the hierarchy in the past traditional governance. Which decision-making method to prioritize depends on the governance paradigm as shown in Table 5. In the traditional government-centered governance, top-down control (hierarchy), in the market-oriented governance, the market mechanism, and in the civil society-centered governance or new governance, participation and network are presented as basic decision-making modes. As mentioned before, however, for good governance, a specific method should not be predetermined without taking into consideration the situation when governance will take place. Flexibility to select or combine various decision-making methods according to the given situation is necessary. In this regard, it is worth noting the discussion of meta-governance raised by Jessop (1997). He termed "meta-governance" to not only govern networks, but to be able to choose between various solutions, such as hierarchy, market, or network. In other words, meta-governance with different governance strategies is needed depending on the situation, and this is nothing but a request for a decision-making method for good governance. It should be added that, as discussed above, regardless of the type of governance, the government plays a leading role to a significant extent (Peters and Pierre 2012). That is, there is no pure market- or citizen-dominated governance without significant government intervention. Thus, it is appropriate to understand the extent and scope of the discussion on the flexibility of governance methods to adjust the roles between the government and other participants. And the understanding of meta-governance should also be understood as adjusting the scope and method of cooperation with the private sector depending on various contexts.

3.4 Micronization of the Governance Unit

For a successful happiness policy, micronization of the governance unit (or policy unit) should be considered important. Happiness is basically a problem at the individual level, and in order to effectively respond to individual demands at the individual level, a small governance unit close to the individual will be advantageous. It is natural that the smaller governance units can better grasp individual demand and respond more properly to individual demand compared to the larger governance units. This signifies that the decentralized system is superior to the centralized system for the implementation of the happiness policy, and at the same time, demands that the center of governance units performing the policy be shifted from the central to the local, and from the local to the community. Such micronization of the governance unit is also important as a measure to increase residents' access to the government and increase the input of residents in the policy process. The smaller the governance unit, the easier it is for residents to participate, and therefore, the input of resident opinions in the policy process becomes more vibrant. As a result, the congruence between government policy and demand for residents increases, and thus, the contribution of the policy to happiness can be increased.

The micronization of the governance unit or the policy unit is closely linked to the "micronization of the policy" presented earlier. It is because the microscopic approach of policy is to effectively respond to individualized demands of citizens as suggested above, and small governance units are superior to large governance units in responding to microscopic policy demand. In other words, local governments rather than central governments, and community-level governments rather than local governments are more advantageous in responding to individualized demand. When it comes to happiness policy, it can be said that small is beautiful, and centrality bias should be avoided. However, the governance unit cannot be reduced indefinitely. This is because governance proceeds for a certain policy or decision unit, district or local or regional level for example. In addition, at least economies of scale and scope of control should be considered. Therefore, the minimum governance unit that works will be the core unit of the happiness policy.

Gerald Suttles (1969)'s seminal work, "The social order of the slum: Ethnicity and territory in the inner city," provides good insight into the probability that such a small governance unit will be able to respond more effectively to individualized demands. His research is a case study of the Addams area in the near West Side of Chicago, suggesting that ethnicity and territory are important factors in determining the social order of the inner city. In this study, he reports the observation that the inhabitants of the Addams area live in the same area while maintaining different cultures of different ethnic groups (Italians, Mexicans, Puerto Ricans, and Blacks) without mixing, which is due to the social conditions of the neighborhood itself (p. 227). Such an observation tells us that the demand for residents varies even at a small regional level, and thus that it is not easy to respond to the demands of various residents with a uniform policy at a large policy unit. This is because the larger the governance unit, the larger the included area, and accordingly, the demand for residents will be more diversified, but the governance capacity that can respond to specific demand will be limited. Yates (1977)'s "the ungovernable city," which points out that it is very difficult for local governments to systematically respond to policies to diversified demands of residents, also supports the argument that small policy delivery units will be relatively effective in responding to diverse demands of residents. Diener and Biswas-Diener (2019)'s argument that local understanding of policymakers is required because family, friends, and meaningful activities are important for happiness to go beyond momentary happiness based on feeling and to become long-term sustainable happiness based on flourishing also supports the need for the micronization of governance units. It is because local understanding can only be secured through a small governance unit that allows practical contact with local residents. In addition, Bevir (2012: 117), who suggested that governance with expanded citizen participation is effective as well as satisfying democratic values, and Nobel laureate E. Ostrom (2000), who argued that polycentric governance is more effective than mono-centric governance in metropolitan governance, present related arguments for the micronization of the governance unit. As such, the micronization of the policy and the governance unit (or the policy unit) are demands that are closely related to each other, and therefore, for the successful implementation of the happiness policy, micronization in both the policy and the governance unit must proceed simultaneously.

3.5 *Summing up*

The prerequisites of the happiness policy suggested so far can be combined into two categories: policy innovation (change of policy paradigm and direction of consumer-centered policy approach) and governance innovation (good governance, strengthening of policy participant competence, and policy unit micronization).

To promote public happiness, first, happiness must be set as an explicit policy goal, and the policy paradigm must be changed from process-based to goal-based. This is because policy is a means to achieve a goal, not an end in itself. Governance should be established as a tool for delivering happiness policies. In order to achieve the goal of the happiness policy, the efforts of the government alone are insufficient, and cooperation with private sector is necessary. Governance is basically a system of cooperation between the government and private sector. However, just linking between the government and the private sector does not ensure that the happiness policy achieves its goal, enhancing public happiness. Substantial governance that contributes to the achievement of goals can be realized only when competent government and civil society are combined beyond formal governance which is simply an encounter between the government and the private actors. Such substantial governance is good governance. In this regard, if an encounter between the government and private actors is a necessary condition for good governance, the cooperation of a competent government and a competent private actor can be the sufficient condition. Therefore, in order to realize good governance and to achieve the goal of enhancing

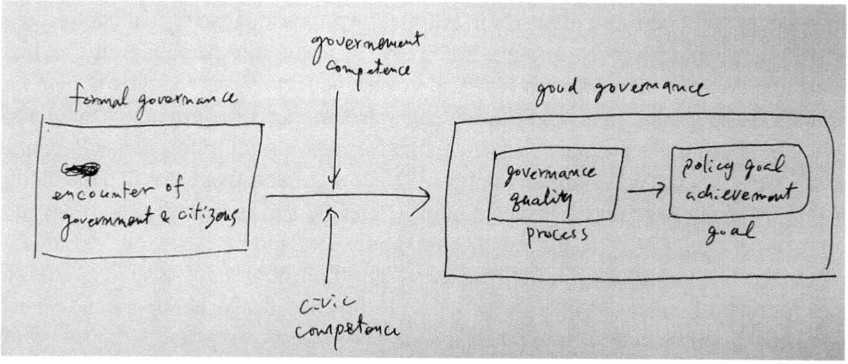

Fig. 1 Conditions for good governance

happiness through it, it is important to strengthen the capacity of the government and the private actors participating in governance. On the other hand, in terms of the spatial aspect, the effective unit of governance is a relatively small spatial unit, and therefore, governance at the local or community level is more important than the central or regional level for the governance of happiness policies. This is why it is necessary to focus on establishing a governance model at the local or community level in the discussion of good governance for strengthening happiness. Figure 1 shows this summary discussion.

References

Azmat, F., & Coghill, K. (2005). Good governance and market-based reforms: A study of Bangladesh. *International Review of Administrative Sciences, 71*(4), 625–638.

Barbalet, J. M. (1988). *Citizenship Minneapolis*. University of Minnesota Press.

Barber, B. R. (2003). *Strong democracy: Participatory politics for a new age*. University of California Press.

Barber, B. R. (2006). *A place for us: How to make society civil and democracy strong*. Hill and Wang.

Barry, B. (1967). The public interest. In A. Quinton (Ed.), *Political philosophy* (pp. 112–126). Oxford University Press.

Berry, F. S. (1994). Innovation in public management: The adoption of strategic planning. *Public Administration Review, 54*(4), 322–330.

Bevir, M. (2012). *Governance: A very short introduction*. Oxford University Press.

Bok, D. (2010). *The politics of happiness: What government can learn from the new research on well-being*. Princeton University Press.

Bovaird, T. E., & Löffler, E. (Eds.). (2009). *Public management and governance*. Routledge

Boyatzis, R. E. (1982). *The competent manager: A model for effective performance*. Wiley.

Campbell, J. L., Hollingsworth, J. R., & Lindberg, L. N. (1991). *Governance of the American economy*. Cambridge University Press.

Carson, L., & Hartz-Karp, J. (2005). Adapting and combining deliberative designs: Juries, polls, and forums. In J. Gastil & P. Levine (Eds.), *The deliberative democracy handbook: Strategies for effective civic engagement in the twenty-first century* (pp. 120–138). Jossey-Bass.
Cho, S. (2005). Rethinking the concept of governance. In: A paper presented at the winter conference held of the Korean Public Administration Association, Seoul, Korea (Korean).
Choi, B. (2002). Governance and citizen participation. In S. Kim, I. Kang, J. Kim, J. Kang, B. MOON, J. Y. Lee, J. H. Lee, T. Yoon, B. Choi, H. Park, & W. Chae (Eds.), *Understanding governance* (pp. 246–252). Daeyoung Publishing (Korean).
Crawford, G. (2006). The World Bank and good governance: Rethinking the state or consolidating neo-liberalism? In A. Paloni & M. Zanardi (Eds.), *The IMF, World Bank and policy reform* (pp. 109–134). Routledge.
Conover, P. J. (1991). Political socialization: Where's the politics? *Political science: Looking to the future* (Vol. 3, pp. 124–152).
Dalton, R. J. (2008). *The good citizen: How a younger generation is reshaping American politics.* CQ Press.
Denhardt, J. V., & Denhardt, R. B. (2003). *The new public service: Serving, not steering.* M. E. Sharpe.
Denhardt, R. B., & Denhardt, J. V. (2000). The new public service: Serving rather than steering. *Public Administration Review, 60*(6), 549–559.
De Sario, J., & Langton, S. (1987). Citizen participation and technocracy. In J. De Sario & S. Langton (Eds.), *Citizen participation in public decision making* (pp. 3–18). Greenwood Press.
Diener, E., & Biswas-Diener, R. (2019). Well-Being interventions to improve societies. In J. Sachs, R. Layard, & J. F. Helliwell (Eds.), *Global happiness and wellbeing policy report 2019* (pp. 95–110). Sustainable Development Solutions Network.
Duley, J. S. (1981). Field experience education. In A. W. Chickering (Ed.), *The modern American college: Responding to the new realities and a changing society* (pp. 600–613). Jossey-Bass.
European Commission. (2001). *European governance—A white paper.* http://eurlex.europa.eu/LexUriServ/site/en/com/2001/com2001_0428en01.pdf
Galston, W. A. (1988). Liberal virtues. *American Political Science Review, 82*(4), 1277–1290.
Ghose, R. (2005). The complexities of citizen participation through collaborative governance. *Space and Polity, 9*(1), 61–75.
Graham, J., Bruce, A., & Tim P. (2003). Principles for good governance in the 21st century. *Policy Brief No.15.* https://www.academia.edu/2463793/Principles_for_good_governance_in_the_21st_century. Accessed May 2, 2020.
Gray, V. (1973). Innovation in the states: A diffusion study. *American Political Science Review, 67*(4), 1174–1185.
Greenberg, E. S. (Ed.). (1983). *The American political system: A radical approach.* Little, Brown & Co.
Gyford, J. (1991). *Citizens, consumers, and councils: Local government and the public.* MacMillan Education Ltd.
Heinrich, C. J., Lynn Jr, L. E., & Milward, H. B. (2010). A state of agents? Sharpening the debate and evidence over the extent and impact of the transformation of governance. *Journal of Public Administration Research and Theory, 20*(suppl_1), i3-i19.
Helliwell, J. F., Sachs, J. D., Adler, A., Bin Bishr, A., de Neve, J. E., Durand, M., ... & Seligman, M. (2019). How to open doors to happiness. In J. D. Sachs, A. Adler, A. B. Bishr, dN. Jan-Emmanuel, M. Durand, E. Diener, J. F. Helliwell, R. Layard, & M. Seligman. *Global happiness and wellbeing policy report 2019* (pp. 9–26). Sustainable Development Solutions Network.
Hyden, G., Court, J. (2002). Governance and development: Sorting out the basics. *World Governance Survey Discussion Paper 1.* https://cdn.odi.org/media/documents/4094.pdf Accessed May 2, 2020.
IMF. (1996, September 29). *Communiqué of the Interim Committee of the Board of Governors of the International Monetary Fund.* Press release no. 96/49.

Jessop, B. (1997). The governance of complexity and the complexity of governance: Preliminary remarks on some problems and limits of economic guidance. In A. Amin & J. Hausner (Eds.), *Beyond market and hierarchy: Interactive governance and social complexity* (pp. 95–128). Edward Elgar.

Kaufmann, D., & Kraay, A. (2008). Governance indicators: Where are we, where should we be going? *The World Bank Research Observer, 23*(1), 1–30.

Kaufmann, D., Kraay, A., & Mastruzzi, M. (2008). Governance matters VII: Aggregate and individual governance indicators, 1996–2007. *Policy Research Working Paper No. 4654.* http://hdl.handle.net/10986/6870. Accessed May 2, 2020.

Kiely, R. (1998). Neoliberalism revised? A critical account of World Bank conceptions of good governance and market friendly intervention. *International Journal of Health Services, 28*(4), 683–702.

Kim, E. (2011). Local good governance: A research framework. *Journal of Korean Politics, 20*(2), 209–234. (Korean).

Kim, M. (2005). Local governance and residents' political participation. *Korean Society and Public Administration, 16(3)*, 325–347. (Korean).

Kim, S., Kang, I., Kim, J., Kang, J., Moon, B., Lee, J. Y., Lee, J. H., Yoon, T., Choi, B., Park, H., & Chae, W. (2002). *Understanding governance.* Daeyoung Publishing (Korean).

Kjær, A. M. (2004). *Governance.* Polity.

Knight, B., Ghigudu, H., & Tandon, R. (2002). *Reviving democracy: Citizens at the heart of governance.* Earthscan.

Kooiman, J. (2003). *Governing as governance.* Sage.

Landell-Mills, P., & Serageldin, I. (1991). Governance and the external factor. In *Proceedings of the World Bank annual conference on development economics.* World Bank.

Lee, J. (2002a). Formation and governance. *Journal of Governmental Studies, 8*(1): 3–91. (Korean).

Lee, M. (2002b). Review article: Conceptualizing governance: Governance as social coordination. *Korean Public Administration Review, 36*(4), 321–339. (Korean).

Lee, S. J. (2004). Policy diffusion in local governments and time: A case study on local acts for administrative information disclosure. *Journal of Local Government Studies, 16*(1), 5–25. (Korean).

Lee, S. J. (2016). Introduction: From process-based governance paradigm to goal-based governance paradigm. *Korean Public Administration Review, 50*(4), 1–10. (Korean).

Lee, S. J., & Kim, H. (2018). *The theory of citizen participation.* Parkyoungsa (Korean).

Lee, S. J., & Oh, Y. (2013). *National happiness and government 3.0: Understanding and application.* Hakjisa (Korean).

Lee, S. J., & Yoon, D. (2005). Conceptualizing the capacity of local governments. *Journal of Local Government Studies, 17*(3), 5–24. (Korean).

Lynn, L. E., Jr. (2010). Has governance eclipsed government? In R. F. Durant (Ed.), *The Oxford handbook of American bureaucracy* (pp. 669–690). Oxford University Press.

Manasan, R. G., Gaffud, R., & Gonzalez, E. T. (1999). Indicators of good governance: Developing an index of governance quality at the LGU level (No. 1999–04). *PIDS (Philippine Institute for Development Studies) Discussion Paper Series.* https://www.econstor.eu/bitstream/10419/187390/1/pidsdps9904.pdf. Accessed May 2, 2020.

March, J. G., & Olsen, J. P. (1995). *Democratic governance.* Free Press.

Mathews, D. (1999). *Politics for people: Finding a responsible public voice.* University of Illinois Press.

McClelland, D. C. (1973). Testing for competence rather than for "intelligence." *American Psychologist, 28*(1), 1–14.

Minogue, M., Polidano, C., & Hulme, D. (1998). Introduction: The analysis of public management and governance. In M. Minogue, C. Polidano, & D. Hulme (Eds.), *Beyond the new public management: Changing ideas and practices in governance* (pp. 1–14). Edward Elgar.

Mirabile, R. J. (1997). Everything you wanted to know about competency modeling. *Training & Development, 51*(8), 73–78.

Mott, S. C. (1993). *A Christian perspective on political thought*. Oxford University Press.

Newman, J. (2001). *Modernizing governance: New labour, policy and society*. Sage.

Nye, J. S., Zelikow, P. D., & King, D. C. (1997). *Why people don't trust government*. Harvard University Press.

O'Conner, J. (1973). *The fiscal crisis of the state*. St. Martin's Press.

OECD. (2007). *Glossary of statistical terms: Good governance*. http://stats.oecd.org/glossary/detail.asp?ID=7237.

Offe, C. (1984). *Contradictions of the welfare state*, J. Keane (ed.), MIT Press.

Osborne, D., & Gaebler, T. (1992). *Reinventing government*. A Plume Book.

Osborne, D., Plastrik, P., & Miller, C. M. (1998). Banishing bureaucracy: The five strategies for reinventing government. *Political Science Quarterly, 113*(1), 168–169.

Ostrom, E. (2000). The danger of self-evident truths. *Political Science & Politics, 33*(1), 33–46.

Peters, B. G. (1996). *The future of governing: Four emerging models*. University Press of Kansas.

Peters, B. G., & Pierre, J. (1998). Governance without government? Rethinking public administration. *Journal of Public Administration Research and Theory, 8*(2), 223–243.

Peters, B. G., & Pierre, J. (2012). Urban governance. In P. John, K. Mossberger, & S. E. Clarke (Eds.), *The Oxford handbook of urban politics* (pp. 71–86). Oxford University Press.

Pierre, J. (Ed.). (2000). *Debating governance: Authority, steering, and democracy*. Oxford University Press.

Pierre, J., & Peters, B. G. (2000). *Governance, politics and the state*. St. Martin's Press.

Ranson, S. (1988). From 1944 to 1988: Education, citizenship and democracy. *Local Government Studies, 14*(1), 1–19.

Rhodes, R. A. W. (1996). The new governance: Governing without government. *Political Studies, 44*(4), 652–667.

Rhodes, R. A. W. (1997). *Understanding governance: Policy networks, governance, reflexivity and accountability*. Open University Press.

Rhodes, R. A. W. (2000). Governance and public administration. In J. Pierre (Ed.), *Debating governance* (pp. 54–90). Oxford University Press.

Robichau, R. W. (2011). The mosaic of governance: Creating a picture with definitions, theories, and debates. *Policy Studies Journal, 39*(1), 113–131.

Rosenau, J. N. (1992). Governance, order, and change in world politics. In J. N. Rosenau & E. O. Czempiel (Eds.), *Governance without government: Order and change in world politics* (pp. 1–29). Cambridge University Press.

Rothstein, B. (2012). Good governance. In D. Levi-Faur (Ed.), *The Oxford handbook of governance* (pp. 143–154). Oxford University Press.

Schachter, H. L. (1995). Reinventing government or reinventing ourselves: Two models for improving government performance. *Public Administration Review, 55*(6), 530–537.

Seligman, M. E. P. (2002a). Positive psychology, positive prevention, and positive therapy. In C. R. Snyder & S. J. Lopez (Eds.), *Handbook of positive psychology* (pp. 3–9). Oxford University Press.

Seligman, M. E. P. (2002b). *Authentic happiness: Using the new positive psychology to realize your potential for lasting fulfillment*. Free Press.

Sen, A. (1999). *Development as freedom*. Anchor Books.

Skocpol, T. (1985). Bringing the state back in: Strategies of analysis in current research. In P. Evans, D. Rueschemeyer, & T. Skocpol (Eds.), *Bringing the state back in* (pp. 3–38). Cambridge University Press.

Smith, B. C. (2007). *Good governance and development*. Macmillan International Higher Education.

Sparrow, P. R. (1996). Competency based pay too good to be true. *People Management*, 22–25.

Stanton, T. K. (1983). *Field study: Information for faculty*. Human Ecology Field Study Office, Cornell University.

Stanton, T. K., Giles, D. E., Jr., & Cruz, N. I. (1999). *Service-learning: A movement's pioneers reflect on its origins, practice, and future*. Jossey-Bass.

Stein, R. M. (1990). *Urban alternatives: Public and private markets in the provision of local services*. University of Pittsburgh Press.

Stoker, G. (2000). Urban political science and the challenge of urban governance. In J. Pierre (Ed.), *Debating governance: Authority, steering, and democracy*. Oxford University Press.

Suttles, G. D. (1969). *The social order of the slum: Ethnicity and territory in the inner city*. University of Chicago Press.

The Commission on Global Governance. (1995). *Our global neighborhood: The report of the commission on global governance*. Oxford University Press.

UNDP. (1997). *Human Development Report*.

United Nations. (1997). *Governance for sustainable human development*. Oxford University Press.

Van Doeveren, V. (2011). Rethinking good governance: Identifying common principles. *Public Integrity, 13*(4), 301–318.

Walker, J. L. (1969). The diffusion of innovations among the American states. *American Political Science Review, 63*(3), 880–899.

Weiss, T. G. (2000). Governance, good governance and global governance: Conceptual and actual challenges. *Third World Quarterly, 21*(5), 795–814.

World Bank. (1989) *Sub-Saharan Africa: From crisis to sustainable growth. A long-term perspective study*. World Bank.

World Bank. (1992). *Governance and development*. World Bank.

World Bank. (1994). Governance: The World Bank's experience. https://doi.org/10.1596/0-8213-2804-2 Accessed March 17, 2009.

Yang, K. (2005). Public administrators' trust in citizens: A missing link in citizen involvement efforts. *Public Administration Review, 65*(3), 273–285.

Yates, D. (1977). *The ungovernable city: The politics of urban problems and policy making*. MIT Press.

Yoo, M. (2012). *Public administration*. Pakyounsa. (Korean)

Chapter 8
Epilogue

In any country, every citizen has the right to pursue happiness, and the state, as a member of the national community, has an obligation to strive for the welfare of its citizens. As such, it is the basic premise of public happiness to view happiness of individual members of the community as a subject of public interest and responsibility beyond the individual level. Such publicness or public responsibility of happiness is fundamentally based on the fact that individual citizens exist as members not isolated but related to the national community, and that individual happiness is not entirely dependent on individual abilities and resources alone but is to a certain extent influenced by public conditions. For this reason, public happiness, unlike individual-level happiness, demands that people not only maintain an appropriate level of happiness but also require everyone to be equally happy.

In order to promote public happiness, active interest in both the happiness policy and the governance as policy executing system is imperative. Nevertheless, most of the happiness studies thus far have heavily focused on individual happiness over public happiness. Relatively, little attention has been given to the overall policies or governance issues while fixating on the measurement and development of the happiness index, identification of happiness causal factors, and fragmentary policies. In order to enhance national happiness, I assert that the efforts to redefine the policy foundations and reconstruct a governance system are necessary beyond the current patchwork of happiness index development, identifying happiness determinants, and fragmented policy prescriptions.

The core elements of the policy efforts required can be summarized in three transformational demands. First, the policy paradigm must be shifted from the conventional process-based policy paradigm to the purpose-based paradigm. Second, policy priorities should shift from macro-, national, and universal policies into micro-, local, and tailored policies. Third, a shift from perfunctory governance to good governance is essential to establish an enabling system for happiness policy that encompasses both the government and the private sector.

It is important to note that public happiness is not at all separate from individual happiness. This is because collective happiness does not exist independent from

S. J. Lee, *Public Happiness*, Community Quality-of-Life and Well-Being,
https://doi.org/10.1007/978-3-030-89643-0_8

individual happiness; public happiness is either based on individual happiness or is related to individual happiness. Thus, this book approaches public happiness as the level and distribution of the happiness of those individual constituents of a group. This responds to the discussion that happiness is a subjective emotion of an individual, and therefore, happiness policy should also prioritize micro-policy over macro-policy. The fact that individual happiness is the basis of public happiness is well documented in the book *The Great Learning* (大學) of Zisi (子思), a Chinese philosopher and the grandson of Confucius. The book introduces the ideology for an ideal society in three core principles and eight articles. In Article 8, a widely known phrase "修身齊家治國平天下 (cultivating oneself, controlling house, governing the country, and pacifying the world) explains that individual attitudes or activities are closely linked to public happiness.[1]

This phrase means that the family, country, and even the world can achieve peace on the basis of self-cultivation. If this is expressed in terms of happiness, the happiness of the family, of the people, and the society can be attained based on individual happiness. In other words, the discourse of public happiness is not to exclude but rather to closely relate to individual happiness. Similarly, the discussion of individual happiness is also related to public happiness. As previously mentioned in *The Great Learning*, individual happiness is related to public happiness as the basis of a larger unit of happiness. Nevertheless, if individual happiness is defined as irrelevant to the happiness of the community, the individual's happiness will be ascribed entirely to individual efforts without any public assistance. This jeopardizes individual happiness and exacerbates the inequality among the levels and distribution of happiness. Therefore, the correlation of individual happiness and public happiness is fundamental in the discussion of happiness. Based on the premise of the relationship between individual happiness and public happiness, I present two unfinished thoughts about happiness as the conclusion of this book. One is the goal of the happiness policy, and the other is the components of happiness.

Opinion on the goals of the happiness policy

Raising the level of happiness is an important goal of the happiness policy. From a public happiness perspective, it is undoubtedly important to improve the distribution of happiness along with the level of happiness. However, the improvement in the distribution becomes inconsequential when the general level of happiness is low. Therefore, it is crucial to increase the level of happiness while not losing interest in the distribution of happiness. We need to ask the question: Is a higher level of happiness as a policy target better?

I look back on my experience of walking the Camino de Santiago in Spain briefly. Camino de Santiago! Many travelers all over the world put it on their bucket lists and

[1] Three basic principles include knowing of true virtue (明明德), loving people (親民), and dwelling in ultimate good (止于至善), and Article 8 is exploring nature (格物), knowing nature (致知), being faithful (誠意), being right-minded (正心), cultivating oneself (修身), controlling home (齊家), governing country (治國), and pacifying the world (平天下). Here, "pacifying the world" is understood as the same as making the world happy.

visit this path. An acquaintance of mine strongly and repeatedly recommended it to me as well, and I finally found an opportunity to walk around 350 km along the path with a backpack for about two weeks in early summer two years ago. The path to Santiago is a pilgrimage route that starts from the French border or southern Spain to Santiago de Compostela. While I did not exactly follow the designated route, I walked on mostly the northern route among the available routes. The northern route is better than the central route to walk, but I would assume the discomfort of midday heat and long-distance walking applies the same. As I walked, I realized that walking with a heavy backpack on a daily basis was not an easy task in itself. There were parts of the path that had good scenery, but there also were quite a few roads that required me to walk amidst the exhaust of passing vehicles. Perhaps, it was because I veered off from the designated route, but it was not pleasant to walk on the asphalt roadway under the burning sun. At times, I would recall many great roads in my own country and wonder why I chose to walk in a foreign land. But I continued to walk one day at a time because I planned for it and wanted to know where the path would take me. After walking for a few days, I began to think. Why am I walking? What's good about walking? What about walking the Camino de Santiago makes people talk in relation to happiness and not pain? I did not reach the final destination and returned halfway due to time constraints, but I would like to recollect my thoughts I had while walking.

Baggage. It was heavy so it needed some unloading. I did not have a lot with me to begin with, but the backpack was heavy and I needed to cut down. First, I threw away books. I took photographs of any highlights or remarks I have made for later and threw away the books. I acknowledged the inconvenience of needing to repurchase the book and to transfer or print my notes out, but I prioritized the need to reduce the weight of my backpack. I thought about abandoning my laptop as well, but I needed to continue using it so I decided to keep it. I downsized my daily necessities to a bare minimum. I even threw away a portion of my underwear to bring down a few grams. There was no new or old, expensive or cheap when it came to the elimination process. Weight was the only consideration. One thing and then another was purged, and my backpack became quite light. I wanted to throw out my backpack itself and prance about, but I needed to keep it to contain my minimal items. Then it occurred to me; if I thought about throwing out my backpack, then it probably meant that I threw out all that I can. I also thought I would regret throwing things away, but was pleasantly surprised to see that there was joy in becoming lighter. "Being light is the best!" I was happier unloading and emptying out my baggage.

Clothing. There was no need to dress particularly well because I did not know anyone and no one would recognize me. I threw away unnecessary extra clothes and only kept lightweight and quick-drying items. I did not need any fancy or stylish clothing. It would have been vain for me to try to look good to others. "Comfortable clothing is the best!" I was happier letting go of good clothes and dressed in comfortable clothes.

Shoes. Nothing is more important than shoes to walk for long hours. Planning for the trip, I contemplated among many shoes I owned. But the shoes that I brought with me were not the right choice. I chose the shoes that were both functional and fashionable, but it was not comfortable after walking for a long time and my feet suffered. I had to buy new shoes. "What's the use for fashionable shoes? Comfortable shoes are the best!" I was happier after letting go of my desire for good design and changed into comfortable shoes.

Food. At first, I wanted to experience and eat the local delicacies. But they were not always available. Sometimes, it was difficult to even find a restaurant if I did not time it right. I could not even carry around food because it was too heavy. Restaurants were not always open. I had to go into any available restaurant when it was time to eat and accepted whatever was available on the menu. I decided to give up my sovereignty over food. I was satisfied if the food was decent, and I was able to get some rest. "Yes, it's best not to be hungry!" I was happier giving up my epicurean desires and eating whatever was available to me.

Scenery. The road to Santiago is known for its scenic beauty. However, the famed scenery did not live up to its expectations. I think the people who had walked the path had an amiable perspective about their experience. The scenery was nice sometimes, but it was also mixed with smoke, asphalt, and steep hills that were not so pleasant. The evaluation of the road to Santiago seemed to be a bit exaggerated. In any case, it was common sense to take the scenic route as much as possible. However, walking required physical strength, and the scenery became a secondary concern. "Scenery is scenery. There is no need to go on a winding path. Easy and fast route is the best!" I was happier after giving up my desire to see the beautiful scenery and simply focused on walking.

Accommodations. The communal accommodation *albergue* was quite well equipped. To stay in an albergue, it required walking a considerable distance and also ensuring to claim a spot while it is still available. I was given quite the scare for possible bed bugs, so I decided to stay in hotels as much as possible instead of a shared space. (I later found out that the fear of bed bugs was exaggerated.) However, I realized that hotels were not always available. When the sun went down and the accommodation was still far away, I started to worry. Actually, the worries kicked in from the moment I woke up in the morning. I had to decide where to stay that night and set it as the destination for the day. However, it was difficult to determine in advance how far I can go before sundown considering the physical strength left in me. So, I had to stop being picky with accommodations. I wanted to stay in a place with a nice view at a good value, at the right timing and in the right place. But that was not always available. Even if it was available, it was not sensible to search for an expensive accommodation. I just needed a comfortable space for sleeping. "Clean and cheap accommodation is the best!" I was happier after giving up my desire to stay in a perfect accommodation.

In retrospect, I think I was happy to finally take everything off a bit. I lightened my baggage and unloaded my desires. After about two weeks of walking, I decided to stop and return to the starting point. As I turned back, I ran into a small port town that just radiated. The town was not too different from other villages I have passed through, but the town had plenty of lodgings, restaurants, and shops. In that town, I ate, dressed, and slept comfortably without having to walk far. It was not an extravaganza, but I was able to address my minimum requirements. Some of my desperate needs while walking were fulfilled, and I felt happiness in simplicity.[2]

I would have certainly appreciated the abundance, but I did not necessarily need it when I found the joy in simplicity. Abundance now became a lavish luxury without discipline. I felt sufficient and relieved of my deficiencies. What I needed was simplicity, not abundance.

It is true. Happiness comes not only from abundance, but also from simplicity. But simplicity and deficiency are different. The journey to Santiago compelled me to eliminate many things for agility and convenience, but still required minimum needs to be met for survival. It was challenging to continue walking in a state of deprivation. I could have endured it to some extent, but knew that it was not sustainable. It is difficult to be happy in a state of deprivation. Deprivation leads to a sense of desperation and will undermine happiness. While my walking journey was demanding, I would not label it as a state of deficiency. I reduced my belongings to a minimum, but I still had a bottle of water for survival and also a towel to wipe my sweat off. I would also eat and recharge when there were restaurants on the way. I also enjoyed the new landscapes and new faces. But I did not have slack. I was not deprived, but often near a state of desperation. However, I was saved from feelings of deprivation once I stepped into the small port town at the end of my walking journey and found the happiness induced by simplicity. The small port town was not an extravaganza but simplicity. The town had humble food, accommodations, and shops. And yet, I found slack and happiness.

Deprivation is to desperation as is simplicity to slack. More precisely, simplicity is a bit of surplus just beyond destitution. However, simplicity implied by small slack is far from the unmoderated extravagance. While walking, I felt desperate at times, but I wanted a bit of slack not luxury. I was content with having a lighter backpack, maintaining a level of comfort, not famished and bathed. It was as simple as that. It comes from unloading excess and greed. That way, you can be fulfilled with one meal, one cup of coffee, and one good night's sleep. Simplicity can be associated with removing unnecessary societal formalities. Backpackers do not have to be bothered by societal formality. People also do not impose unnecessary expectations onto backpackers. However, in the society we live in, we impose excessive demands beyond the simple living requirements and burden each other with the overwhelming weight of the uploaded backpack in our lives. If we can identify the unnecessary restraints and sort them out one by one, we can all find a way to be happy together within a simplicity society.

Abundance and simplicity. They are two different paths to happiness. Of course, both are equally important. The problem is that until now, we have only emphasized abundance and have forgotten simplicity. We pursue abundance thinking "more is

[2] Simplicity here expresses "so-bak (素樸)" in English. Originally, so (素) refers to the unpainted base, and the bak (樸) refers to the natural wood untouched with planers or knives. Therefore, simplicity(so-bak) would mean a humble and natural thing without adornment. This is contrary to excessive greed (Lao, 2007: 97). The verse of 知足者富 (Those who know what they have enough are rich) or 知足常樂 (He who knows what they have enough is always happy) can be said to be a happiness perspective that leads to simplicity (Yao, 2018).

better, more is more." But from my short walking journey, I am now aware that it can actually be "less is more, less is better." I acknowledge that having this new insight after such a short walk can be excessive, but a long walk is not required to reach an organized thought. I am lucky to be enlightened with this realization without walking longer. Of course, anyone can share such thoughts regardless of walking. Anyway, this thought became clear to me as I walked. I also found such thought to be meaningful for the successful delivery of the happiness policy. One of the core issues in executing the happiness policy is that there is no limit to human desires, and there are limits to public resources to satisfy and support these desires. In this regard, recognizing the meaning of simplicity rather than focusing on abundance only can be an important foundation for overcoming such a problem.

In relation to this perception, it is helpful to compare the eastern and the western views of happiness. In the East, the religious and psychocultural approach, in which people believe that happiness can be achieved by controlling human desires to a minimum, prevails as there is a limit to what humans can acquire from nature and social environment. In the West, the secular and material approach, in which people believe that happiness can be achieved by maximizing acquisition from the surrounding environment, prevails as human desires are not only impossible to control but rather, such suppression is seen as a violation of human dignity—freedom and reason. In other words, "minimizing desires" is at the root of the eastern view of happiness, while "maximization of achievement" is at the root of the western view of happiness. As a result, the East has succeeded in constructing a religious and ethical culture, but experienced relative material poverty. On the other hand, the West celebrated the development of science and technology, industrialization, political democratization, and material civilization, but undermined the sustainability of the global environment. The above is a summary of the diagnosis of Han (2000: 45) and Choi (2006: 73). In my opinion, there are aspects of the diagnoses that seem to be simplified or exaggerated for the purpose of contrasting the happiness paradigm of the East and the West. However, the diagnosis of the relative tendency to emphasize the restraint of desire in the East and the expansion of resources in the West in general seems reasonable. It would be ideal to strengthen the advantages and supplement the disadvantages through balance and harmony of both viewpoints. The direction is indeed to balance and reconcile the limits of unlimited human desires and resource input. At this time, the key to balancing the two perspectives lies in "simplicity." Harmony of desires and resources requires the control of desires and resources, because simplicity enables the moderation of desires and consequently saving of resource input. Simplicity should be a reflection of people's daily lives in both the East and the West, regardless of the region. Whether it be prioritizing material or spirit, an approach that focuses on simplicity and does not interfere with the daily lives is a starting point for resolving the differences in views on happiness between the East and the West.

Opinion on the Components of Happiness

Many scholars have identified the components of happiness as affect, life evaluation, and eudaimonia (OECD, 2013: 29–32). Some scholars presented happiness components by classifying affect into positive and negative affect. For example, Diener et al. (1985) presented positive affect, negative affect, and life evaluation as three "separable" components. This approach is to understand the positive and negative affect as concepts of mutually independent dimensions (Diener & Emmons, 1985). As an extension of this perception, Diener et al. (2010) classified positive and negative feelings and presented the difference between the two as a measure of happiness. (A combined score is calculated by subtracting the negative score from the positive score.) This idea is also in line with the early traditional viewpoints of Bentham (1789, from Veenhoven, 2015) who viewed happiness as the sum of pleasures and pains. However, directly subtracting the score difference between positive feelings and negative feelings assumes that pleasant feelings are always a positive factor of happiness, and unpleasant feelings are always a negative factor of happiness. Therefore, the net happiness is measured by calculating the difference between the scores. The understanding of happiness for most people, whether they are experts or not, is like this.

Is this really the case? Are positive feelings and negative feelings truly independent factors? This question needs to be asked. The first thing to admit is that happiness comes from pleasant feelings. When I say pleasant feelings, I am referring to "petty pleasures." Petty pleasure is happiness that arises from small events that occur in everyday life for everyone. No explanation is needed that small positive and pleasant things in everyday life are the source of happiness. What about great pleasure? Naturally, a big positive event will bring more pleasure. But great pleasure does not happen very often on a daily basis, it is practically incidental. The state of great pleasure (euphoria) following a great event is difficult to sustain, and in some cases, great pleasure may be the cause of unhappiness. Simple pleasures are things that happen on a daily basis, such as socializing with friends, and are easy to enjoy with little effort, but great pleasures such as winning the lottery do not happen on a daily basis, nor are they ensured through one's own efforts. It can make you unhappy if when you want it you do not get it. In addition, even when acquired, one may become unhappy when the result of acquisition does not meet expectations or when one fails to adapt to a new situation. It is a common story that not a few lottery winners suffer misfortune. As much as the joy was great, the damage of the loss would also be great. Expected or unexpected, great pleasure is always questionable whether it is possible and how long it will last (Brickman et al., 1978). This is also a key point emphasized in set point theory, which states that emotional states return to their original state after a certain period of time. Of course, the set point theory is not fully supported. Depending on the event, the time it takes to return to the normal state will vary, and even if the period is short, positive emotions in the meantime may be meaningful. Even so, it is also recognized as a fact that in many cases, the adaptation effect suggested by set point theory works to some extent. Therefore, for the stable maintenance of happiness, it is more important that simple pleasures from everyday conditions (events or states) continue rather than one-time great pleasures.

With this in mind, I recommend it to myself and to others around me. Do not spare pennies on simple pleasures. A cup of delicious coffee, a book you want to read, a fun movie, snacks with acquaintances, small giving .... In many cases, pennies are consumption for experiences or memories (Choi, 2018: 117) or relational goods for maintaining relationships with people (Bruni & Zamagni, 2007: 239) compared to consumption of material goods for possession. Since such consumption is advantageous in magnitude and durability in terms of the happiness effect compared to consumption of material goods, my recommendation is probably not wrong. I do not recommend saving pennies to accumulate a large pile of money. Saving pennies does not necessarily accumulate to a large sum of money, the process of collecting is painful, and when you do not achieve it even if you try, you are likely to get frustrated. Just because you save a lot of money and spend it big does not mean it will bring you stable happiness in life. Therefore, rather than the great pleasure that may or may not be present, it seems that small pleasures that occur every day should be emphasized as the essence of happiness. From this point of view, the study of Diener et al. (1991) that happiness depends on the frequency, not the intensity of positive or negative emotions, seems basically valid.

If pleasure brings happiness, negative affect or unpleasant feeling is a component of unhappiness. But in fact, it is not. Happiness does not mean the absence of worries (Choi, 2018: 45). Of course, great anxiety cannot but be an element of unhappiness. It is impossible to be happy with the death of an acquaintance, loss of a job, or serious illness. Moreover, the effects of such negative events are long lasting (Brickman et al., 1978). But simple worries are different. Simple worry is as much a factor of happiness as simple pleasure. To be anxious is to express the desire to get out of the situation of worry. Wanting to get out of a situation where you should be worried means you have the will to live. Therefore, if you do not have simple worries in your daily life, you are not interested in life, and it is like being alive but dead. Just as simple pleasures stem from the desire to enjoy a good life, so too simple worries stem from the desire to manage a good life. Both are not different in that they are "vitality of being." The only difference is that the former seeks to pursue a good life by enjoying a given state and the latter by overcoming the given state. The fact that simple pleasure and simple worry are happiness factors at the same time can be seen from the fact that, for example, when exercising, it is tiring and enjoyable. From another perspective, happiness is a work–life balance. In general, work–life balance refers to the balance between work life and life outside work. Between the two, a boundary is assumed between the workplace and outside of the workplace. However, in the true sense of work and life balance, there should be no barriers between work and life. A true work–life balance is when a work–life balance is achieved in everyday life, moment by moment, irrespective of boundaries between work and life. Such an integrated and balanced life is a happy life. Just as there is both a negative feeling and a positive feeling while exercising, a happy life is a life in which simple pleasures and simple worries are well harmonized and overcome in everyday life. Then, it becomes clear that the above-mentioned argument in the study of Diener et al. (1991) that happiness depends on the frequency, not the intensity of positive versus negative emotions, is not entirely correct. Initially, it seems reasonable to say that happiness depends on frequency rather than intensity of emotion. This is because happiness will depend on simple daily routines rather than one-time big events. However, it is difficult to agree that happiness depends on the difference between positive and negative emotions. This is because, as much as simple pleasures, simple worries are a factor of happiness. That is, the approach that sees happiness as the difference between positive and negative emotions needs to be revised.

In theory, there could be a life of only pleasure or a life of only worry. But such a life is not common. A life in which enjoyment and anxiety intersect is a daily aspect of life, and everyone lives with pleasure and worry on a daily basis. Indeed, joy and sorrow are with us as brothers and sisters. A life in which one element is utterly absent, daily in pleasure or worry, is difficult to exist, and even if it does exist, it is not the life of simple joy and simple worry that I am talking about here. An imperfect human with fundamentally changing emotions cannot consistently be in a state of constant pleasure or anxiety, regardless of the conditions of the changing world. Therefore, rather than looking at positive and negative as opposed to each other, it is necessary to recognize that both are important components of life, and that the value of pleasure increases with anxiety and that anxiety decreases with pleasure. In addition, it is necessary to reflect on the "virtuous mean" view of happiness. As is well known, the virtuous mean, which refers to an intermediate or appropriate state that is neither excessive nor insufficient, is a virtue that has been emphasized in the traditional oriental philosophy and the Aristotelian ethics, and helps us to understand that simplicity is not only a practical necessity but also a normatively valid request in life. This thinking raises a question about the conventional wisdom that positive affect is beneficial to a happy life but negative affect is detrimental to a happy life. In other words, the fact that both positive and negative affects can be positive factors for happiness needs to be considered in happiness research and practice. Of course, this idea can be equally applied not only to affect, but also to life satisfaction or meaning, which is another element of happiness, because such factors are also feelings of individuals.

The idea that a simple life in which small pleasures and small worries intersect can be the source of happiness raises questions about the perspective that prioritizes only abundance. Generally, the prevailing perception is that good living conditions (events and states) bring pleasure, but that poor living conditions cause anxiety and hinder happiness, and therefore, both individuals and countries strive to accumulate good living conditions. It is considered that the better the living conditions, the more happiness, and this idea is based on the affluence-priority principle. Of course, good living conditions are necessary conditions that can contribute to happiness, and poor living conditions are factors that can hinder happiness. However, when we come to realize that small (simple) pleasures are the source of happiness, and that a life in which small worries and small pleasures intersect can be a happy life, we have doubts about the one-sided view of pursuing only good conditions. In other words, the maximization of good living conditions (or social conditions) is not a condition for happiness, but a moderate living condition can be the condition for happiness.

Simplicity and happiness policy

So far, I have talked about two opinions about happiness, and my thoughts that connect these two are in simplicity. Although great pleasure or great anxiety is an important factor related to happiness, it is generally necessary to pay attention to the happiness that arises from small pleasures or small worries that occur on a daily basis for everyone. "Simplicity." It is commonplace and relevant to everyone. Thus, simplicity related to the general people is the basis of individual happiness and becomes related to public happiness. Simplicity is in line with "安分知足 (satisfaction with moderated life)," which has been emphasized by the old scholarly society of Korea. Such a life with contentment without being too greedy is contrasted with the life of Pahom, the main character in a widely known short story of Leo Tolstoy (1886), where he eventually loses his life because of his desire to occupy more land.

Recognition of such simplicity has an important meaning in relation to the direction of the happiness policy. As already mentioned, with the beginning of the twenty-first century, a new interest in happiness has emerged from the practical and academic aspects. This change is basically a movement to shift or supplement the view of development from an economic-centered toward a non-economic aspect, and it is characterized as a beyond GDP movement. At its nature, these changes are related to the qualitative aspect of development, and there has been a lot of discussion about it. On the other hand, in the new interest in development, there is no adequate discussion on the quantitative aspect of development. Why? In the past, economic-centered development perspective did not require a separate discussion on the quantitative aspect of development. If the economy was the standard for development, of course, the larger the total size of the economy, the better. For example, a larger GDP is better, and a smaller one is worse. This is also true in the discussion of economic inequality. This is because the discussion of economic inequality is also aimed at a small gap at a large income level, not a small gap at a small income level. However, in a situation where the development perspective is shifting to increased interest in happiness rather than income, there should be a discussion about whether a large amount of happiness is good.

Despite this necessity, although there have been relatively many discussions about the qualitative change of the transition from GDP to happiness, the quantitative change of happiness itself has not yet been seriously discussed. Instead, it has been considered that the greater the happiness, the better, by implicitly applying the perspective in the past looking at the total amount when evaluating economic performance. Announcing rankings through the comparison of the level of happiness between countries and paying attention to it is the definite evidence for this. However, it is necessary to question whether happiness is as good as in the total amount of the economy. In this regard, if the discussion of simple pleasures and simple worries, or the moderate view of a good life, is valid, maximizing the total amount of happiness may not be the correct answer.

Basically, the maximization of happiness is limited as a goal to be pursued. First of all, as aforementioned, maximizing happiness is an unrealizable goal, considering the infinity of human desires and the limitations of resources. Also, seeing from the perspective of public happiness that considers the distribution of happiness along with the level of happiness, not from the isolated individual level, maximizing the total amount of happiness cannot be the optimum, because the level and distribution of happiness are not exactly proportional. In addition, the endless pursuit of happiness exhausts the capabilities of individuals and governments, and overlooks the possibility of happiness based on a balance between pleasure and worry. In other words, while promoting happiness is good, maximizing happiness is neither feasible nor desirable. Rather, the optimization of happiness by balancing limitless human desires and resource limits is a more feasible and desirable direction in the pursuit of happiness. Also, in order to increase the effectiveness of the happiness policy, it is necessary to pursue the optimization of happiness instead of maximizing happiness which is infeasible.

What is the optimization of happiness? First, it is a heightened concern for the simplicity discussed before in relation to the level of happiness. It is the promotion of happiness related to social conditions at a level that eliminates deprivation but excludes luxury. Second, an equitable distribution of happiness among community members is ensured. In other words, the optimization of happiness is the balance between an appropriate level of happiness and the distribution happiness. The former is the basis of the latter. This is because the enhanced interest in simplicity provides the conditions for sharing happiness equally. If you pursue the maximization of happiness, it is difficult to realize the simple happiness you enjoy together due to unlimited desires and limited resources. On the other hand, it is possible to realize simple but integrated happiness that can be enjoyed together only by optimizing happiness. From a public point of view, happiness should not be the subject of an endless chase with greed, ignoring the limitations of resources. Happiness should not be subject to the renunciation of passive reception to external conditions. Happiness should be an object of enjoyment based on active adaptation and reaction to external conditions. Happiness should be recognized as an object that is achieved by pursuing simplicity as a balance point between the pursuit of luxury and the resolution of deficiency. In this regard, the happiness policy should be considered a policy that can actually contribute to public happiness only when it is delivered on the basis of supporting this simple happiness.

As mentioned in the previous chapter, the ultimate concern of happiness policies is to promote happiness per se, but its basic goal is to support the happiness pursuant activity of individuals by the amelioration of social conditions. An important question in this regard is what level of social conditions to pursue as a goal. I suggest some directions for it below based on the discussion above.

First, happiness policy should include the relief of people's urgent needs as the minimum goal. Urgent needs are induced from deficiency. Deficiency signifies the status of lacking the minimum condition for maintaining human dignity. People cannot enjoy happiness under such a situation, and accordingly, the happiness policy should aim at resolving deficiency as its priority and minimum necessity.

Second, happiness policy should pursue securing the social condition of simplicity beyond resolving deficiency. A simple level of social condition is the level that permits the enjoyment of a modest surplus, i.e., slack between the luxury of abundance and the urgency of deficiency. Such a goal is feasible and can be achieved in a balanced consideration of both the infinity of individual desires and the limit of resource mobilization. Simple social conditions do not suppress happiness to a low level, because the level of happiness is not necessarily in a positive relation with the level of social condition. This has been consistently emphasized in the set point theory, which emphasizes individual disposition prior to external conditions. Basically, it seems clear that a consistent correlation between the two will not be found because an individual's disposition and response to external conditions are involved in the process of connecting external conditions to happiness. Of course, social conditions at the deprivation level will have a negative effect on happiness, but it should also be recognized that social conditions beyond a certain level of threshold will not have a significant impact on happiness. This can be explained by the fact that the characteristics of social conditions with respect to happiness are more of the hygiene factor than the motivation factor, borrowing from the motivation and hygiene factor model suggested by Herzberg et al. (1959). That is, social conditions at the deprived level act as a barrier to happiness, but the effect of high or low social conditions on happiness at the level at which the deprivation is resolved may not be significant. As discussed before, external conditions of simplicity lead to low levels of happiness. But it can invite the abundance of happiness. This is because simple social conditions enable balanced and stable happiness, wherein small pleasures and small worries intersect. When I walked the road to Santiago, the conditions were simple, but I was very happy. Now arising feelings of mine wanting to walk the same path again when given another opportunity can be a good example of the abundance of happiness that simplicity brings. As such, the establishment of simple social conditions can be an appropriate goal of the happiness policy.

Third, it is necessary to take a cautious approach as to whether the happiness policy can be aimed at securing affluent social conditions. Abundance implies a level of social condition that goes beyond simplicity. However, there is a clear limit to the pursuit of prosperity as the primary goal of the happiness policy. This is because the creation of affluent conditions is not only practically infeasible, but also has undesirable aspects. First of all, considering the realistic constraint factors of the infinity of human needs and the limitations of resources, purporting abundance is unlikely to be achieved and highly likely to be limited to political rhetoric. In addition, in a society where social inequality exists and serious deprivation of some groups remains a problem and pursuing affluence first is a problematic norm because there is a risk of becoming a discriminatory policy. Also, excessive government intervention in the pursuit of abundance may lead to distortion of resource allocation or violation of individual autonomy. Basically, a society that expects happiness to be determined by affluent social conditions without individual voluntary effort or temperance is undesirable. Therefore, it is both realistic and normatively better to prioritize simplicity over abundance in pursuing happiness policy. Of course, just because a happiness policy should aim for simplicity does not mean that affluence should be completely rejected. This is because simplicity has an aspect that responds to the request for restraint of excessive desire, but also an inevitable limit due to resource constraints. Therefore, if everyone demands abundance and resources are abundant, the establishment of affluent living conditions can be pursued as the goal of the happiness policy. The problem is that it is difficult to achieve the affluent condition, and even if affluence is achieved, there is a possibility that the level of happiness under the condition of abundance will not be significantly higher than the level of happiness under the condition of simplicity. This is because, in addition to the uncertainty of the connection between happiness and external conditions, happiness from abundance can be one time and exceptional. Then, in a situation where a meaningful level of differential happiness effect is not expected, the authenticity of a happiness policy that seeks affluence prior to resolving deprivation or simplistic social conditions may be questioned. Fundamentally, it is necessary to recognize that the goal of maximizing social conditions is not necessary for the promotion of happiness. Ultimately, government should focus its happiness policy on creating simple social conditions as the minimum social foundation for all citizens to enjoy stable happiness.

It is difficult to dismiss the simple happiness policy as an excuse for neglecting efforts to improve inferior social conditions. The pursuit of simplicity does not mean abandoning or pursuing destitute conditions. Simplicity is not the same as deficiency; rather, it is associated with slack or some surplus—not excessive or luxury. Simplicity social conditions should be understood as seeking to create living conditions suitable for individuals as community members to pursue happiness, and pursuing social conditions of a decent level that are neither excessive nor deficient. Decency is not an expression of infinite desire or despair of paucity, but a state in which temperance and enjoyment are properly balanced. Therefore, the pursuit of simple social conditions is connected with the restoration of civic dignity. In addition, the happiness policy with this orientation will be interested in policy which pays close attention to the citizens' daily lives in the locality or community, as much as or more than the establishment of a material base or a macro-level economic policy at the national or regional level. This is also related to the restoration of civic dignity that is respected and communicated with the government in close proximity. Simplicity. It should be an important recognition base to support a policy oriented toward happiness, unlike the conventional economy-oriented policy.

References

Bentham, J. (1789). *An introduction to the principles of morals and legislation*. Printed for T. Payne and son.

Brickman, P., Coates, D., & Janoff-Bulman, R. (1978). Lottery winners and accident victims: Is happiness relative? *Journal of Personality and Social Psychology, 36*(8), 917–927.

Bruni, L., & Zamagni, S. (2007). *Civil economy: Efficiency, equity, public happiness*. Peter Lang.

Choi, H. (2006). *Development administration*. Shinwon Culture Co. (Korean).

Choi, I. (2018). *Good life*. Book21 (Korean).

Diener, E., & Emmons, R. A. (1985). The independence of positive and negative affect. *Journal of Personality and Social Psychology, 47*(5), 1105–1117.
Diener, E., Emmons, R. A., Larsen, R. J., & Griffin, S. (1985). The satisfaction with life scale. *Journal of Personality Assessment, 49*(1), 71–75.
Diener, E., Sandvik, E., & Pavot, W. (1991). Happiness is the frequency, not the intensity, of positive versus negative affect. In F. Strack, M. Argyle, & N. Schwarz (Eds.), *Subjective well-being: An interdisciplinary perspective* (pp. 213–231). Pergamon Press.
Diener, E., Ng, W., Harter, J., & Arora, R. (2010). Wealth and happiness across the world: Material prosperity predicts life evaluation, whereas psychosocial prosperity predicts positive feeling. *Journal of Personality and Social Psychology, 99*(1), 52–61.
Han, Y. (2000). *The theory development administration.* Asian Culture Publishing (Korean).
Herzberg, F., Mauser, B., & Snyderman, B. (1959). *The motivation to work.* Wiley.
Lao, T. (2007). *Lao Tzu* (G. S. Lee, Trans. (2007)). Publisher Gil (Korean).
OECD. (2013). *OECD guidelines on measuring subjective well-being.* OECD Publishing.
Veenhoven, R. (2015). The overall satisfaction with life: Subjective approaches (1). In W. Glatzer, L. Camfield, V. Møller, & M. Rojas (Eds.), *Global handbook of quality of life* (pp. 207–238). Springer.
Yao, K. (2018). *Lecture on Lao Tzu* (S. H. Son, Trans. (2010)). Kimyoungsa (Korean).

Index

S. J. Lee, *Public Happiness*, Community Quality-of-Life and Well-Being,
https://doi.org/10.1007/978-3-030-89643-0

Printed by Printforce, the Netherlands